Symptoms, Diagnosis and Treatment of Kidney Diseases

Symptoms, Diagnosis and Treatment of Kidney Diseases

Editor: Donald Moore

AMERICAN
MEDICAL PUBLISHERS
www.americanmedicalpublishers.com

AMERICAN
MEDICAL PUBLISHERS
www.americanmedicalpublishers.com

Cataloging-in-Publication Data

Symptoms, diagnosis and treatment of kidney diseases / edited by Donald Moore.
p. cm.
Includes bibliographical references and index.
ISBN 979-8-88740-225-3
1. Kidneys--Disease. 2. Kidneys--Disease--Diagnosis. 3. Kidneys--Diseases--Treatment.
4. Kidneys--Diseases--Etiology. 5. Nephrology. I. Moore, Donald.
RC902 .S96 2023
616.61--dc23

American Medical Publishers,
41 Flatbush Avenue,
1st Floor, New York,
NY 11217, USA

ISBN 979-8-88740-225-3 (Hardback)

Contents

Preface

It is often said that books are a boon to mankind. They document every progress and pass on the knowledge from one generation to the other. They play a crucial role in our lives. Thus I was both excited and nervous while editing this book. I was pleased by the thought of being able to make a mark but I was also nervous to do it right because the future of students depends upon it. Hence, I took a few months to research further into the discipline, revise my knowledge and also explore some more aspects. Post this process, I begun with the editing of this book.

The kidneys are vital organs in the body that play a crucial role in filtering the waste products and excessive fluid from the blood. The conditions that affect the kidney function are referred to as kidney diseases. There are several types of conditions and diseases, which affect the kidneys including kidney cancer, chronic kidney disease, acute kidney disease, cysts, kidney stones and kidney infections. Most of these diseases affect the ability of the nephrons to perform their functions effectively. Some common symptoms of kidney diseases are fatigue, weakness, hypertension, loss of appetite, nausea and vomiting, chest pain, and shortness of breath. Genetic problems, injuries and medications are the main factors that lead to the development of kidney diseases. Diagnostic methods that are used for diagnosing kidney conditions and diseases include urine tests, renal ultrasonography, biopsy of the kidney, and blood tests. The treatments involve the management of disease progression by relieving the symptoms. Dialysis and kidney transplantation are the treatment methods for end-stage kidney disease. This book presents recent studies on the symptoms, diagnosis and treatment of kidney diseases. With state-of-the-art inputs by acclaimed experts of this field, it targets students and professionals.

I thank my publisher with all my heart for considering me worthy of this unparalleled opportunity and for showing unwavering faith in my skills. I would also like to thank the editorial team who worked closely with me at every step and contributed immensely towards the successful completion of this book. Last but not the least, I wish to thank my friends and colleagues for their support.

Editor

1

Public attitudes towards screening for kidney cancer

Laragh L. W. Harvey-Kelly[1], Hannah Harrison[2], Sabrina H. Rossi[3], Simon J. Griffin[2], Grant D. Stewart[4] and Juliet A. Usher-Smith[2*]

Abstract

Background: Kidney cancer is often asymptomatic, leading to proposals for a screening programme. The views of the public towards introducing a new screening programme for kidney cancer are unknown. The aim of this study was to explore attitudes towards kidney cancer screening and factors influencing intention to attend a future screening programme.

Methods: We conducted an online population-based survey of 1021 adults aged 45–77 years. The main outcome measure was intention to attend four possible screening tests (urine, blood, ultrasound scan, low-dose CT) as well as extended low-dose CT scans within lung cancer screening programmes. We used multivariable regression to examine the association between intention and each screening test.

Results: Most participants stated that they would be 'very likely' or 'likely' to undergo each of the screening tests [urine test: $n = 961$ (94.1%); blood test: $n = 922$ (90.3%); ultrasound: $n = 914$ (89.5%); low-dose CT: $n = 804$ (78.8%); lung CT: $n = 962$ (95.2%)]. Greater intention to attend was associated with higher general cancer worry and less perceived burden/inconvenience about the screening tests. Less worry about the screening test was also associated with higher intention to attend, but only in those with low general cancer worry (cancer worry scale ≤ 5). Compared with intention to take up screening with a urine test, participants were half as likely to report that they intended to undergo blood [OR 0.56 (0.43–0.73)] or ultrasound [OR 0.50 (0.38–0.67)] testing, and half as likely again to report that they intended to take part in a screening programme featuring a low dose CT scan for kidney cancer screening alone [OR 0.19 (0.14–0.27)].

Conclusion: Participants in this study expressed high levels of intention to accept an invitation to screening for kidney cancer, both within a kidney cancer specific screening programme and in conjunction with lung cancer screening. The choice of screening test is likely to influence uptake. Together these findings support on-going research into kidney cancer screening tests and the potential for combining kidney cancer screening with existing or new screening programmes.

Keywords: Attitudes, Kidney cancer, Cancer, Screening, Survey

Background

Internationally, there is great interest in evaluating the potential for a screening programme for kidney cancer [1–3]. Half of all patients with kidney cancer have asymptomatic disease and up to a quarter of individuals have evidence of metastases at diagnosis [4]. Survival is strongly related to stage at diagnosis [4]. A screening

*Correspondence: jau20@medschl.cam.ac.uk
[2] The Primary Care Unit, Department of Public Health and Primary Care, University of Cambridge, Cambridge CB2 0SR, UK
Full list of author information is available at the end of the article

programme, potentially in a selected higher risk population, may down-stage the disease, reduce the prevalence of metastatic tumours at diagnosis, improve survival and decrease the expenditure related to systemic therapies [5].

The two currently available potential screening modalities are ultrasound and CT scan. Our group reported a detailed cost-effectiveness analysis of ultrasound scan-based screening. This suggested that screening may have acceptable cost-effectiveness in men aged 50–60y (£18–22k/QALY) and in women aged 60 if the prevalence of kidney cancer is at least 0.2% [6]. When combined with other CT scan-based screening programmes, such as current lung cancer screening pilots [7], additional screening for kidney cancer by CT scan has the potential to provide health and economic benefits. Research into new urinary (i.e. perilipin 1 and aquaporin 2 [8]) and blood based markers (i.e. KIM-1 [9]) is also on-going and these may provide additional options for screening in the future.

Whichever screening modality is used, the benefits will only be realised if sufficient numbers of the target population undergo screening. This requires consideration of the views of the population on the acceptability and potential engagement with future programmes [10]. To our knowledge, no studies have addressed these issues for kidney cancer. We aimed to explore the attitudes of the public towards potential future screening programmes for kidney cancer with different tests and to understand the individual and system-level factors influencing intention to take up screening.

Methods

Study design

We conducted an online population-based survey. The survey was conducted and is reported in line with the checklist for Reporting Results of Internet E-Surveys (CHERRIES) [11].

Participants and recruitment

We aimed to recruit 1000 participants (50% female) through Prolific (www.prolific.ac), an online platform in which individuals volunteer to take part in studies and are compensated for their time at an hourly rate (£6/hour). Participants were eligible if they were between 45–79 years of age and, in line with accepted practice [12], had a Prolific approval rating $\geq$ 95%. The approval rating reflects the percentage of studies that participants have completed that have been approved by researchers. We chose the age range 45–79 years because it is unlikely that a future kidney cancer screening programme would screen individuals younger than 45 and we wanted to be able to capture any differences in attitudes in older groups. We did not prevent participants with a history of kidney cancer from completing the survey but their data were subsequently excluded from the analysis.

When the survey was launched, a random subset of eligible participants were invited to complete the survey via email through the Prolific platform (Additional file 1). The survey then remained open to new participants until recruitment was complete. After starting the survey, all participants had the option to 'return' their submission at any point. This allowed them to stop part way through the study without affecting their Prolific rating. Data from participants who returned their submission were deleted and not analysed. Cookies were not used to identify each participant computer. Duplicate entries were prevented within the Prolific platform through use of unique participant identification numbers.

Survey

The survey was developed by the study team and piloted with two patient and public representatives to check that the questions were comprehensible and being interpreted correctly. Validated questions were used wherever possible. A complete version of the survey is provided in Additional file 2. Briefly, participants first provided socio-demographic details including age, lifestyle, highest level of education, employment and socioeconomic status (assessed via the occupation of the household's chief income earner [13, 14]). They were then asked questions about their medical screening history, perception of cancer risk, cancer worry [15], knowledge of kidney cancer symptoms and risk factors for kidney cancer [16]. Participants were then given brief summary information about kidney cancer and the estimated benefits and harms of four potential screening methods using data from the literature [5]. A series of questions followed about beliefs and attitudes concerning kidney cancer and screening [17] and whether, based on the information provided, participants would take part in screening. Finally, participants were asked about how much influence various other factors, identified from the literature [18], would have on their decision to undergo screening. Written online consent was obtained from each participant before they began the survey.

Data collection

The questions and scenarios were embedded within an online questionnaire and two studies (one for men and one for women) run in parallel on the Prolific website to enable us to achieve a sample with equal numbers of men and women. All questions except those inviting free text responses were mandatory for all participants. The questions were distributed over 22 pages with between one and seven questions per page to enable completion on tablets or smartphones with small screens. It was not possible for participants to go back through the pages and change their answers. The technical functionality of the electronic questionnaire was tested by the study team. We included an instructional manipulation check to identify inattentive participants and increase the validity and reliability of the responses [19]. Participants who failed to answer this question correctly were excluded from the study.

Analysis

We used descriptive statistics to characterise the participants and their overall attitudes towards, and intention to take-up, kidney cancer screening. Socioeconomic status (SES) was classified as higher (ABC1) and lower (C2DE). For awareness of kidney cancer symptoms and risk factors participants were categorised into two groups (high/low) based on whether their overall score was above or below the median (see Additional file 2 for details).

We used a linear regression model to analyse differences between the burden/ inconvenience and worry associated with each screening test. The null hypothesis of no difference between the four groups was tested using an F-test, followed by the estimation of four pairwise contrasts between the screening tests: (1) urine vs blood; (2) urine vs ultrasound; (3) urine versus CT; and (4) ultrasound vs CT. Confidence intervals (98.75%, based on a Bonferroni corrected significance threshold of 1.25%) are presented for these analyses to acknowledge that four pairwise comparisons were performed.

Logistic regression was then used to examine the influence of the different screening tests and participant characteristics on intention to take up screening. For these analyses, cancer beliefs about treatment was treated as a continuous variable from 1–5, 1 reflecting the view that most cancer treatment is worse than the cancer itself. Cancer beliefs about outcomes was similarly treated as a continuous variable, computed by combining responses from the relevant questions 1, 4 and 6 using published coefficients [17] (see Additional file 2 for details).

To enable us to compare the intention to take up each of the five screening test modalities, we included the screening test as an independent variable as well as adjusting for participant characteristics (age, sex, education level, ethnicity, self-reported general health, country of residence, income group, body mass index (BMI), smoking status, prior history of cancer, family history of kidney cancer), cancer worry, perceived risk of cancer, beliefs about cancer outcomes and treatments, the mean burden/inconvenience and the mean worry associated with all of the tests combined for each participant. The analysis was adjusted for the clustering of responses by participant using the—cluster—command in Stata.To enable comparison of participant characteristics associated with intention to take up each of the screening tests separately, we repeated the analysis for each screening test with the burden/inconvenience and worry associated with each specific test. We checked for collinearity between the covariates in the regression models by calculating the variance inflation factors (vif) for each covariate using the command –collin- in Stata. All variables had vif values less than 4.20, suggesting no evidence of substantial collinearity. We also separately assessed for interactions between cancer worry, perceived risk of cancer and beliefs about cancer outcomes, and burden/inconvenience of the screening tests and worry about the screening tests by adding interaction terms into the regression. The hypothesis being tested was that worry about the screening tests and the perceived burden/inconvenience of screening may have less of an impact on intention to take up screening among those individuals with higher cancer worry, higher perceived risk of cancer or stronger negative beliefs about the outcomes of cancer. Interactions were considered significant if $p<0.05$. Where the interaction was significant we additionally stratified by high (> 5) and low (≤ 5) cancer worry and estimated the association between worry about screening tests and intention to take up screening separately in these two groups. All results from these analyses are presented as odds ratios (OR) with 95% confidence intervals.

All analyses were performed using Stata Version 14.

Patient and public involvement

Two members of the public contributed, through face-to-face discussions and email, to the development of the survey and participant information sheet. They also provided comments on the final manuscript prior to submission.

Results

At the time of recruitment, 7767 participants were registered with Prolific and met the eligibility criteria for the study. Based on demographic data on the Prolific website, approximately 80% of these were White/Caucasian, 34% male, 53% lived in the UK, 33% lived in the US, 15% were current smokers and 43% had a university level education. 51% considered themselves to be in the top five deciles of socioeconomic status. The survey was live for eight hours. During this time 1190 participants clicked through to view the participant information leaflet and consent form. 1077 (90.5%) started the survey. 29 failed the instructional manipulation check and so were excluded. A further 22 returned their submission. 1025 (86%) completed the survey. Four of those 1025 participants reported a history of kidney cancer and so were excluded from analysis. The characteristics of the remaining 1021 participants are shown in Table 1.Participants were aged from 45–77 years, 513 (50.2%) were female. Reflecting the eligible participant pool, the majority were from the UK (668, 65.4%) or USA (183, 17.9%), 46% had a university level education and 16.1% were current smokers. Men were over-represented amongst the study participants due to our sex-specific recruitment strategy. The proportion of participants of White ethnicity (95.3%) and those of higher SES (76.2%) were also higher among the study participants than the eligible population. A previous diagnosis of any cancer was reported by 63 (6.2%) and a family history of kidney cancer by 29 (2.8%). The majority (835, 81.8%) knew nothing about kidney cancer or had only heard of the condition before participating in the survey.

Table 1 Participant characteristics

Participant characteristic	n (%) or mean (± s.d.)
Age	
45–54	590 (57.7)
55–64	328 (32.1)
> 65	103 (10.1)
Mean (± s.d.)	54.3 (± 7.1)
Sex (n, % female)	513 (50.2)
Country	
UK	668 (65.4)
US	183 (17.9)
Europe	77 (7.5)
University level education	471 (46.1)
Ethnicity (n, % White)	973 (95.3)
General health measure	
Excellent, very good, good	811 (79.4)
Fair, poor	210 (20.6)
Smoking status	
Non-smoker	512 (50.1)
Ex-smoker	345 (33.8)
Current smoker	164 (16.1)
BMI (kg/m^2) (mean ± s.d)	27.4 (± 5.7)
Previous diagnosis of cancer	63 (6.2)
Family history of kidney cancer	29 (2.8)
Social group*	
ABC1	778 (76.2)
C2DE	188 (18.4)
Kidney cancer knowledge	
I am very familiar with it	6 (0.6)
I have only heard of the term before	497 (48.7)
I know a little about the disease	180 (17.6)
Nothing at all	338 (33.1)
Cancer worry (mean ± s.d)**	5.6 (± 2.3)
Cancer risk perception (mean ± s.d)***	34.1 (± 23.2)
Kidney cancer symptom awareness****	
High symptom awareness (≥ 5)	547 (53.6)
Low symptom awareness (< 5)	474 (46.4)
Kidney cancer risk factor awareness****	
High risk factor awareness (≥ 43)	585 (57.3)
Low risk factor awareness (< 43)	436 (42.7)

*ABC1 = higher SES, C2DE = lower SES

**On a scale of 3–15 where 3 = no worry, 15 = maximum worry

***On a scale of 1–100 from unlikely to likely

****Where high/low awareness was defined as above/below the median score. The breakdown for each risk factor/symptom can be found in Additional file 3: Supplementary Table 1, and the scoring system in Additional file 2

Cancer beliefs and attitudes towards kidney cancer screening

Table 2 shows the participants' general cancer beliefs and their attitudes towards kidney cancer screening. The majority of participants were positive about cancer outcomes, only 6.7% expressed cancer fatalism. Attitudes towards screening were also positive, the majority (91.8%) agreed with the statement that screening could reduce the chance of dying from kidney cancer.

Intention to attend screening

Intention to take-up screening was high overall (Table 3), with over 90% reporting that they would accept the invitation for screening by urine testing, blood testing or low-dose CT combined with lung screening. Intention was lower for ultrasound (89.5%) and low-dose CT of kidneys alone (78.8%).

Fig. 1 shows the pattern of responses at an individual level across the five modalities. A majority (771, 76%) reported that they would attend screening by all five modalities, 20 (2%) said they would not attend screening by any method and 28 (27%) reported they would only attend screening by the combined lung and kidney CT scan and not by the other methods. 217 (21%) participants would not attend screening by CT scan of the kidneys alone, but 181 of these 217 (83%) participants would attend kidney cancer screening by CT scan if lung cancer screening was also included.

The mean burden/inconvenience and the mean worry for each of the four screening tests are given in Table 3. Both were measured on a scale from 1–5. There were significant differences between the screening tests in both burden/inconvenience and worry, with significantly higher values for ultrasound, blood test and low-dose CT than for urine test [mean difference 0.38 (0.32–0.44) and 0.16 (0.12–0.19) for burden/inconvenience and worry respectively for ultrasound, 0.33 (0.28–0.37) and 0.11 (0.07–0.15) for blood test and 0.69 (0.62–0.75) and 0.47 (0.41–0.53) for low-dose CT]. Additionally, both burden/inconvenience and worry were significantly higher for low-dose CT than ultrasound (mean difference 0.31 (0.26–0.35) and 0.36 (0.31–0.41)).

Table 2 General cancer beliefs and attitudes towards kidney cancer screening

	Strongly agree /agree (n, %)	Neither agree nor disagree (n, %)	Disagree or Strongly disagree (n, %)
General cancer beliefs			
"These days, many people with cancer can expect to continue with normal activities and responsibilities"*	704 (69.0)	206 (20.2)	110 (10.9)
"Cancer can often be cured"*	740 (72.5)	199 (19.5)	82 (8.1)
"Some people think a diagnosis of cancer is a death sentence. To what extent do you agree or disagree that cancer is a death sentence?"*	138 (13.5)	310 (30.4)	573 (56.1)
Beliefs about cancer treatment: "Most cancer treatment is worse than the cancer itself"	406 (40.1)	343 (33.6)	272 (26.6)
Cancer fatalism: "I would NOT want to know if I have cancer"	68 (6.7)	109 (10.7)	844 (82.7)
Attitudes towards kidney cancer screening			
"I would be so worried about what might be found at kidney cancer screening that I would prefer not to have it."	72 (7.1)	83 (8.1)	866 (84.8)
"Kidney cancer screening is only necessary if I have symptom"	80 (7.8)	149 (14.6)	792 (77.6)
"I don't think there is any point going for kidney cancer screening because it won't affect the outcome"	13 (1.3)	71 (7)	937 (91.8)
"Kidney cancer screening could reduce my chance of dying from kidney cancer."	937 (91.8)	45 (4.4)	39 (3.8)

*Questions that were combined using published coefficients to form "Beliefs about cancer outcomes"

Table 3 Intention to take up screening and the burden/inconvenience and worry associated with each screening test

Screening test	Mean Burden/ inconvenience (mean ± sd)*	Worry (mean ± sd)*	Intention to take up screening	
			Unlikely n (%)	Likely n (%)
Urine test	1.2 (± 0.5)	1.2 (± 0.6)	60 (5.9)	961 (94.1)
Blood test	1.6 (± 0.7)	1.4 (± 0.7)	99 (9.7)	922 (90.3)
Ultrasound scan	1.6 (± 0.8)	1.3 (± 0.7)	107 (10.5)	914 (89.5)
Low dose CT scan	1.9 (± 0.9)	1.7 (± 0.9)	217 (21.3)	804 (78.8)
Low dose CT scan combined with lung screening**	–	–	49 (4.8)	962 (94.2)

*1=none and 5=very great; **10 participants did not answer this question.

After adjusting for participant characteristics (age, sex, education level, ethnicity, self-reported general health, country of residence, income group, BMI, smoking status, prior history of cancer, family history of kidney cancer), cancer worry, perceived risk of cancer, beliefs about cancer outcomes and treatments, and the burden/inconvenience and worry associated with the tests, and clustering of response by participant, there were significant differences between the different tests in intention to take up screening (Fig. 2). In particular, compared with intention to take up screening with a urine test, participants were half as likely to report that they intended to undergo blood [OR 0.56 (0.43–0.73)] or ultrasound [OR 0.50 (0.38–0.67)] testing compared to urine testing, and half again as likely to report that they intended to take part in a screening programme featuring a low dose CT scan [OR 0.19 (0.14–0.27)).

Participants with higher BMI and higher general cancer worry were more likely to report intention to attend screening (Fig. 3). Being more worried about the screening tests or associating more burden and inconvenience were associated with decreased odds of intending to take up screening overall in the study population. There was, however, an interaction between general cancer worry and worry about the screening tests, with worry about screening tests associated with reduced odds of intending to attend only in those with low cancer worry (cancer worry scale ≤ 5) (OR 0.67 (0.48–0.94)) and not in than those with high cancer worry (OR 0.98 (0.69–1.40)). There was no evidence of an interaction ($p>0.05$) for the other potential interactions assessed. Although not statistically significant as a result of the small numbers with a family history of kidney cancer, having a family history of kidney was also associated with an increased odds of intending to take up screening (OR 4.70 (0.41–53.7), with

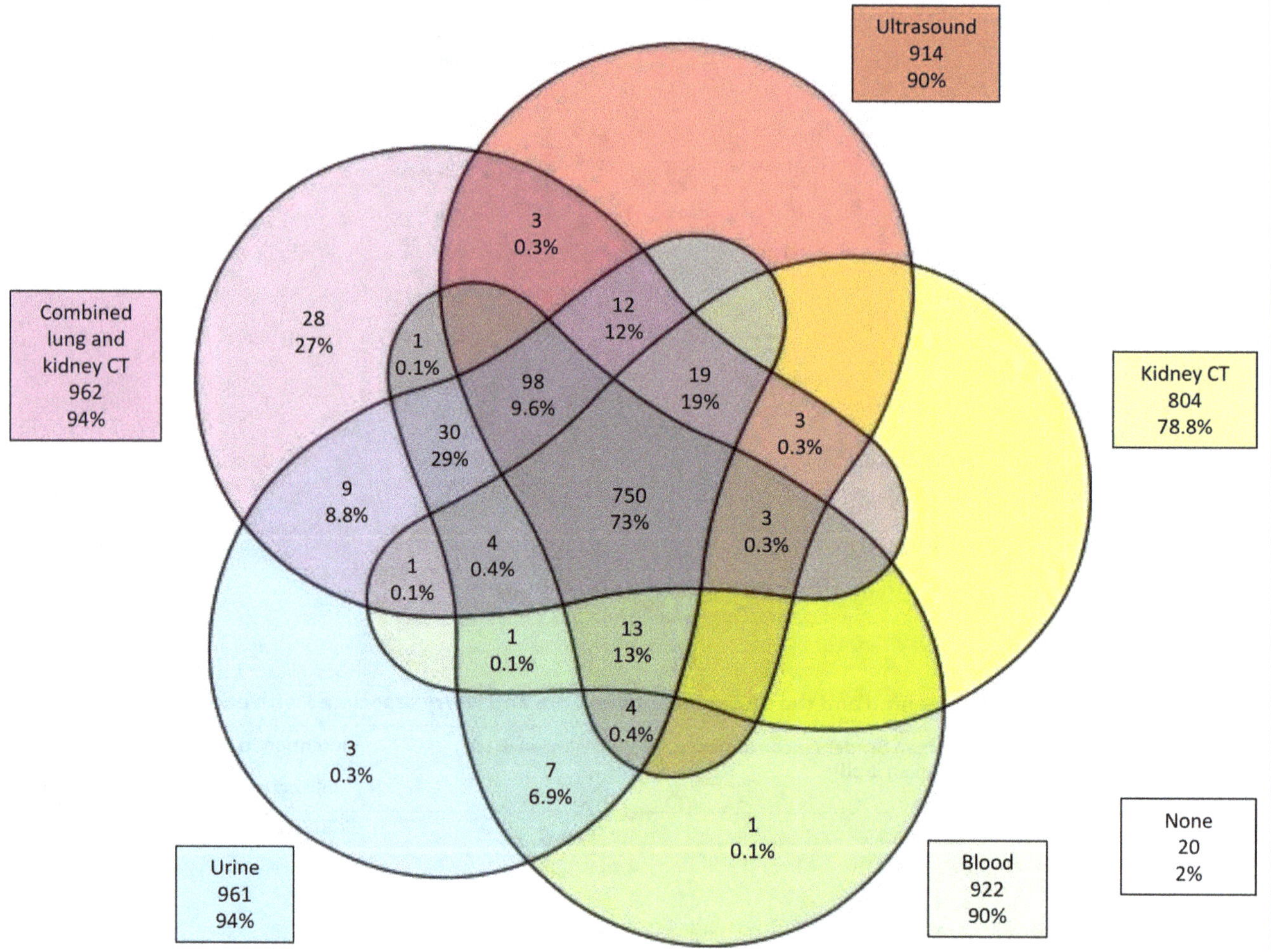

Fig. 1 Participants expressing intention to take up screening across each of the five screening modalities. Blank areas indicate 0 participants. n=1021

27 of the 29 participants with a family history of kidney cancer likely to take up all four screening tests. These findings were similar when each screening option was considered separately (Additional file 3: Supplementary Table 2 and Additional file 4: Supplementary Fig. 1a-e). Notably all those with a family history of kidney cancer reported they would take up screening with an ultrasound scan, 28 out of 29 would take up screening with urine or blood testing, and 27 out of 29 would take up low-dose CT scanning.

The reported influence of other factors on intention to attend kidney cancer screening are reported in Table 4. Having symptoms of kidney cancer and a recommendation by their GP were the most influential factors.

Discussion

To the best of our knowledge, this study is the first to assess public attitudes towards potential kidney cancer screening programmes. Participants expressed high levels of intention to take-up kidney cancer screening, both within kidney cancer specific screening programmes and in conjunction with lung cancer screening. This was despite over 80% knowing nothing about kidney cancer or having only heard of the condition before participating in the survey. There were significant differences in intention between screening modalities, with a preference for urine testing or low-dose CT combined with lung cancer screening over a blood test, ultrasound scan or low-dose CT alone. Participants were also more likely to intend to undergo screening if they reported higher general cancer worry or less burden/inconvenience associated with the screening test, and if they had symptoms of kidney cancer or their GP had recommended screening. Less worry about the screening test was also associated with higher intention to attend, but only in those with lower general cancer worry. For those with higher general cancer worry, the general worry about cancer appeared to dominate any worry associated with the screening test itself.

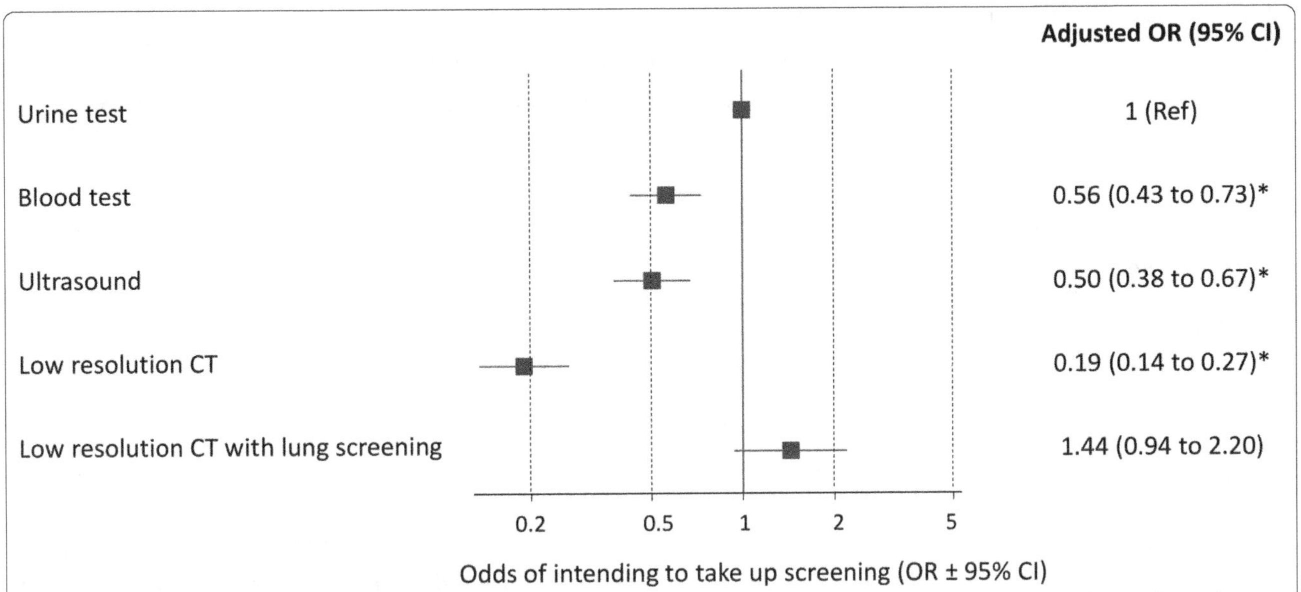

Fig. 2 Odds (OR ± 95% confidence intervals) of intending to take up screening with each of the five screening modalities, adjusting for participant characteristics, the burden/inconvenience and worry associated with each test, and clustering of response by participant. *significantly lower than urine test ($p<0.05$)

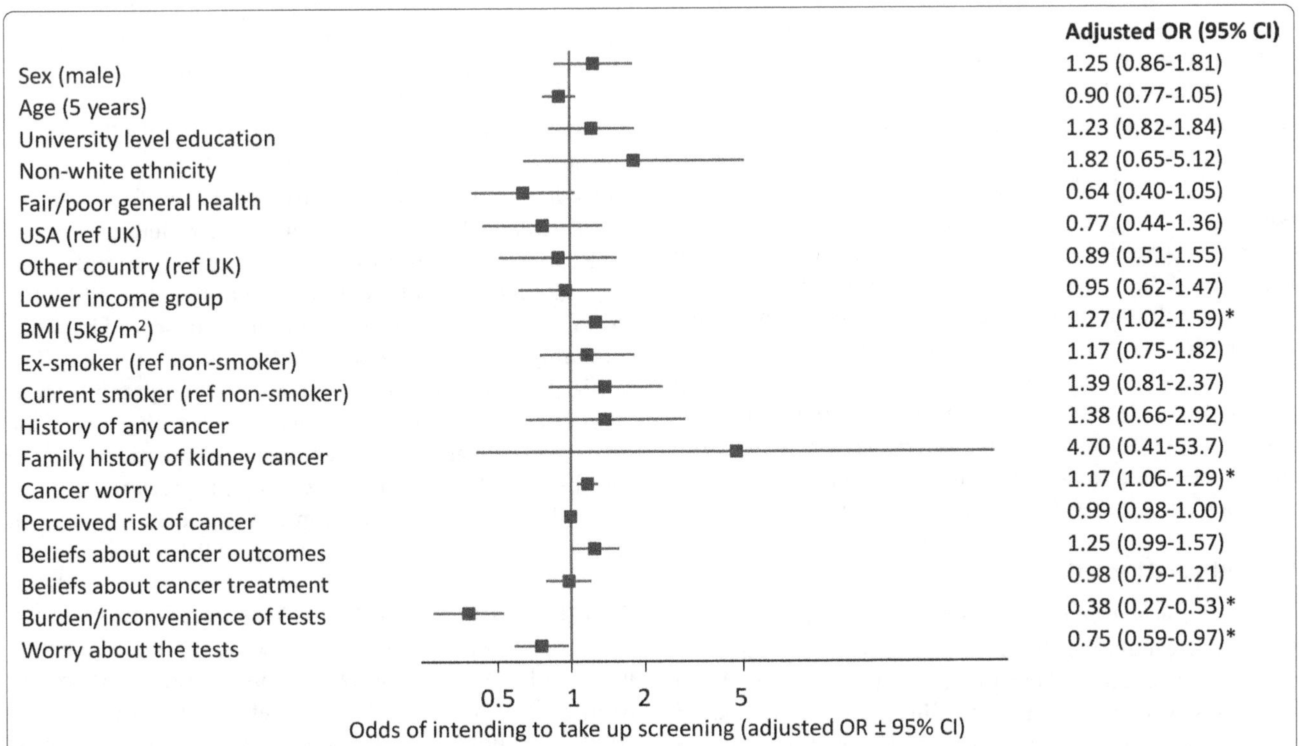

Fig. 3 The association between participant characteristics and intention to attend screening across all screening modalities. Odds ratios (OR) are adjusted for all factors in the figure. Cancer worry is measured on a scale from 3 to 15, perceived risk of cancer from 0 to 100, beliefs about cancer outcomes from 1.3 to 6.6, beliefs about cancer treatment from 1 to 5, burden/inconvenience and worry about the tests from 1 to 5.* $p < 0.05$

Table 4. Factors influencing intention to take up screening

	Influence on intention to take up screening		
	Much/slightly less likely (n, %)	No influence (n, %)	Much/slightly more likely (n, %)
If it was recommended by my GP?	11 (1.1)	129 (12.6)	881 (86.3)
If I had symptoms of kidney cancer?	13 (1.3)	45 (4.4)	963 (94.3)
If I could do the test at home?	26 (2.5)	277 (27.1)	718 (70.3)
If I could do the test at the GP?	20 (2)	278 (27.2)	723 (70.8)
If I had to go to the hospital for the test?	244 (23.9)	377 (36.9)	400 (39.2)
If I could make an appointment at the weekend or in the evenings?	28 (2.7)	465 (45.5)	528 (51.7)
If I had to leave work early?	179 (17.5)	657 (64.3)	185 (18.1)
If I could book the appointment online?	19 (1.9)	449 (44)	553 (54.2)

Comparison with literature

The overall positive attitude towards a screening programme for kidney cancer mirrors the general enthusiasm for cancer screening seen in population based surveys [20] and findings of a similar study on a potential lung cancer screening programme [13]. In that study over 90% of survey respondents believed that there was benefit to lung cancer screening, with the majority agreeing that lung screening could reduce chances of lung cancer death and only a small minority endorsing avoidance of lung cancer screening due to fear of what might be found or low perceived effectiveness of screening.

The observed differences between tests in intention to take part in a screening programme, with a preference for urine testing over a blood test, ultrasound scan or low-dose CT alone, is also consistent with existing literature which reports a preference for non-invasive tests requiring no preparation and causing no pain or long-term harm [21–23]. The greater intention seen for low-dose CT in combination with lung cancer screening likely reflects greater acceptability for combination screening, as seen in the context of a 'One Stop' cancer screening programme [24]. Given the low prevalence of kidney cancer, such a 'bolt on' screening programme may well be the most cost-effective as well as the most acceptable. It may also increase uptake of existing programmes [25].

Strengths and limitations

The survey was developed with the support of patient and public representatives in order to maximise participants' understanding and, where possible, previously validated questions were used. The main limitation is our use of an online recruitment platform. Although the platform we used has been developed specifically for research and enabled us to rapidly recruit participants of different ages and from different socio-economic backgrounds, compared with the UK and US population, the participants in this study were more likely to have university level education (46% in this study compared with 40% in the UK [26] and 35% in the US [27]) and be of White ethnicity (95% in this study compared with 86% in the UK [28] and 76% in the US [29]) and high socioeconomic status (76% in social group ABC1 in this study compared with 54% in England [30]). Uptake of other cancer screening programmes is known to be around 5–15% higher amongst these groups than those without university education, of ethnic minority groups and in lower social classes [31, 32]. The high proportion of participants expressing an intention to attend screening observed in this study may therefore be an over-estimation of intention in the wider population. Additionally, Prolific members are experienced in completing online tasks and their views may not be representative of those of the general population [33]. However, while these differences might lead to over-estimation of levels of intention and affect the absolute levels of worry and burden reported by the respondents as a whole, the differences observed between screening tests and the associations between worry and burden and other participant socio-demographic characteristics and intention to take up screening would be expected to be generalizable to other populations [34]. In the absence of an existing screening programme we were also only able to measure intention and not attendance at screening. Although there is an established relationship between screening intention and screening attendance [35], there is known to be an 'intention-behaviour gap' which is modified by various factors [36, 37]. The actual uptake of any future screening programme is therefore likely to be lower than the estimates of intention in this study. The uptake of any future screening programme will also likely depend on the information provided to eligible individuals. As data are currently not available on all the potential benefits and harms of kidney cancer screening, the information provided to participants in this study was based on estimates from the best available evidence and provided in less detail that would likely be included in any future screening programme. In particular, although we mentioned the possibility of both false positive and false negative findings as a result of screening, we did not provide participants with specific details on the possibility of detecting benign small renal masses or data on the growth rate of small incidentally detected tumours. With on-going research in this area, especially surrounding potential blood and urine biomarkers and approaches to the management of small renal masses, these estimates may change, making screening either more or less favourable to individuals.

Conclusion

Among the participants in our study, we found that there is an overall enthusiasm for kidney cancer screening, with high potential uptake rates. Our findings also highlight the influence of screening modality, with particular support for urine and low-dose CT combined with lung cancer screening, as well as individual-level and system-level factors that are likely to influence uptake. Together these findings support on-going research into kidney cancer screening tests and the potential for combining kidney cancer screening with existing or new screening programmes.

Supplementary information

Additional file 1. Participant invitation email.

Additional file 2. Exploring attitudes towards kidney cancer screening survey.

Additional file 3. Supplementary Tables.

Additional file 4. Supplementary Figures.

Abbreviations

BMI: Body mass index; CT: Computed tomography; OR: Odds ratio; QALY: Quality adjusted life year; SD: Standard deviation; SES: Socioeconomic status; USS: Ultrasound scan.

Acknowledgements

We would like to thank Dr Katie Mills for help with setting up the study, Dr Catherine Saunders for statistical advice, all the participants who took part and our two patient and public representatives Phil Alsop and Philip Dondi for their input and advice throughout this study and comments on this manuscript.

Authors' contributions

LHK, HH, SHR, SJG, GDS and JUS were involved in the design of the study. JUS completed data collection. JUS and LHK completed the initial data analysis. LHK, HH, SHR, GDS and JUS contributed to the final analysis and interpretation of the data. LHK and JUS wrote the first draft of the manuscript. HH, SHR, SJG and GDS critically reviewed the manuscript and have approved the final version. All authors read and approved the final manuscript.

Author details

[1] University of Cambridge School of Clinical Medicine, Addenbrooke's Hospital, Hills Road, Cambridge CB2 0SP, UK. [2] The Primary Care Unit, Department of Public Health and Primary Care, University of Cambridge, Cambridge CB2 0SR, UK. [3] Department of Oncology, University of Cambridge, Addenbrooke's Hospital, Cambridge Biomedical Campus, Hills Road, Cambridge CB2 0QQ, UK. [4] Department of Surgery, University of Cambridge, Addenbrooke's Hospital, Cambridge Biomedical Campus, Hills Road, Cambridge CB2 0QQ, UK.

References

1. Motzer RJ. Perspective: what next for treatment? Nature. 2016;537:S111.
2. Rossi SH, Blick C, Handforth C, Brown JE, Stewart GD. Essential research priorities in renal cancer: a modified delphi consensus statement. Eur Urol Focus. 2019;6:991–8.
3. Rossi SH, Fielding A, Blick C, Handforth C, Brown JE, Stewart GD. Setting research priorities in partnership with patients to provide patient-centred urological cancer care. Eur Urol. 2019;75:891–3.
4. Kidney cancer statistics | Cancer Research UK. https://www.cancerresearchuk.org/health-professional/cancer-statistics/statistics-by-cancer-type/kidney-cancer. Accessed 30 May 2019.
5. Rossi SH, Klatte T, Usher-Smith J, Stewart GD. Epidemiology and screening for renal cancer. World J Urol. 2018;36:1341–53.
6. Rossi SH, Klatte T, Usher-Smith JA, Fife K, Welsh SJ, Dabestani S, et al. A decision analysis evaluating screening for kidney cancer using focused renal ultrasound. Eur Urol Focus. 2019. https://doi.org/10.1016/j.euf.2019.09.002.
7. The Yorkshire Lung Screening Trial: ISRCTN42704678. https://www.isrctn.com/ISRCTN42704678. Accessed 20 Mar 2020.
8. Morrissey JJ, Mellnick VM, Luo J, Siegel MJ, Figenshau RS, Bhayani S, et al. Evaluation of urine aquaporin-1 and perilipin-2 concentrations as biomarkers to screen for renal cell carcinoma. JAMA Oncol. 2015;1:204.
9. Scelo G, Muller DC, Riboli E, Johannson M, Cross AJ, Vineis P, et al. KIM-a blood-based marker for early detection of kidney cancer: a prospective nested case-control study. Clin Cancer Res. 2018;24(22):5594–601.
10. Mühlbacher AC, Juhnke C. Patient preferences versus physicians' judgement: does it make a difference in healthcare decision making? Appl Health Econ Health Policy. 2013;11:163–80.
11. Eysenbach G. Improving the quality of web surveys: The Checklist for Reporting Results of Internet E-Surveys (CHERRIES). J Med Internet Res. 2004;6:1–6.
12. Peer E, Vosgerau J, Acquisti A. Reputation as a sufficient condition for data quality on Amazon Mechanical Turk. Behav Res Methods. 2014;46:1023–31.
13. Smits SE, McCutchan GM, Hanson JA, Brain KE. Attitudes towards lung cancer screening in a population sample. Health Expect. 2018;21:1150–8.
14. Social Grade | National Readership Survey. https://www.nrs.co.uk/nrs-print/lifestyle-and-classification-data/social-grade/. Accessed 30 May 2019.
15. Lerman C, Trock B, Rimer BK, Jepson C, Brody D, Boyce A. Psychological side effects of breast cancer screening. Health Psychol. 1991;10:259–67.
16. Cancer Awareness Measure toolkit version 2.1 Cancer Research UK Cancer Awareness Measure (CAM) Toolkit (version 2.1). 2007. https://www.cancerresearchuk.org/sites/default/files/health_professional_cancer_awareness_measure_toolkit_version_2.1_09.02.11.pdf.
17. Simon AE, Forbes LJL, Boniface D, Warburton F, Brain KE, Dessaix A, et al. An international measure of awareness and beliefs about cancer: development and testing of the ABC. BMJ Open. 2012;2:e001758.
18. Ali N, Lifford KJ, Carter B, McRonald F, Yadegarfar G, Baldwin DR, et al. Barriers to uptake among high-risk individuals declining participation in lung cancer screening: a mixed methods analysis of the UK Lung Cancer Screening (UKLS) trial. BMJ Open. 2015;5:e008254.
19. Oppenheimer DM, Meyvis T, Davidenko N. Instructional manipulation checks: detecting satisficing to increase statistical power. J Exp Soc Psychol. 2009;45:867–72.
20. Waller J, Osborne K, Wardle J. Enthusiasm for cancer screening in Great

Britain: a general population survey. Br J Cancer. 2015;112:562–6.
21. Marshall DA, Johnson FR, Phillips KA, Marshall JK, Thabane L, Kulin NA. Measuring patient preferences for colorectal cancer screening using a choice-format survey. Value Health. 2007;10:415–30.
22. Hawley ST, Volk RJ, Krishnamurthy P, Jibaja-Weiss M, Vernon SW, Kneuper S. Preferences for colorectal cancer screening among racially/ethnically diverse primary care patients. Med Care. 2008;46(9 Suppl 1):S10-6.
23. Mansfield C, Tangka FK, Ekwueme DU, Smith JL, Guy GPJ, Li C, et al. Stated preference for cancer screening: a systematic review of the literature, 1990–2013. Prev Chronic Dis. 1990;13:150433.
24. Bobridge A, Price K, Gill TK, Taylor AW. Influencing cancer screening participation rates—providing a combined cancer screening program (a 'one stop' shop) could be a potential answer. Front Oncol. 2017;7:308.
25. Labeit A, Peinemann F. Breast and cervical cancer screening in Great Britain: Dynamic interrelated processes. Health Econ Rev. 2015;5:32.
26. Office of National Statistics. Labour Market Profile - Great Britain. 2019. https://www.nomisweb.co.uk/reports/lmp/gor/2092957698/report.aspx#defs. Accessed 15 Dec 2019.
27. United States Census Bureau. Educational Attainment in the United States. 2018. https://www.census.gov/data/tables/2018/demo/education-attainment/cps-detailed-tables.html. Accessed 15 Dec 2019.
28. Office of National Statistics. Population of England and Wales. https://www.ethnicity-facts-figures.service.gov.uk/uk-population-by-ethnicity/national-and-regional-populations/population-of-england-and-wales/latest. Accessed 15 Dec 2019.
29. United States Census Bureau. QuickFacts United States. 2019. https://www.census.gov/quickfacts/fact/table/US/PST045219. Accessed 15 Dec 2019.
30. Office of National Statistics. 2011 Census: Approximated social grade, local authorities in England and Wales. 2011. https://www.ons.gov.uk/file?uri=/peoplepopulationandcommunity/populationandmigration/populationestimates/datasets/2011censusquickstatisticsforenglandandwalesonnationalidentitypassportsheldandcountryofbirth/r24ewrttableqs611ewladv1_tcm77-304378(2).xls. Accessed 15 Dec 2019.
31. Hirst Y, Stoffel S, Baio G, McGregor L, von Wagner C. Uptake of the English Bowel (Colorectal) Cancer Screening Programme: an update 5 years after the full roll-out. Eur J Cancer. 2018. https://doi.org/10.1016/j.ejca.2018.07.135.
32. Ricardo-Rodrigues I, Jiménez-García R, Hernández-Barrera V, Carrasco-Garrido P, Jiménez-Trujillo I, López de Andrés A. Social disparities in access to breast and cervical cancer screening by women living in Spain. Public Health. 2015;129:881–8.
33. Palan S, Schitter C. Prolific.ac—A subject pool for online experiments. J Behav Exp Finance. 2018;17:22–7.
34. Collins R. What makes UK Biobank special? Lancet. 2012;379:1173–4.
35. Cooke R, French DP. How well do the theory of reasoned action and theory of planned behaviour predict intentions and attendance at screening programmes? A meta-analysis. Psychol Health. 2008;23:745–65.
36. Vrinten C, Waller J, Von Wagner C, Wardle J. Cancer Fear: Facilitator and Deterrent to Participation in Colorectal Cancer Screening. Cancer Epidemiol Biomarkers Prev. 2015;24:400–5.
37. Sheeran P. Intention—behavior relations: a conceptual and empirical review. Eur Rev Soc Psychol. 2002;12:1–36.

2

Do organic substances act as a degradable binding matrix in calcium oxalate kidney stones?

Adi Adelman[1†], Yaniv Shilo[1†], Jonathan Modai[1], Dan Leibovici[1], Ishai Dror[2] and Brian Berkowitz[2*]

Abstract

Background: Calcium oxalate (CaOx) stones are considered to be highly resistant to chemolysis. While significant organic matter has been identified within these stones, which is presumed to bind (inorganic) CaOx particles and aggregates, most chemolysis efforts have focused on methods to attack the CaOx components of a stone. We examine the feasibility of inducing chemolysis of CaOx kidney stones, within hours, by specifically attacking the organic matrix present in these stones.

Methods: In contrast to previous studies, we focused on the possible "brick and mortar" stone configuration. We systematically tested, via in vitro experiments, the ability of an extensive range of 26 potential chemolysis agents to induce relatively fast disintegration (and/or dissolution) of a large set of natural CaOx stone fragments, extracted during endourological procedures, without regard to immediate clinical application. Each stone fragment was monitored for reduction in weight and other changes over 72 h.

Results: We find that agents known to attack organic material have little, if any, effect on stone chemolysis. Similarly, protein and enzymatic agents, and oral additive medical treatments, have little immediate effect.

Conclusions: These findings suggest that the organic and inorganic constituents present in CaOx stones are not structured as "brick and mortar" configurations in terms of inorganic and organic components.

Keywords: Chelating agents, Enzymes, Organic compounds, Chemolysis

Background

The phenomenon of nephrolithiasis afflicts approximately 10% of the population globally, and its prevalence is rising continuously [1, 2]. Of the main types of kidney stones—calcium oxalate (CaOx), uric acid, struvite, hydroxyapatite, brushite and cystine—calcium-containing stones are by far the most prevalent, comprising as much as 80% of all stones.

*Correspondence: brian.berkowitz@weizmann.ac.il
†Adi Adelman and Yaniv Shilo have contributed equally to this article
[2] Department of Earth and Planetary Sciences, Weizmann Institute of Science, 7610001 Rehovot, Israel
Full list of author information is available at the end of the article

Kidney stones have been the target for chemolysis for many years though with only limited success. Of the various kidney stones, CaOx stones in particular are considered to be the most resistant to chemolysis. Studies of oral intake treatments find little evidence of successful dissolution of existing CaOx stones (or, even of inhibiting stone formation [3–5]). In vivo chemolysis of kidney and bladder stones began seriously with the use of Renacidin, which appeared effective as a powerful dissolution agent for calcium phosphate, calcium carbonate, and magnesium ammonium phosphate (struvite) stones, but not for CaOx stones [6]; see also, e.g., [7] for calcium phosphate stones. If appropriate agents could be identified, the principal of in vivo chemolysis of CaOx kidney stones remains attractive [8, 9].

In efforts to investigate chemolytic behavior of CaOx stones, several in vitro studies have considered various potential agents. These agents have generally demonstrated poor efficacy in terms of percentage dissolved and relatively long times required for disintegration, for both real and synthetic stone types. Studies using artificial, *synthesized* "kidney stones", consisting of relatively pure calcium oxalate aggregates and calcium phosphate crystals [9–11], yielded disappointing results of up to 10% stone weight loss over several hours, and 13–47% stone weight loss over days using enzymatic disintegration (oxalate decarboxylase and oxalate oxidase) to attack oxalate [10]. Moreover, in vitro studies that test chemolysis of *real* CaOx kidney stones harvested from human patients are similarly limited, particularly in terms of (1) the actual number of studies, and (2) the small number and type of chemolysis agents and stones tested in each study. For example, one report focused mostly on snake venom thrombin-like enzyme with the addition of antibiotics [12], while another [9] investigated natural and synthetic chelating reagents (citrate and EDTA) together with an antibiotic. These studies on real stones, too, demonstrated overall poor efficacy in terms of percentage disintegrated and/or time required for disintegration, e.g., ~ 10–50% disintegration by weight after 5 days [12], and up to ~ 10% over several (2–10) hours [9].

Significantly, though, with the partial exception of one investigation of an enzyme to specifically target proteins in the stone matrix [12], essentially all of these studies investigate agents that are expected to attack the CaOx (inorganic) components of a stone. And yet, a range of studies have identified significant organic matter, even as a matrix structure, within these stones, which is presumed to bind CaOx particles and aggregates [13–25]. Indeed, scanning electron microscope images (from these and other studies) show that CaOx stones are highly heterogeneous, containing layered, amorphous, and crystalline material. In this context, too, over 1000 proteins have been identified in kidney stones [20], which may form an organic protein matrix [13, 14]. However, while the literature mentions the *presence* of organic matter, it does not generally give *quantitative* measures of the relative amount of organic matter [13–21]; one series of studies yielded estimates of ~ 2.5% organic matrix by weight [22, 23]. Identification and quantification of *organic* constituents, whether from surface analysis or total sample analysis, remains difficult. Moreover, the precise nature and influence of organic matter remains uncertain, and the amount and type of organic matter varies among different stones, patient pathologies, and other factors. Given the assumption that the organic "matrix" in stones may act to bind inorganic components (such as CaOx particles), the overall stone structure may be that of a "brick and mortar" configuration, wherein the organic matter is the "mortar" and the inorganic constituents being the "bricks"; if so, then regardless of the specific stone configuration (e.g., containing layered, amorphous, and/or crystalline regions), it might be possible to achieve fast stone disintegration by attacking organic components.

In light of the highly limited information available on disintegration properties of real CaOx kidney stones, and to evaluate potential new routes for, ultimately, in vivo chemolytic treatments, the objectives of this study were to systematically analyze potential chemolysis agents on real kidney stones, effective within hours, and without regard to immediate clinical application. For the first time, we focus specifically on the question of whether CaOx stones can be treated as "brick and mortar" aggregates, which would enable chemolysis targeted to attack the organic material within CaOx stones [13–25]. We note that in all such studies, it is important to differentiate between "dissolution" and "disintegration"—while pure synthetic CaOx particles dissolve to various extents, CaOx kidney stones (which are aggregates of inorganic and organic materials) may also disintegrate into fragments when binding material is affected—so that the term "chemolysis" encompasses all processes of stone decomposition.

Methods

Collection and analysis of stones

Patients arriving to a medical institution for elective endourological procedures to remove kidney stones during March–May 2019 were invited to take part in this research. Written informed consent was obtained from all patient participants. Multiple stone *fragments* (hereafter referred to as "stones")—as obtained from laser lithotripsy and percutaneous nephrolithotomy, without further treatment—removed during each endourological procedure were used in this research. The stone weights were in the range 10–165 mg (3–7 mm length along the major axis). One stone from each patient was analyzed to confirm that it was calcium-oxalate based (all containing mixtures (e.g., [16]) of monohydrate (> 70%) and dihydrate (< 30%) calcium oxalates), via x-ray diffraction. Overall, more than 100 stones collected from 15 patients were used.

Chemolysis protocol

We surveyed, via in vitro experiments, a broad range of 26 potential chemolysis agents, divided into four groups (Table 1). These agents were selected specifically to target, in particular, organic binding material reported to be present in stone fragments, with the aim

Table 1 Selected potential chemolysis agents and concentrations

Type of chemolysis agent	Agent* (Supplier)	Concentration (Purity %)
Organic solvents	Toluene (Bio Lab, Israel)	Neat (99.7%)
	Ethanol (J.T. Baker, Holland)	Neat (99.5%)
	Acetone (Bio Lab, Israel)	Neat (99.8%)
	Acetonitrile (Bio Lab, Israel)	Neat (99.97%)
	Dimethylformamide, DMF (Merck)	Neat (99.8%)
	Tetrahydrofuran, THF (Sigma-Aldrich)	Neat (99.9%)
	Dimethylsulfoxide (Sigma-Aldrich)	Neat (99.5%)
Degradation of organic "cement" (binding agents)	H_2O_2 (Bio Lab, Israel)	8.8 M (30%)
	Copper nanoparticles + H_2O_2 (synthesized[26], in house)	0.24 mM CuNP + 1.5% H_2O_2 (30%)
	Fenton: pH 2–4, Fe^{2+}, H_2O_2 (synthesized[27], in house)	1 mM Fe, 11 mM H_2O_2 (30%)
	Macerozyme R-10 plant digestion enzyme (Sigma-Aldrich)	20–40 enzyme units
	Drain cleaner (commercial, enzyme-based; HG, Israel)	As received
	Barbecue grill cleaner (commercial, enzyme-based; HG, Israel)	As received
Chelating agents and other agents	Potassium citrate, $K_3C_6H_5O_7 \cdot H_2O$ (Sigma, USA)	16 mM (98%)
	EDTA (Sigma, USA)	0.1 M, 1 M, 2.5 M (99%)
	SDS (Ridel-de-Haen, Germany)	0.1 mM (90%)
	Triton X (Sigma, USA)	0.15 mM (> 99%)
	NH_4OH (Merck, Germany)	Concentrated 16.7 M (25%)
Organic acids	Citric acid (Sigma-Aldrich)	0.1 M (99%)
	Ascorbic acid, vitamin C (Sigma, USA)	0.1 M (> 99%)
	Nicotinic acid (Sigma-Aldrich)	0.1 M (> 98%)
	Lactic acid (Sigma-Aldrich)	0.1 M (> 85%)
	Oxalic acid (Sigma-Aldrich)	0.3 M (> 85%)
	Acetic acid (Bio Lab, Israel)	0.1 M, concentrated 16.7 M (99.8%)
	Apple (cider) vinegar (commercial, food store)	5%
	Formic acid (J.T. Baker, Holland)	0.1 M, concentrated 21.7 M (98%)

* All agents were as received from manufacturers without further purification or modification

of achieving fast disintegration. The agents were chosen on the basis of existing medical literature and current clinical practice, folk remedies, and knowledge of known dissolution and digestion techniques of both inorganic and organic matter used in biogeochemical studies in the earth sciences.

We emphasize that the solutions examined here are not generally appropriate for use in clinical applications; our intent here, before attempting to reach a translational approach at the clinical level, was to first understand whether focusing on the organic components of CaOx stones offers a potential avenue for further study. The justifications for these solution choices are as follows.

First, we investigated the potential dissolution of small organic molecules by strong organic solvents. These solvents might be expected to dissolve the cementing agent that is presumed to hold the inorganic debris (including CaOx particles which generally occur at sizes of up to about 20 microns) in the stone together [13–23]. If true, then stones might disintegrate into small (micron size) fragments that in turn could be flushed out.

The second group of chemolytic agents tested here were strong oxidation agents—copper nanoparticles with H_2O_2 [26] and Fenton reaction (pH 2–4, Fe^{2+}, H_2O_2) [27]—both of which have been shown highly effective in degrading organic matter in complex matrices. These agents were applied to check their ability to degrade the organic substances and thus weaken or disintegrate the stone. Enzymatic mixtures to degrade organic matter—Macerozyme R-10 plant digestion pectinase enzyme [28], and even commercial drain cleaner and commercial barbecue grill cleaner—containing protease and other enzymes [10])—were similarly tested.

The third group we tested comprised potassium citrate, a chelator prescribed ubiquitously in clinical practice [3–5], EDTA, a chelating agent that was reported to effectively disintegrate CaOx [9, 11], anionic (SDS) and nonionic (Triton X) surfactants, and NH_4OH. The underlying assumption in these cases was that strong chelators or surfactants could reverse chemical precipitation processes by shifting the equilibrium toward higher aqueous concentrations. In other words, it was expected that increasing the solution carrying capacity for calcium (and other metals) or particulate matter in solution would result in partitioning of calcium from CaOx to the solution and to stone disintegration. It was further assumed here that the strong chelating/complexing capacity of these compounds would replace or break existing bonding between organic substances and the CaOx (inorganic crystals), and in turn lead to stone chemolysis.

The fourth group comprised eight organic acids that can target a broad spectrum of inorganic and organic components. Organic acids also have chelating capabilities that can react with the CaOx. The rationale for testing this group is based on standard geochemical dissolution protocols applied for the disintegration or dissolution of stones and minerals, which have proven effective in other biogeochemical contexts [29, 30]. The organic acids were tested also because they include oft-suggested folk remedies via oral consumption, including citric acid, ascorbic acid (vitamin C), and acetic acid (particularly apple cider vinegar).

The experiments were performed in controlled conditions and in a comparative framework. Each stone was weighed and placed in a test tube containing a potential chemolysis agent solution at room temperature (24 °C), with some replicate tests performed with samples at 37 °C. In all cases, the same ratio of stone fraction mass to dissolving solution was employed; a relatively large relative volume of solution (1 mL of solution per 10 mg of stone) ensured a chemical excess of each potential chemolysis agent, and each sample was mixed periodically by gentle shaking. Note, too, that because stone *fragments* were tested, both the outer stone and internal surfaces were exposed to the solutions. Two replicates of stones (pairs of larger and smaller stones from the available set) with each potential agent in separate test tubes were tested. The samples were monitored for reduction in weight and any visual change. During the experiments, the stones were removed from solution, dried (by quickly removing excess solution with absorbent tissues), and weighed every hour for the first 3 h, and again after 12, 24, 48 and 72 h. Control experiments were performed in parallel, with several stones samples exposed in the same conditions to double deionized water.

Finally, for additional support and interpretation of the measurements, according to a standard geochemical method [29, 30], separate experiments were performed to determine stone dissolution properties by exposure to strong acids. In this context, HCl (8.8 M; Bio Lab, Israel, 37% purity) and HNO_3 (11.1 M; Sigma-Aldrich, 70% purity) were used according to the same protocols as above to examine dissolution behavior. As a benchmark, similar experiments were also performed with pure, synthetic CaOx crystals (Sigma-Aldrich, > 99.9% purity). Synthetic kidney stones were not tested as they are known to be unrepresentative of real stones, particularly in terms of the binding material (e.g., [9–11]).

Results

We examined four groups of chemolysis agents (Table 1) on CaOx stones. It was found that none of these agents had any measurable impact (no change in weight) on stone disintegration, at least over the time frame of the experiments (72 h). Moreover, SEM analysis (Fig. 1) of some of these stone samples, before and after treatment, indicated essentially no significant modification of surface morphology. The only exception was the (oft-prescribed) agent potassium citrate, which indicated up to 30% disintegration (weight loss) of stone samples over this 72 h period; moreover, in addition to notable loss of stone mass, the remaining samples displayed changes in surface morphology, as seen from SEM images (Fig. 1e,f).

It is noted, too, that no change in the stones was observed in control experiments with double deionized water. Replicate tests performed with samples at 24 °C and at 37 °C showed that temperature had essentially no effect on the results.

We emphasize that concentrations of solutions were chosen to maximize possible chemolytic effects of each candidate agent. For illustration (Table 1), a potassium citrate at 16 mM is equivalent to 48 meq. This corresponds to a citrate concentration at least an order of magnitude higher than in urine [31]; to compare, oral potassium citrate therapy of 60–90 meq/d can increase urinary citrate by 30–115% [31].

Discussion

Here, we assessed the potential of different solutions to dissolve or disintegrate CaOx stones within hours. In contrast to previous in vitro studies that focused on dissolution of (inorganic) CaOx components, we hypothesized—on the basis of numerous studies analyzing stone content and structure—that the organic matrix in the stones [13–23] may lead to a "brick and mortar" configuration, and thus serve as an "Achilles heel", enabling fast stone disintegration by attacking organic components. We stress again that we use the term "brick and mortar" to differentiate between the two kinds of components—inorganic and organic—which in some embodiments may appear as distinct regions or layers of calcium oxalates and organic substances. In this context, we considered four groups of solutions to examine different possible modes of chemolytic processes of kidney stones that can attack (principally) organic constituents (see Table 1 and Methods above for the rationale of testing these agents).

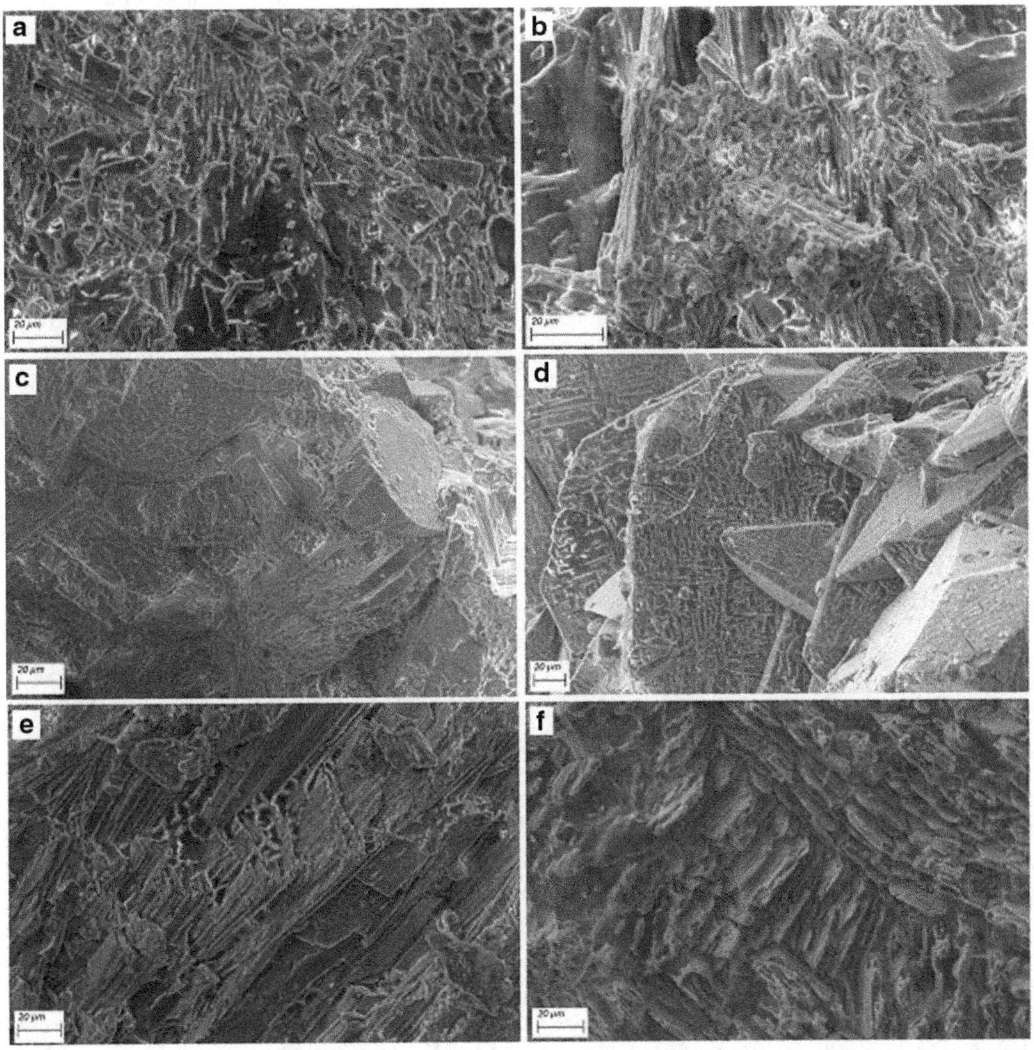

Fig. 1 Representative SEM images of CaOx stone fragment (internal surfaces)—**a** before and **b** after, 24 °C, **c** before and **d** after, 37 °C—exposure to potential chemolysis agents, showing little change (similar images were found over a range of samples and at both temperatures); and **e** before and **f** after treatment at 37 °C with the potassium citrate solution, which displayed measured weight loss and chemolytic effects on the stone samples. Scale bars indicate 20 μm

We argue that the lack of change in stone weight—essentially no dissolution and certainly no fragmentation/disintegration of the stone fragments—is a clear indication that the stones do not consist of a "brick and mortar" configuration. Given the usual structure of kidney stone fragments, which contain layered materials and amorphous aggregates of CaOx crystals and organic matter (see Fig. 2), it is therefore deeply significant that none of the agents known to attack organic matter by direct chemolysis and/or chelation—organic solvents, degraders of organic binding material, chelating agents—had any noticeable effect on disintegration (or dissolution) of the stones. Moreover, none of the folk remedies had noticeable impact, at least at the concentrations we tested. As a consequence, it appears infeasible to quickly disintegrate stones by attempting to attack, specifically, the organic material in the stones.

We attribute these results to the recognition that a distinct organic matrix is not present, so that organic and inorganic constituents are not structured as "brick and mortar" configurations. Rather, it appears that real CaOx stone structures involve aggregates and inclusions that interweave inorganic and organic constituents having a wide range of (sub)crystal structures. This conclusion is further supported by analysis of dissolution properties by mineral acids that target a broad spectrum of both organic and inorganic materials: parallel tests using the above protocols with concentrated HCl (8.8 M) and

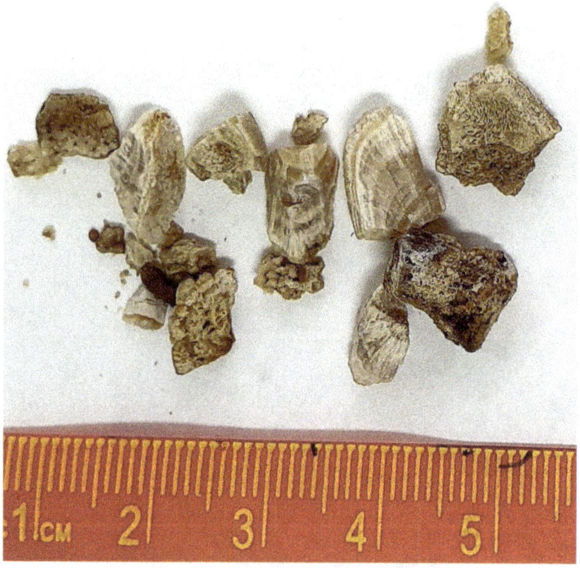

Fig. 2 Example of CaOx stone fragments from a single patient. Note the various external and internal views of the stone fragments, some showing regions with visible internal layering, and others showing more heterogeneous or amorphous internal structures

HNO_3 (11.1 M) yielded up to 100% dissolution within 0.5–3 h, with no detectable (visually, and following filtration on Whatman GF/A (Sigma-Aldrich) filters) particulate matter in solution. In contrast, similar tests using pure synthetic CaOx crystals show dissolution rates at least 1–2 orders of magnitude faster than human CaOx stones. The same acids at lower concentration—0.1 M—showed negligible dissolution even after 72 h; for comparison, HCl at 0.1 M is similar to that of gastric acid (100 meq). Detailed comparisons showing such behavior, between synthetic CaOx crystals and powdered real CaOx stones, appear elsewhere [32]. Thus, it appears that only strong agents that can simultaneously attack inorganic and organic components lead to fast stone dissolution.

We emphasize here that the findings from this systematic survey do not rule out the possibility (1) that some agents, such as potassium citrate or EDTA, may have a softening or slow dissolution effect on existing CaOx kidney stones, over longer time periods, and/or (2) that some of these agents, as well as others, may be beneficial in inhibiting or preventing formation of entirely new stones. [We note parenthetically, too, but in a different context, that natural, in vivo dissolution may occur over thin, nanometer layers of CaOx stones, with estimated time scales of hours [18].]

A unique feature of this study—systematic analysis of the effects of a wide range of potential dissolution agents on actual CaOx kidney stones—has an inherent limitation, namely, the lack of uniform stone size, structure, and composition among real stone samples even from the same patient. On the other hand, synthetically-grown kidney stones are relatively homogeneous, and in particular do not contain the potentially critical impurities, including organic matter, present in real stones. To reduce the uncertainty and variability in our survey, stone fragments from the same patient were tested where possible, in parallel. We also mediated the size differences by keeping a constant ratio of solution to stone mass. We emphasize, too, that stone *fragments* were employed, so that possible dissolution—a surface phenomenon—was maximized by solution exposure to both internal and external portions of each stone. In spite of the inherent variability in surface area, and use of replicates, similar behavior (essentially no dissolution or disintegration) was found among treatments.

Conclusions

Our study is the first to examine the feasibility of inducing chemolysis of CaOx kidney stones, within hours, by specifically attacking the organic matrix present in CaOx stones. This matrix is often reported to be a possible binding agent between CaOx particles. In contrast to previous studies, we focused on the possible "brick and mortar" stone configuration, in an effort to gain basic insight into disintegration behavior of these stones. We systematically tested, via in vitro experiments, the ability of an extensive range of 26 potential chemolysis agents to induce relatively fast disintegration (and/or dissolution) of a large set of natural CaOx stone fragments, extracted during endourological procedures, without regard to immediate clinical application.

Within time periods of up to 72 h, we find—notably—that a broad range of biogeochemical agents known to attack organic material have little, if any, effect on the stones. Similarly, protein and enzymatic agents, and oral additive medical treatments (primarily potassium citrate pills and lemon juice), have little effect. These findings suggest that the organic and inorganic constituents present in CaOx stones are not structured as "brick and mortar" configurations, so that stone disintegration does not occur readily by attacking organic components. Rather, CaOx stones represent more complex aggregates that interweave inorganic and organic constituents, with wide ranges of (sub)crystal structures and inclusions.

To reach a translational approach at the clinical level, one must first understand the disintegration behavior of kidney stones and potential/perceived prospects for fast, in vivo disintegration. It remains to evaluate new routes for fast in vitro breakdown, and ultimately, in vivo, CaOx chemolytic treatments.

Abbreviations

CaOx: Calcium oxalate.

Acknowledgements

The authors thank Prof. Itay Halevy and Nir Galili for x-ray diffraction analysis of the kidney stone samples.

Authors' contributions

All authors contributed to the study conception and design. Material preparation, data collection, and analysis were performed by AA, ID YS and BB. The first draft of the manuscript was written by BB, with key input from AA and ID, and all authors commented on previous versions of the manuscript. All authors read and approved the final manuscript.

Author details

[1] Department of Urology, Kaplan Medical Center, 7661041 Rehovot, Israel.
[2] Department of Earth and Planetary Sciences, Weizmann Institute of Science, 7610001 Rehovot, Israel.

References

1. Chen Z, Prosperi M, Bird VY. Prevalence of kidney stones in the USA, The National Health and Nutrition Evaluation Survey. J Clin Urol. 2018. https://doi.org/10.1177/2051415818813820.
2. López M, Hoppe B. History, epidemiology and regional diversities of urolithiasis. Pediatr Nephrol. 2010;25:49–59. https://doi.org/10.1007/s00467-008-0960-5.
3. Sinha M, Prabhu K, Venkatesh P, Krishnamoorthy V. Results of urinary dissolution therapy for radiolucent calculi. Int Braz J Urol. 2013;39:103–7. https://doi.org/10.1590/S1677-5538.IBJU.2013.01.13.
4. Kim D, Rimer JD, Asplin JR. Hydroxycitrate: a potential new therapy for calcium urolithiasis. Urolithiasis. 2019;47:311–20. https://doi.org/10.1007/s00240-019-01125-1.
5. Morgan MSC, Pearle MS. Medical management of renal stones. BMJ. 2016;352:i52. https://doi.org/10.1136/bmj.i52.
6. Gonzalez RD, Whiting BM, Canales BK. The history of kidney stone dissolution therapy: 50 years of optimism and frustration with Renacidin. J Endourol. 2012;26:110–8. https://doi.org/10.1089/end.2011.0380.
7. Xiang-bo Z, Zhi-ping W, Jian-min D, Jian-zhong L, Bao-liang M. New che molysis for urological calcium phosphate calculi—a study in vitro. BMC Urol. 2005;5:9. https://doi.org/10.1186/1471-2490-5-9.
8. Kachrilas S, Papatsoris A, Bach C, Bourdoumis A, Zaman F, Masood J, Buchholz N. The current role of percutaneous chemolysis in the management of urolithiasis: review and results. Urolithiasis. 2013;41:323–6. https://doi.org/10.1007/s00240-013-0575-6.
9. Kustov AV, Shevyrin AA, Strel'nikov AI, Smirnov PR, Trostin VN. Chemolysis of calcium oxalate stones: study in vitro and possible clinical application. Urol Res. 2012;40:205–9. https://doi.org/10.1007/s00240-011-0429-z.
10. Thalji NK, Richards NG, Peck AB, Canales BK. Enzymatic dissolution of calcium and struvite crystals: in vitro evaluation of biochemical requirements. Urology. 2011;78:721.e13-721.e17. https://doi.org/10.1016/j.urology.2011.04.046.
11. Chutipongtanate S, Chaiyarit S, Thongboonkerd V. Citrate, not phosphate, can dissolve calcium oxalate monohydrate crystals and detach these crystals from renal tubular cells. Euro J Pharmacol. 2012;690:219–25. https://doi.org/10.1016/j.ejphar.2012.06.012.
12. Zhou X-J, Zhang J, Zhang C, Xu C-G. In vitro dissolution of calcium oxalate stones with ethylenediaminetetraacetic acid and snake venom thrombin-like enzyme. Urol Int. 2014;92:349–55. https://doi.org/10.1159/000353096.
13. Stapleton AMF, Dawson CJ, Grover PK, Hohmann A, Comacchio R, Boswarva V, Tang Y, Ryall RL. Further evidence linking urolithiasis and blood coagulation: urinary prothrombin fragment 1 is present in stone matrix. Kidney Int. 1996;49(3):880–8. https://doi.org/10.1038/ki.1996.121.
14. Durrbaum D, Rodgers AL, Sturrock ED. A study of crystal matrix extract and urinary prothrombin fragment 1 from a stone-prone and stone-free population. Urol Res. 2001;29:83–8. https://doi.org/10.1007/s002400000163.
15. Wesson JA, Ward MD. Pathological biomineralization of kidney stones. Elements. 2007;3:415–21. https://doi.org/10.2113/GSELEMENTS.3.6.41.
16. Cloutier J, Villa L, Traxer O, Daudon M. Kidney stone analysis: "give me your stone, I will tell you who you are!" World J Urol. 2015;33:157–69. https://doi.org/10.1007/s00345-014-1444-9.
17. Khan SR, Pearle MS, Robertson WG, Gambaro G, Canales BK, Doizi S, Traxer O, Tiselius H-G. Kidney stones. Nat Rev Dis Primers. 2016;2:16008. https://doi.org/10.1038/nrdp.2017.1.
18. Sivaguru M, Saw JJ, Williams JC Jr, Lieske JC, Krambeck AE, Romero MF, Chia N, Schwaderer AL, Alcalde RE, Bruce WJ, Wildman DE, Fried GA, Werth CJ, Reeder RJ, Yau PM, Sanford RA, Fouke BW. Geobiology reveals how human kidney stones dissolve in vivo. Sci Rep. 2018;8:13731. https://doi.org/10.1038/s41598-018-31890-9.
19. Grover PK, Thurgood LA, Fleming DE, van Bronswijk W, Wang T, Ryall RL. Intracrystalline urinary proteins facilitate degradation and dissolution of calcium oxalate crystals in cultured renal cells. Am J Physiol-Renal. 2008;294:F355–61. https://doi.org/10.1152/ajprenal.00529.2007.
20. Witzmann FA, Evan AP, Coe FL, Worcester EM, Lingeman JE, Williams JC Jr. Label-free proteomic methodology for the analysis of human kidney stone matrix composition. Proteome Sci. 2016;14:4. https://doi.org/10.1186/s12953-016-0093-x.
21. Rez P. What does the crystallography of stones tell us about their formation? Urolithiasis. 2017;45:11–8. https://doi.org/10.1007/s00240-016-0951-0.
22. Boyce WH, Garvey FK. The amount and nature of the organic matrix in urinary calculi: a review. J Urol. 1956;76(3):213–27. https://doi.org/10.1016/S0022-5347(17)66686-2.
23. Boyce WH. Organic matrix of human urinary concretions. Am J Med. 1968;45(5):673–83. https://doi.org/10.1016/0002-9343(68)90203-9.
24. Daudon M, Dessombz A, Frochot V, Letavernier E, Haymann J-P, Jungers P, Bazin D. Comprehensive morpho-constitutional analysis of urinary stones improves etiological diagnosis and therapeutic strategy of nephrolithiasis. C R Chim. 2016;19(11–12):1470–91. https://doi.org/10.1016/j.crci.2016.05.008.
25. Grases F, Costa-Bauzá A, Ramis M, Montesinos V, Conte A. Simple classification of renal calculi closely related to their micromorphology and etiology. Clin Chim Acta. 2002;322:29–36. https://doi.org/10.1016/S0009-8981(02)00063-3.
26. Kalidhasan S, Dror I, Berkowitz B. Atrazine degradation through PEI-copper nanoparticles deposited onto montmorillonite and sand. Sci Rep. 2017;7:1415. https://doi.org/10.1038/s41598-017-01429-5.
27. Koppenol WH. The centennial of the Fenton reaction. Free Radic Biol Med. 1993;15:645–51. https://doi.org/10.1016/0891-5849(93)90168-T.
28. Jiménez-Lamana J, Wojcieszek J, Jakubiak M, Asztemborskac M, Szpunar J. Single particle ICP-MS characterization of platinum nanoparticles uptake and bioaccumulation by: *Lepidium sativum* and *Sinapis alba* plants. J Anal At Spectrom. 2016;31:2321–9. https://doi.org/10.1039/C6JA00201C
29. Chao TT. Use of partial dissolution techniques in geochemical exploration. J Geochem Explor. 1984;20:101–35. https://doi.org/10.1016/0375-6742(84)90078-5.
30. Eby N. Principles of environmental geochemistry. San Diego: Cengage Learning, Inc.; 2003.
31. Zuckerman JM, Assimos DG. Hypocitraturia. Pathophysiology and medical management. Rev Urol. 2009;11(3):134–44. https://doi.org/10.3909/riu0424.
32. White DJ, Coyle-Rees M, Nancollas GH. Kinetic factors influencing the dissolution behavior of calcium oxalate renal stones: a constant composition study. Calcif Tissue Int. 1988;43:319–27. https://doi.org/10.1007/BF02556642.

3

Risk factors of kidney stone disease: A cross-sectional study in the southeast of Iran

Parvin Khalili[1], Zahra Jamali[2], Tabandeh Sadeghi[3], Ali Esmaeili-nadimi[2], Maryam Mohamadi[4], Amir Moghadam-Ahmadi[5], Fatemeh Ayoobi[2*] and Alireza Nazari[2]

Abstract

Background: The prevalence of kidney stones in the world is increasing and environmental factors seem to play a major role in this issue. The aim of the present study was to investigate the prevalence of risk factors of kidney stones in the adult population of Rafsanjan city based on the data of the Rafsanjan Cohort Study (RCS).

Methods: In the baseline phase of this study, 10,000 people aged 35 to 70 years are enrolled in the RCS, as one of the prospective epidemiological research studies in Iran. From this population, 9932 participants completed related demographic questionnaires as well as reported a history of diabetes mellitus, kidney stone, and hypertension diseases. The obtained data were analyzed using univariable and multivariable logistics regression.

Results: According to the obtained results, 46.54% of the studied population were male and 53.46% were female. The mean age of the participants was 49.94 ± 9.56 years. 2392 people accounting for 24.08% of the population had kidney stones. After adjustment of the variables, six variables of gender, WSI, no consumption of purified water, BMI, and history of hypertension and diabetes were found to be significant related factors of kidney stone disease.

Conclusions: Gender, hypertension, obesity, diabetes, and personal habits like alcohol consumption, opium use and, cigarette smoking are effective in the development of kidney stones. So, by identifying the susceptible patients and teaching them, the burden of the disease on society and the individual can be reduced. The results of this study are helpful to health care providers for preventive planning for kidney stone disease.

Keywords: Kidney stone, Risk factors, Prospective epidemiological research studies in Iran (PERSIAN)

Background

The prevalence and incidence of kidney stones is rising worldwide [1]. Kidney stones are hard deposits of minerals (calcium, oxalate and phosphate) which are formed from dissolved minerals in the urine and are usually excreted in the urethra [2]. Kidney stones are the third most common urinary tract problem after urinary tract infections and prostate disorders [3]. Kidney stones are classified into calcium oxalate, calcium phosphate, uric acid, cysteine, struvite, and mixed stones types, depending on the material of the stones. Calcium stones account for almost 70–80% of all kidney stones [4].

Risk factors related to kidney stones are different among different population groups and environmental factors have a key role in their pathogenesis [5]. Research on urological patients has shown that the incidence of kidney stones can be associated with sex, race, geographic region, occupation, hot climate, positive family history, unhealthy diet (excessive intake of caffeine, salt, dairy products, animal proteins and fat) [6], smoking, alcohol consumption, physical activity, obesity, low fluid intake, dehydration [2] socioeconomic status, education [5], water quality [7], high intake of vitamins D and C [8], genetic background [9] and comorbid metabolic

*Correspondence: ayoobi.fatemeh@gmail.com
[2] Non-Communicable Diseases Research Center, Rafsanjan University of Medical Sciences, Rafsanjan, Iran
Full list of author information is available at the end of the article

disorders (diabetes mellitus, hypertension, chronic kidney disease, and cardiovascular disease) [1].

Epidemiologically, about 5% of women and 12% of men experience kidney stones during their lives [9]. Basiri et al. which conducted a study on the prevalence of urinary stones among 24 provinces of Iran, reported an average age of 41.5 years for the patients [7]. In another study, Safarinejad et al. found that the average cumulative recurrence of kidney stones was 16% after 1 year, 33% after 5 years and 53% after 10 years [5].

Iran is located on the kidney stone belt and this health issue is of high prevalence (5.7%) in this country [5' 10]. Kidney stone disease is a costly disease because it imposes a major financial burden to the patient and society [11]. Epidemiological evaluation of the issue, particularly assessment of the related risk factors, may result in finding appropriate approaches that reduce the risk of the development of kidney stones. Also, previous studies have shown that interventions in nutrition and water composition can prevent the occurrence of kidney stones [6, 12]. In some studies, contradictory results have been obtained about the risk factors associated with the formation of kidney stone [1, 2, 5–8], and additional studies should be performed to resolve the existing ambiguities. On the other hand, limited studies in Iran have reported demographic factors affecting the kidney stones and the prevalence of kidney stones among probabilistic samples in a population-based study. Accordingly, the present study was aimed to investigate the related factors of kidney stone disease in the adult population of Rafsanjan city, based on the data of the Rafsanjan Cohort study (RCS).

Methods

Study population

The population of this study was actually the population of the RCS, one of Prospective Epidemiological Research Studies in Iran (PERSIAN). In the RCS, it was designed to recruit a total of 10,000 participants of both genders aged 35–70 years from four pre-determined districts (2500 participants from each site) of Rafsanjan city (in the Southeast of Iran) including both urban and suburban areas. Of all the participants, 9932 had a complete medical questionnaire and entered our study using census sampling method. Those who had incomplete medical questionnaire met our exclusion criterion and so were excluded [13]. The following inclusion criteria were considered in the selection of the population: (1) inclusion of areas with minimum migration rates in order to limit loss to follow-up rate (2) inclusion of populations with different socio-economic levels, as well as environmental and occupational exposures [13]. The protocol of the present study was designed in accordance with the Persian cohort study and also was approved by the Ethics Committee of Rafsanjan University of Medical Sciences with the Ethical code of IR.RUMS.REC.1399.029.

Outcome assessment

Expert interviewers interviewed each participant and completed the related questionnaires about his/her socioeconomic status, demography, occupational status, personal habits, history of disease, biochemical tests, blood pressure, physical activity and body mass index (BMI). All of the questionnaires were previously validated in the PERSIAN cohort study [14].

Based on the self-administered questionnaire, kidney stone, hypertension and diabetes was identified and included in the history of diseases if the disease was previously diagnosed by a doctor. Also, the expert interviewers asked questions about the signs of the diseases and the treatments used was overweight and obesity, intake of purified water, habits and lifestyle were also self-reported by the participants [13].

Education level was coded as (1) Illiterate, (2) Elementary, (3) Guidance school and Diploma, (4) College education [13]. It is noteworthy that the informed consent was obtained from the legal guardians of the illiterate participants.

The daily physical activity of the participants was weighted based on its relative metabolic cost, known as a metabolic equivalent (MET), and MET-h/day for 24 h is derived in this way [14, 15].

Data on the personal habit including cigarette and hookah smoking, alcohol drinking, and opium consumption were coded as yes (currently or formerly) and no (never) [13].

The wealth score index (WSI) was classified into four categories: low income (1st quartile: ≤ -0.6069), low-middle income (2nd quartile: -0.607 to 0.0349), middle-high income (3rd quartile: 0.035 to 1.169) and high income (4th quartile: ≥ 1.170) [14].

The source of drinking water was also questioned; whether purified water was consumed or not [13].

Statistical analyses

Related factors for kidney stones including sociodemographic characteristics, life style and history of chronic disease were identified using relevant epidemiological texts and based on subject matter knowledge. For describing the distribution of the data, the frequency (percentage) of the categorical variables and the mean ± standard deviation of the quantitative variables were reported and their distribution among the case and control groups were compared using chi-square and independent t-test tests, respectively. The strength of the association between histories of kidney stones and relevant related factors was evaluated using odds ratios (ORs) and confidence intervals (CIs). We used univariable and multivariable logistics regression analyses to estimate odds ratios with 95% confidence intervals. For this purpose, separate models at bivariate level were run to obtain variables associated with kidney stone, at first. Afterwards, variables with a p value < 0.25 were included in the multivariable logistic regression model to calculate the adjusted odds ratio (OR) and 95% confidence interval (CI). The goodness-of-fit of the adjusted model was assessed using Hosmer–Lemeshow test. To clarify how kidney stone can be identified by gender, age, education level, WSI, cigarette smoking, alcohol drinking, opium consumption, hookah smoking, BMI, and history of chronic disease (diabetes and hypertension), receiver operating characteristic (ROC) curve analysis was applied. According to the method suggested by Swets [16] the area under the ROC curve follows: less accurate ($0.5 < \text{AUROC} < 0.7$), moderately accurate ($0.7 < \text{AUROC} < 0.9$), highly accurate ($0.9 < \text{AUROC} < 1$), and perfect tests ($\text{AUROC} = 1$). All of the analyses were performed using State V.12. All p values were two-sided, and p values < 0.05 and 95% confidence intervals were considered as statistically significant.

Results

This study included 9932 participants, 4622 men (46.54%) and 5310 women (53.46%) with the mean age of 49.94 ± 9.56 years.

The details of the demographic characteristics including age, gender, education level, habits and WSI were presented in Table 1. As one can see, the distribution of these characteristics was different in the case (with kidney stone) and the control (without kidney stone) groups. In addition, we compared the distribution of lifestyle-related variables, as well as, history of diabetes and high blood pressure between the two groups.

The prevalence of kidney stone was associated with alcohol drinking, opium consumption, and hookah smoking. Moreover, kidney stone was more prevalent in the people with middle-high WSI, high BMI, and with a history of diabetes and blood pressure.

Majority of the case group (people with kidney stone) was male and had significantly higher alcohol consumption, higher opium use, Hookah smoking and middle to higher WSI in comparison to the control group (people without kidney stone). Consumption of purified drinking water was considerably lower in the case group compared with the control group. In addition, the cases were more likely to have a high BMI, history of diabetes and high blood pressure compared with the study controls (Table 1).

Table 2 represents the association of patient factors and kidney stone, using the univariate and multivariate analyses. The related factors associated with kidney stone in Univariate analysis were also assessed and the subjects with kidney stone were compared with the normal subjects (Table 2). The odds of having kidney stone were estimated for twelve factors: gender, age, education level, WSI, cigarette smoking, alcohol drinking, opium consumption, hookah smoking, BMI, consumption of purified water in lifetime, and history of chronic disease (diabetes and hypertension) (Table 2). It was found that all of these factors with the exception of cigarette smoking were significantly associated with kidney stone in the Univariate analysis.

After adjustment, only six variables of gender, 3 levels of the WSI (low, low-middle and middle-high), consumption of purified water in lifetime, BMI, history of hypertension and diabetes were shown to be significantly associated with kidney stone (Table 2). In the crude regression model, the odds of kidney stone was higher (odds ratio (OR): 1.38, 95%CI 1.26 to 1.52) among men compared with women and the odds increased after adjustment for confounders (adjusted model) (OR: 1.57, 95% CI 1.39 to1.76). In the crude regression model, the odds of kidney stone was slightly higher for all categories of WSI except high (low-middle OR: 1.16, 95% CI 1.02 to 1.32 and middle-high OR: 1.23, 95% CI 1.09 to 1.40) and this association persisted after adjustment for the confounders (low-middle OR: 1.14, 95% CI 1.01 to 1.30 and middle-high OR: 1.25, 95% CI 1.10 to 1.42). Also, in the crude regression model the odds of kidney stone were slightly higher in overweight and obese people (25 to 29.9 kg/m^2 OR: 1.24, 95% CI 1.11 to 1.40 and ≥ 30 kg/m^2 OR: 1.25, 95% CI 1.14 to 1.41), in comparison to normal-weight people and this association persisted after adjustment for the confounders (25 to 29.9 kg/m^2 OR: 1.24, 95% CI 1.11 to 1.40 and ≥ 30 kg/m^2 OR: 1.30, 95% CI 1.14 to 1.48). Regarding history of high blood pressure and diabetes, in the crude regression model, the odds of kidney stone was higher in people with history of high blood pressure (OR: 1.48, 95% CI 1.33 to 1.64) and diabetes (OR: 1.45, 95% CI 1.29 to1.61), in comparison to healthy people. Although, the odds of kidney stone was slightly reduced after adjustment for the confounders, the association persisted for high blood pressure (OR: 1.33, 95% CI 1.18 to 1.50) and diabetes (OR: 1.26, 95% CI 1.12 to1.43). In addition, no consumption of purified water in lifetime was associated with kidney stones (OR: 1.20, 95% CI 1.08 to 1.35) after adjustment for the confounders. Assessment of goodness-of-fit of the adjusted model using Hosmer–Lemeshow test showed that the model fits well ($p = 0.\ 0811$). After adjustment, ROC

Table 1 Baseline characteristics of the Rafsanjan cohort participants with and without kidney stone

Characteristics	Total (n = 9932)	Kidney stone (n = 2392)	No kidney stone (n = 7540)
Age—years (Mean ± SD)	49.94 ± 9.56	51.02 ± 9.48	49.59 ± 9.56
Age—no. (%)			
35–44	3433 (34.57)	725 (30.31)	2708 (35.92)
45–54	3028 (30.49)	723 (30.23)	2305 (30.57)
55–64	2745 (27.64)	735 (30.73)	2010 (26.66)
≥ 65	726 (7.31)	209 (8.74)	517 (6.86)
Gender—no. (%)			
Female	5310 (53.46)	1132 (47.32)	4178 (55.41)
Male	4622 (46.54)	1260 (52.68)	3362 (44.59)
Education—no. (%)			
Illiterate	948 (9.55)	245 (10.24)	703 (9.33)
Elementary	2537 (25.56)	640 (26.76)	1897 (25.18)
Guidance school and Diploma	4820 (48.55)	1102 (46.07)	3718 (49.34)
College	1622 (16.34)	405 (16.93)	1217 (16.15)
Physical activity (mean ± SD)	38.79 ± 6.32	38.85 ± 6.30	38.77 ± 6.33
Alcohol consumption—no. (%)			
Yes	1352 (13.64)	361 (15.13)	991 (13.17)
No	8599 (86.36)	2025 (84.87)	6534 (86.83)
Cigarette smoking—no. (%)			
Yes	2542 (25.59)	628 (26.25)	1914 (25.38)
No	7390 (74.41)	1764 (73.75)	5626 (74.62)
Hookah smoking—no. (%)			
Yes	1718 (17.30)	466 (19.48)	1252 (16.60)
No	8214 (82.70)	1926 (80.52)	6288 (83.40)
Opium consumption—no. (%)			
Yes	2378 (23.94)	616 (25.75)	1762 (23.37)
No	7554 (76.06)	1776 (74.25)	5778 (76.63)
Drinking of purified water in lifetime—no. (%)			
Yes	4692 (47.47)	1005 (42.16)	3687 (49.16)
No	5192 (52.53)	1379 (57.84)	3813 (50.84)
Hypertension—no. (%)			
Yes	2235 (22.50)	668 (27.93)	1567 (20.78)
No	7697 (77.50)	1724 (72.07)	5973 (79.22)
BMI—no. (%)			
< 25	2865 (28.87)	610 (25.51)	2255 (29.94)
25–29.9	4069 (41.01)	1025 (42.87)	3044 (40.41)
≥ 30	2989 (30.12)	756 (31.62)	2233 (29.65)
Diabetes mellitus—no. (%)			
Yes	1933 (19.46)	576 (24.08)	1357 (18.00)
No	7999 (80.54)	1816 (75.92)	6183 (82.00)
WSI—no. (%)			
Low	2720 (27.41)	600 (25.09)	2120 (28.15)
Low-middle	2462 (24.81)	608 (25.43)	1854 (24.62)
Middle-high	2780 (28.02)	720 (30.11)	2060 (27.35)
High	1960 (19.75)	463 (19.36)	1497 (19.88)

BMI body mass index, *WSI* wealth score index

Table 2 Patient factors and the odds of having kidney stone (n = 9932)

Patient factors	Univariable OR (95% CI)	Multivariable OR (95% CI)
Age—year		
35–44	1	1
45–54	1.17 (1.04–1.32)	1.04 (0.92–1.19)
55–64	1.37 (1.21–1.54)	1.10 (0.95–1.28)
≥65	1.51 (1.26–1.82)	1.15 (0.93–1.42)
Gender		
Female	1	1
Male	1.38 (1.26–1.52)	1.57 (1.39–1.76)
Alcohol consumption		
No	1	1
Yes	1.18 (1.03–1.34)	1.12 (0.96–1.31)
Cigarette smoking		
No	1	1
Yes	1.05 (0.94–1.16)	0.80 (0.70–0.93)
Hookah smoking		
No	1	1
Yes	1.22 (1.08–1.37)	1.16 (1.02–1.32)
Opium consumption		
No	1	1
Yes	1.14 (1.02–1.26)	1.02 (0.88–1.17)
Drinking of purified water in lifetime		
Yes	1	1
No	1.33 (1.21–1.46)	1.20 (1.08–1.35)
Hypertension		
No	1	1
Yes	1.48 (1.33–1.64)	1.33 (1.18–1.50)
BMI		
<25	1	1
25–29.9	1.24 (1.11–1.40)	1.24 (1.11–1.40)
≥30	1.25 (1.11–1.41)	1.30 (1.14–1.48)
Diabetes mellitus		
No	1	1
Yes	1.45 (1.29–1.61)	1.26 (1.12–1.43)
WSI		
Low	1	1
Low-middle	1.16 (1.02–1.32)	1.14 (1.01–1.30)
Middle-high	1.23 (1.09–1.40)	1.25 (1.10–1.42)
High	1.09 (0.95–1.25)	1.08 (0.94–1.25)

BMI body mass index, *WSI* wealth score index

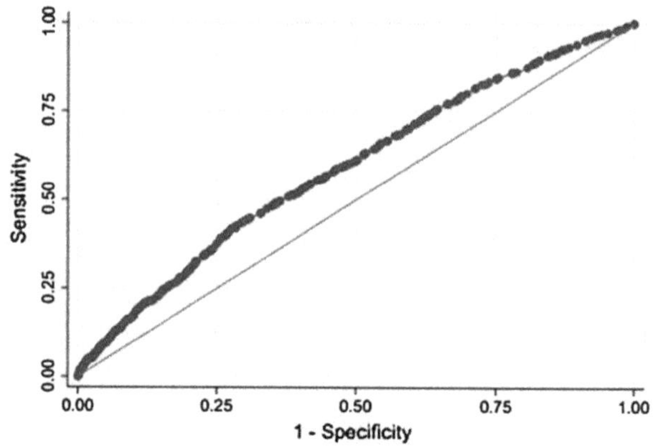

Fig. 1 ROC curve of the related factors for the identification of kidney stone

curve analysis was also employed to clarify how kidney stone can be identified by the variables previously listed. According to the ROC analysis, the AUROC was obtained to be 0.59 (95% CI = 0.586–0.61), for the presence of six variables of gender, WSI, consumption of purified water in lifetime, BMI, history of hypertension and diabetes (Fig. 1).

Discussion

According to the obtained results, significant differences were observed when comparing the case and the control groups based on some demographic variables. Our results showed the highest risk of kidney stone development for male. In contrast, Rafiei et al. reported that women were at the higher risk kidney stone development [8]. However, Curhan found that kidney stone was more prevalent among men in the United States [17]. Shirazi et al., also reported that the majority of cases of kidney stones in Tehran in Iran are men (66.5%) [18]. There are other similar studies in Iran and abroad that confirmed our finding [5, 19–21]. The effects of sex hormones (estrogens and androgens) on urinary oxalate and calcium can be responsible for the higher risk of kidney stone development in men. Estrogen prevents the formation of kidney stones by increasing the production of citric acid [22]. Therefore, recommendations in terms of diet and physical activity for the prevention of kidney stone development in men seem necessary and also, follow-up of them is suggested.

Based on our results, subjects in the case group had higher alcohol consumption (15.13% vs 13.17%), opium use (25.75% vs 23.37), hookah smoking (19.485 vs 16.60) and cigarette smoking (26.25% vs 25.38%) compared with the control group. In this regard, Ketabchi et al. reported higher rate of opium dependency among people with recurrent kidney stone, in Iran [23]. In another study by Nalini et al. [2] 36.03% of the patients with kidney stone had the habits of smoking and 41.59% of them had the habits of alcohol consumption, which are higher than our results. In consistence with the results of the present work, the study conducted by Tamadon et al. showed that the proportion of smokers in nephrolithiasis patients was significantly higher than normal subjects. The relation between cigarette smoking and the formation of kidney stone may be explained by the high levels of cadmium and lead in smokers' body. Cigarette smoking may result in the induction of urolithiasis by reducing urinary flow and increasing the concentration of serum cadmium [2]. However, these associations were examined in the adjusted model and the obtained results showed that there was no association between cigarette smoking, alcohol consumption and opium use with kidney stones after adjusting for other related factors.

According to the results, cases were more likely to have a high WSI and BMI, history of diabetes and high blood pressure compared with the study controls. Even after adjustment for potential confounders, we found that high WSI and BMI, as well as, history of diabetes and high blood pressure increased odds of kidney stones. Similarly, Taylor et al. reported a positive correlation of the risk of kidney stones development with BMI and waist circumference (WC) [24]. Also, Nowfar et al. found that the incidence of nephrolithiasis was directly associated with obesity in both genders [25]. Moreover, the study of Curhan et al. revealed a positive association between the prevalence of calcium oxalate stone disease and BMI [17]. It can be proposed that, weight control and dietary interventions are preventive methods against the development kidney stones.

In our study, 27.93% of the case group had hypertension. In the study of Kalani et al. [26] 29.7% of patients with nephrolithiasis had hypertension, which is consistent with our results. Also, Shang et al. [27] showed that the risk of nephrolithiasis was directly associated with hypertension incidence. In addition, it has been shown that patients with hypertension as a related factor of the metabolic syndrome are more susceptible to kidney stones [5]. Accordingly, these findings are possibly of warning signs for these patients.

Our results showed that 24.08% of the cases had diabetes and the odds of kidney stone in diabetic cases was 1.26 compared with non-diabetic cases, after adjustment for the potential confounders. In this regard, Weinberg et al. [11] found that the severity of Type 2 diabetes was an important risk factor for kidney stone disease. Also Chung et al. reported that patients with kidney stones were at increased risk of diabetes after 5 years of follow-up [28]. However, Kabeya et al. [29] showed that there was no significant relationship between insulin resistance parameters and kidney stone risk, which is inconsistent with our study. Therefore, further studies are needed to clarify this possible relationship.

Based on the results of our study, odds of consumption of purified water in the case group was lower in comparison to the control group, and this parameter was a significantly association of kidney stone. In this regard and in contrast to our results, the results of a study by Basiri et al. on various capitals of Iran showed that the total hardness of tap water was not significantly associated with the regional prevalence of urinary calculus [7]. Also, Pubali et al. reported no considerable association between water quality and the occurrence of kidney stones [30]. Similarly our results, the results of the studies by Barkers and Donnan [31] and Churchill et al. [32] demonstrated a positive association between urinary calculus and the total hardness of drinking water.

Finally, ROC analyses revealed that variables of gender, WSI, no consumption of purified water in lifetime, BMI, and history of hypertension and diabetes are "less accurate" for the identification of kidney stones.

This study has strengths and limitations. One of the main strengths of our study is its population-based nature with a large sample size, and extensive data collection for the related factors of interest (e.g. age, sex, variables related to lifestyle and etc.). However, the study has some limitations too. For instance, cross-sectional design of the present study does not allow deriving any causal inferences. Or this fact that, cross-sectional studies are weak in predicting the risk factors of a model, because the temporality sequence between the related factors and kidney stones in these studies is not clear. In addition, it is possible that a number of the participants have not completely report the status of their kidney stones. On the other hand, there may have been some degrees of non-differential misclassification due to self-reporting and recall biases. Accordingly, it is suggested that the relationships reported here be reconsidered in the follow-up phase of the RCS. In addition, further research is recommended to determine the variables and to be able to suggest efficient ways to reduce the incidence of kidney stones in the general population.

Conclusion

According to the results of the present study, factors such as gender, hypertension, obesity, diabetes and personal habits like alcohol consumption, opium use and cigarette smoking are related with the development of kidney stones. So, by identifying the susceptible patients and teaching them, the burden of the disease on society and the individual can be reduced. The results of this study are helpful to health care providers for preventive planning for kidney stone disease.

Abbreviations

RCS: The Rafsanjan Cohort Study; PERSIAN: Prospective epidemiological research studies in Iran; BMI: Body mass index; CIs: Confidence intervals; OR: Odds ratio; WC: Waist circumference; MET: Metabolic equivalent; WSI: Wealth score index.

Acknowledgements

We thank the people who participated in the study, the study-site personnel, and members of the Rafsanjan cohort center in Rafsanjan, Iran.

Authors' contributions

PK contributed to design of the study, analysis and drafting of the manuscript. ZJ contributed to data collection, drafting of the manuscript. TS contributed to data collection, drafting of the manuscript. AE contributed to the design of the study, data collection. MM contributed to critical review of the draft manuscript. AM contributed to the design of the study, data collection. FA contributed to the design of the study, data collection and critical review of the draft manuscript. AN contributed to the design of the study. All authors read and approved the final manuscript.

Author details

[1]Department of Epidemiology, School of Public Health, Social Determinants of Health Research Centre, Rafsanjan University of Medical Sciences, Rafsanjan, Iran. [2]Non-Communicable Diseases Research Center, Rafsanjan University of Medical Sciences, Rafsanjan, Iran. [3]Department of Pediatric Nursing, School of Nursing and Midwifery, Non-Communicable Diseases Research Center, Rafsanjan University of Medical Sciences, Rafsanjan, Iran. [4]Occupational Safety and Health Research Center, NICICO, World Safety Organization and Rafsanjan University of Medical Sciences, Rafsanjan, Iran. [5]Department of Neurology, School of Medicine, Non-Communicable Diseases Research Center, Rafsanjan University of Medical Sciences, Rafsanjan, Iran.

References

1. Romero V, Akpinar H, Assimos DG. Kidney stones: a global picture of prevalence, incidence, and associated risk factors. Rev Urol. 2010;12(2–3):e86.
2. Sofia NH, Walter TM, Sanatorium T. Prevalence and risk factors of kidney stone. Glob J Res Anal. 2016;5(3):183–7.
3. Delfan B, Baharvand-Ahmadi B, Bahmani M, Mohseni N, Saki K, Rafieian-Kopaei M, et al. An ethnobotanical study of medicinal plants used in treatment of kidney stones and kidney pain in Lorestan province, Iran. J Chem Pharm Sci. 2015;8(4):693–9.
4. Nikpay S, Moradi K, Azami M, Babashahi M, Otaghi M, Borji M. Frequency of kidney stone different compositions in patients referred to a Lithotripsy Center in Ilam, West of Iran. J Pediatr Nephrol. 2016;4(3):102–7.
5. Safarinejad MR. Adult urolithiasis in a population-based study in Iran: prevalence, incidence, and associated risk factors. Urol Res. 2007;35(2):73–82.
6. Salmeh F, Yaghoubi T, Zakizadeh M, Yaghoubian M, Shahmohammadi S. Evaluation of health behaviours in patients with kidney stones in Sari/Iran. Int J Urol Nurs. 2012;6(1):17–21.
7. Basiri A, Shakh SN, Khoushdel A, Pakmanesh H, Radfar MH. Drinking water composition and incidence of urinary calculus introducing a new index. 2011.
8. Rafiei H, Malekpoor F, Amiri M, Rahimi Madiseh M, Lalegani H. Kidney stone development among older adults in Iran. J Indian Acad Geriatr. 2014;10:10–3.
9. Li D, Liu J, Ren J, Yan L, Liu H, Xu Z. Meta-analysis of the urokinase gene 3′-UTR T/C polymorphism and susceptibility to urolithiasis. Biomed Rep. 2013;1(3):369–74.
10. Farshid S, Aghdashi A, Fallahi H, Valizadeh R, Rahimi MM. Evaluation of osteoporosis frequency in patients with recurrent kidney stones. Acta Med Iran. 2020;58(10):494–9.
11. Weinberg AE, Patel CJ, Chertow GM, Leppert JT. Diabetic severity and risk of kidney stone disease. Eur Urol. 2014;65(1):242–7.
12. Frassetto L, Kohlstadt I. Treatment and prevention of kidney stones: an update. Am Fam Phys. 2011;84(11):1234–42.
13. Hakimi H, Ahmadi J, Vakilian A, Jamalizadeh A, Kamyab Z, Mehran M, et al. The profile of Rafsanjan cohort study. Eur J Epidemiol. 2020;36:1–10.
14. Eghtesad S, Mohammadi Z, Shayanrad A, Faramarzi E, Joukar F, Hamzeh B, et al. The PERSIAN cohort: providing the evidence needed for healthcare reform. Arch Iran Med. 2017;20(11):691–5.
15. Aguilar-Farias N, Brown WJ, Skinner TL. Peeters GGJJoPA, Health. Metabolic equivalent values of common daily activities in middle-age and older adults in free-living environments: a pilot study. J Phys Act Health. 2019;16(3):222–9.
16. Swets JA. Measuring the accuracy of diagnostic systems. Science. 1988;240(4857):1285–93.
17. Curhan GC. Epidemiology of stone disease. Urol Clin North Am. 2007;34(3):287–93.
18. Shirazi F, Shahpourian F, Khachian A, Hosseini F, Heidari S, Sanjari M. Personal characteristics and urinary stones. Hong Kong J Nephrol. 2009;11(1):14–9.
19. Healy KA, Hubosky SG, Bagley DH. 24-hour urine collection in the metabolic evaluation of stone formers: is one study adequate? J Endourol. 2013;27(3):374–8.
20. Noshad H, Ahmadpour F, Soltanpour B, Ghojazadeh M. Study of renal stones complications in 200 patients in Tabriz, Iran. J Res Clin Med. 2014;2(4):187–92.
21. Hadian B, Zafar-Mohtashami A, Ghorbani F. Study of urine composition of patients with recurrent nephrolithiasis in Lorestan, Iran. Iran J Kidney Dis. 2018;12(1):22–6.
22. Altaf J, Arain AH, Kella NL, Rehman SU. Chemical analysis of urinary stones and its locations associated to urinary tract. J Liaquat Univ Country: Pakistan. 2013;12(3):203–7.
23. Ketabchi AA, Ebad-Zadeh MR, Parvaresh S, Moshtaghi-Kashanian GR. Opium dependency in recurrent painful renal lithiasis colic. Addict Health. 2012;4(1–2):73.
24. Taylor EN, Stampfer MJ, Curhan GC. Obesity, weight gain, and the risk of kidney stones. JAMA. 2005;293(4):455–62.
25. Nowfar S, Palazzi-Churas K, Chang DC, Sur RL. The relationship of obesity and gender prevalence changes in United States inpatient nephrolithiasis. Urology. 2011;78(5):1029–33.
26. Kalani L, Rashidi N, Mehranfard S, Bahrami H, Majidipour N, Moghaddam AS, et al. Epidemiology of the urinary stones: a 6-year retrospective study at Dezful-Iran. Int J Pharm Phytopharmacol Res. 2020;10(4):79–85.
27. Shang W, Li Y, Ren Y, Yang Y, Li H, Dong J. Nephrolithiasis and risk of hypertension: a meta-analysis of observational studies. BMC Nephrol. 2017;18(1):1–6.
28. Chung S-D, Chen Y-K, Lin H-C. Increased risk of diabetes in patients with urinary calculi: a 5-year followup study. J Urol. 2011;186(5):1888–93.
29. Kabeya Y, Kato K, Tomita M, Katsuki T, Oikawa Y, Shimada A, et al. Associations of insulin resistance and glycemic control with the risk of kidney stones. Intern Med. 2012;51(7):699–705.
30. Mitra P, Pal DK, Das M. Does quality of drinking water matter in kidney stone disease: a study in West Bengal, India. Investig Clin Urol. 2018;59(3):158.
31. Barker D, Donnan S. Regional variations in the incidence of upper urinary tract stones in England and Wales. Br Med J. 1978;1(6105):67–70.
32. Churchill D, Bryant D, Fodor G, Gault MH. Drinking water hardness and urolithiasis. Ann Intern Med. 1978;88(4):513–4.

4

Elevated MTA1 induced the migration and invasion of renal cell carcinoma through the NF-κB pathway

Cai Lv[1], Yuan Huang[2], Qingqing Lei[1], Zhenxiang Liu[1], Shixing Shen[3*] and Wenxia Si[4*]

Abstract

Background: The metastasis-associated gene 1 (MTA1) has been extensively reported as a crucial oncogene, and its abnormal expression has been associated with the progression of numerous cancers. However, the role of MTA1 in renal cell carcinoma (RCC) progression and metastasis remains unclear. Herein, we investigated the expression of MTA1 and its role in RCC.

Methods: 109 matched clear cell RCCs (ccRCCs) and corresponding normal tissue samples were analyzed via immunohistochemistry to test the expression of MTA1. Human A498 cell lines were transfected with pcDNA3.1-Flag (control) or Flag-MTA1 to overexpress MTA1 or with specific interfering RNA (si-MTA1) or specific interfering negative control to knockdown MTA1 expression. Transfected cells were used in wound healing and transwell invasion assay. Quantitative real time polymerase chain reaction was used to assess the effect of MTA1 on MMP2/MMP9 and E-cadherin gene expression. Western blot was used to qualify the phosphorylation of p65.

Results: Herein, we found a significantly increased expression of MTA1 in 109 ccRCCs, compared to the corresponding normal tissue. In addition, the overexpression of MTA1 in A498 cells facilitated cell migration and invasion, while the down-regulation of MTA1 expression using specific interfering RNA sequences could decrease cell migration and invasion. Furthermore, we showed that MTA1 is up-regulated in ccRCCs, which contributes to the migration and invasion of human kidney cancer cells by mediating the expression of MMP2 and MMP9 through the NF-κB signaling pathway. Similarly, we found that MTA1 could regulate E-cadherin expression in RCCs.

Conclusions: MTA1 is overexpressed in RCC and is involved in the progression of RCC through NF-κB.

Keywords: MTA1, RCC, Cell migration and invasion, NF-κB, MMP2/MMP9, E-cadherin

Background

Renal cell carcinoma (RCC) is annually increasing worldwide, often with the lack of early-warning signs, as only up to 10% of RCC patients present characteristic clinical symptoms [1]. Kidney cancer is a highly heterogeneous malignancy, and clear cell RCC (ccRCC) is the most common pathologic type, accounting for 75% of all renal malignancies [2]. The five-year survival rates of RCC patients with stage I, II, III, and IV renal cancer are reported to be 94.7%, 88.9%, 68.8%, and 19.3%, respectively [3]. Thus, earlier detection of RCC places a greater emphasis on the preservation of kidney function and treatment of RCC. With the understanding of the molecular mechanisms underlying RCCs, targeted therapies with small molecules, such as sorafenib and sunitinib, have been effective in treating RCCs [4]. Therefore, further understanding of the underlying mechanisms of

*Correspondence: Hainan2050@163.com; siwenxia1573@163.com
[3] Department of Urology, Danzhou People's Hospital, Danzhou 571799, Hainan, China
[4] Hubei Key Laboratory for Kidney Disease Pathogenesis and Intervention, Huangshi Central Hospital of Edong Healthcare Group, Hubei Polytechnic University School of Medicine, Huangshi, China
Full list of author information is available at the end of the article

RCC development and search for new therapeutic targets dependent on these mechanisms are needed.

The metastasis-associated gene 1 (MTA1) is a crucial gene involved in cancer metastasis and is overexpressed in many cancers, including gastric, ovarian, prostate, and breast cancer [5–9]. MTA1 has been reported as a key component of the nuclear remodeling and deacetylation complex, which regulates metastasis-associated gene expression, including cell migration and invasion [10]. Moreover, MTA1 could mediate the migration and invasion of cancers by regulating the phosphorylation of various intracellular proteins involved in signaling pathways, such as AKT, hypoxia, and hedgehog signaling [7, 8, 11]. MTA1 has been reported to promote cancer cell invasion by depressing the E-cadherin expression [12, 13]. Recently, MTA1 has been recognized as a prognostic biomarker in lung cancer and is associated with poor prognosis in these patients [5]. However, the role of MTA1 in kidney cancer and its molecular mechanisms are currently unknown.

This study aimed to examine the relationship between MTA1 and RCC as well as the MTA1 expression and prognosis of RCC patients. Based on the clinical results, we further performed in vitro experiments to investigate the effects of MTA1 expression on the metastasis of RCC cell line and its molecular mechanisms.

Methods

Patients and tissue samples

The 109 matched ccRCC and adjacent normal tissue specimens were obtained from the Haikou Municipal Hospital (Haikou, China).This study was approved by the Ethics Committee of Haikou Municipal Hospital and by Hubei Polytechnic University. Written informed consent was obtained from all patients.

Cell culture and reagents

The human kidney cancer cell line A498 was purchased from the China Center for Type Culture Collection (Wuhan, China). Cells were cultured in DMEM (Hyclone) with 10% FBS (GIBCO) and incubated in a cell incubator at 37 °C and 5% CO_2.

A498 cells were transfected with Flag-MTA1, specific interfering RNA (siRNA), and their respective controls pcDNA3.1-Flag and siNC using Lipo2000 (Invitrogen). MTA1 siRNA (si-MTA1) and siNC were purchased from Ribobio (Guangzhou, China). The NF-κB inhibitor, pyrrolidine dithiocarbamate (PDTC), was purchased from MedChemEepress.

Immunohistochemistry

The ccRCC and adjacent tissues were treated following our previous report [14]. Briefly, tissues were fixed with formalin (Beijing Suolebao Biotechnology), sectioned, deparaffinized, and hydrated following endogenous peroxidase inactivation and antigen recovery. Sections ware incubated with MTA1 antibody (14682–1-AP, Proteintech) at 4 °C overnight, followed by the secondary antibody (GB23303; Servicebio) at 37 °C for 30 min. After washing, the sections were then treated with diaminobenzidine reagent (DAB horseradish peroxidase color development kit; Beyotime) and visualized at 200× and 400× magnification with a light microscope (Olympus) in a double-blind analysis by two pathologists. For each specimen, the number of positive cells was randomly counted and was scored based on the average percentage of positive cells in five high-power fields (≤ 5%, 0 points; 6–25%, 1 point; 26–50%, 2 points; 51–75%, 3 points; and > 75%, 4 points). In addition, the specimens were scored according to the intensity of staining: no staining, 0 points; light yellow, 1 point; brown, 2 points; light brown, 3 points; and dark brown, 4 points. Finally, the two scores were added and categorized as follows: 0–2, negative; 3–5, weak positive; and 6–8, strong positive. To facilitate statistical analysis, a score of ≥ 3, points was classified as positive.

Quantitative real time polymerase chain reaction

Total RNA was isolated using the TRIzol kit (Takara) as previously described [15]. A total of 2 μg RNA was used to transcribe cDNA using reverse transcription kit (Promega). Quantitative real time polymerase chain reaction (qRT-PCR) was performed using ABI QuantStudio version 5 (Applied Biosystems; Thermo Fisher Scientific, Inc.). The results were analyzed using the $2^{-\Delta\Delta Ct}$ method and GAPDH as an internal reference.

The primers used in the study were as follows:

GAPDH-F	ATCGTGGAAGGACTCATGACC
GAPDH-R	AGGGATGATGTTCTGGAGAGC
MMP2-F	CCCACTGCGGTTTTCTCGAAT
MMP2-R	CAAAGGGGTATCCATCGCCAT
MMP9-F	AGACCTGGGCAGATTCCAAAC
MMP9-R	CGGCAAGTCTTCCGAGTAGT
E-cadherin-F	CGAGAGCTACACGTTCACGG
E-cadherin-R	GGGTGTCGAGGGAAAAATAGG

Western blot assay

Western blot assay was performed as previously described [16]. In brief, the treated A498 cells were lysed with RIPA lysis buffer containing proteinase inhibitors and phosphatase inhibitors (Roche). Then, the obtained cell lysates were used for western blot analysis. The MTA1 (BA2749) was from BOSTER, and β-actin (10230-1-AP) antibodie was purchased from Proteintech,

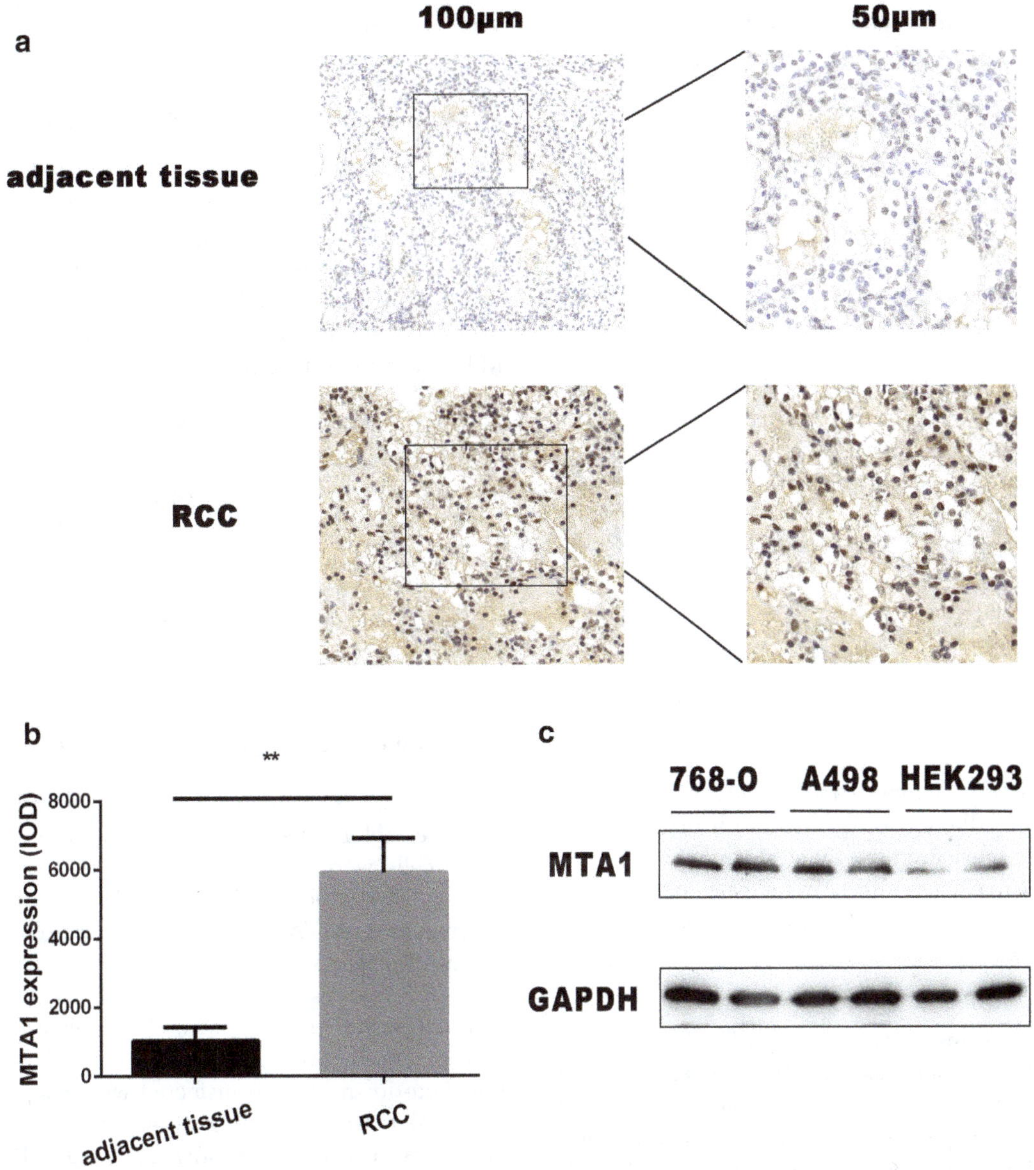

Fig. 1 The expression of MTA1 is up-regulated in RCCs. **a** Immunohistochemistry was used to characterize the expression of MTA1 in RCC and adjacent tissues. MTA1 was highly expressed in ccRCCs, compared to very weak staining in adjacent tissue. **b** Image Pro Plus was used for the statistical analysis of the positive signal (IOD) of MTA1 expression in ccRCCs and the adjacent tissue. The expression of MTA1 was significantly up-regulated in ccRCCs. $^{**}p < 0.01$; scale bar: 100 μm and 50 μm. **c** The expression of MTA1 in RCC cell lines. Normal renal cell line HEK293T and RCC cell lines A498 and 768-O cell lysates were used in western blotting analysis with MTA1 and GAPDH antibodies. The bands of MTA1 were from Additional file 1: Fig. 1 and gapdh were from Additional file 1: Fig. 1

Table 1 MTA1 expression in 109 pairs of RCC and adjacent tissues

Tissue type	MTA1		χ^2 value	*p* value
	Positive	Negative		
Renal cell carcinoma	81	28	44.114	0.000
Adjacent tissue	32	77		

Note: MTA1, metastasis-associated gene 1; RCC, renal cell carcinoma

and p65 (AF5006) and p-p65 (AF2006) antibodies were obtained from Affinity Biosciences.

Cell migration assay: wound healing

Cultured A498 cells (at 80% confluence) were transfected with Flag-MTA1, si-MTA1, and their relative control vectors pcDNA3.1-Flag and siNC using Lipo2000 (Invitrogen). After 12 h, a wound (scratch) was artificially created

Table 2 Relationship between MTA1 expression and clinical-pathological data in ccRCC patients

Clinical-pathological feature	MTA1		χ^2 value	*p* value
	Positive, n	Negative, n		
Age, year				
<60	29	16	3.909	0.048*
≥60	52	12		
Sex				
Male	56	16	1.335	0.248
Female	25	12		
T stage				
T1	18	13	6.159	0.046*
T2	38	10		
T3	25	5		
Grade				
G1	20	14	6.813	0.033*
G2	27	8		
G3	34	6		
Lymph node metastasis				
With	19	4	1.051	0.305
Without	62	24		

*$p < 0.05$

using the tip of a 10 μl pipette in the center of middle well containing the adherent cells. The width of the scratch was regularly measured under 100 × magnification to measure the gap closure rate as an indicator of cell migration data on wound healing (Olympus microscope).

Cell invasion assay

A498 cells were transfected with Flag-MTA1, pcDNA3.1-Flag, si-MTA1, and siNC as described above. After 24 h, cells from each condition were transferred in to the upper part of matrigel-coated (rehydrated with medium, 1:8) transwell chambers with 200 μL serum-free DMEM, while the lower part of the chamber contained 500 μL DMEM with 10% FBS. After culturing for 12 h in the incubator, the invaded cells on the outer surface of the filter screen were fixed with methyl alcohol for 10 min and were stained by 0.1% crystal violet for 10 min; then, they were photographed using an Olympus light microscope using a 40 × objective and counted using Image J.

Statistical analysis

All statistical analyses were performed using SPSS version 17.1. The correlations between the MTA1 expression and the clinical-pathological characteristics were determined using the χ^2 test. Data are expressed as the mean ± standard deviation. Statistical significance was analyzed using the Student's *t*-test between the two groups and ANOVA for multiple groups. A *p* value < 0.05 was considered significant.

Results

MTA1 was highly expressed in RCC cells and tissues

To explore the relationship between the MTA1 expression and RCC progression, the expression of MTA1 in 109 pairs of ccRCCs and adjacent tissues was analyzed by immunohistochemistry. As shown in Fig. 1a, b, MTA1 was highly expressed in ccRCCs, while it was poorly expressed in adjacent tissues. In addition, we compared MTA1 expression in corresponding normal tissues and in ccRCC cell lines. In A498 and 768-O RCC cell lines, the MTA1 expressions were higher than those of normal HEK293T cells (Fig. 1c). Further analysis of 109 ccRCCs and adjacent tissue pairs showed that 74.3% (81/109) of ccRCCs had a positive expression of MTA1 (Table 1). As shown in Table 2, the MTA1 expression was associated with the age, tumor (T) stage, and grade in ccRCC patients ($p < 0.05$; Table 2). These clinical data suggest MTA1 may play a crucial role in RCC progression.

MTA1 promotes the migration of RCC cells

As MTA1 plays an important role in migration and invasion, we explored its effect on the migration of RCC cells. A498 cells were engineered to overexpress MTA1 following transfection with Flag-MTA1 or MTA1 knockdown with si-MTA1 and the respective control vectors pcDNA3.1-Flag and negative control (siNC). After 48 h, cells were harvested for WB to test the MTA1 protein levels. As shown in Fig. 4a, the expression of MTA1 was markedly overexpressed in control conditions or knocked-down when transfected with Flag-MTA1 or si-MTA1. For wound healing assay using A498 cells, similar transfections were performed using pcDNA3.1-Flag, Flag-MTA1, Flag-MTA1, siNC, and si-MTA1. After 12 h of transfection, cells were subjected to the wound healing assay for 12 h and 36 h. The wound healing assays showed that overexpression of MTA1 significantly increased migration of A498 cells (Fig. 2; lines 1, 2), whereas the knockdown of MTA1 expression decreased migration of A498 cells (Fig. 2; lines 3, 4).

MTA1 supports A498 cell invasion

To identify whether MTA1 has an effect on the invasion of RCC cells, A498 cells were again transfected with Flag-MAT1, si-MTA, and the negative controls (pcDNA3.1-Flag and siNC) as indicated above. After 36 h of transfection, cells were used in transwell matrigel invasion assays (in vitro). The results are shown in Fig. 3. Compared to the negative control, the overexpression of MTA1 increased the invasion of A498 cells. While the

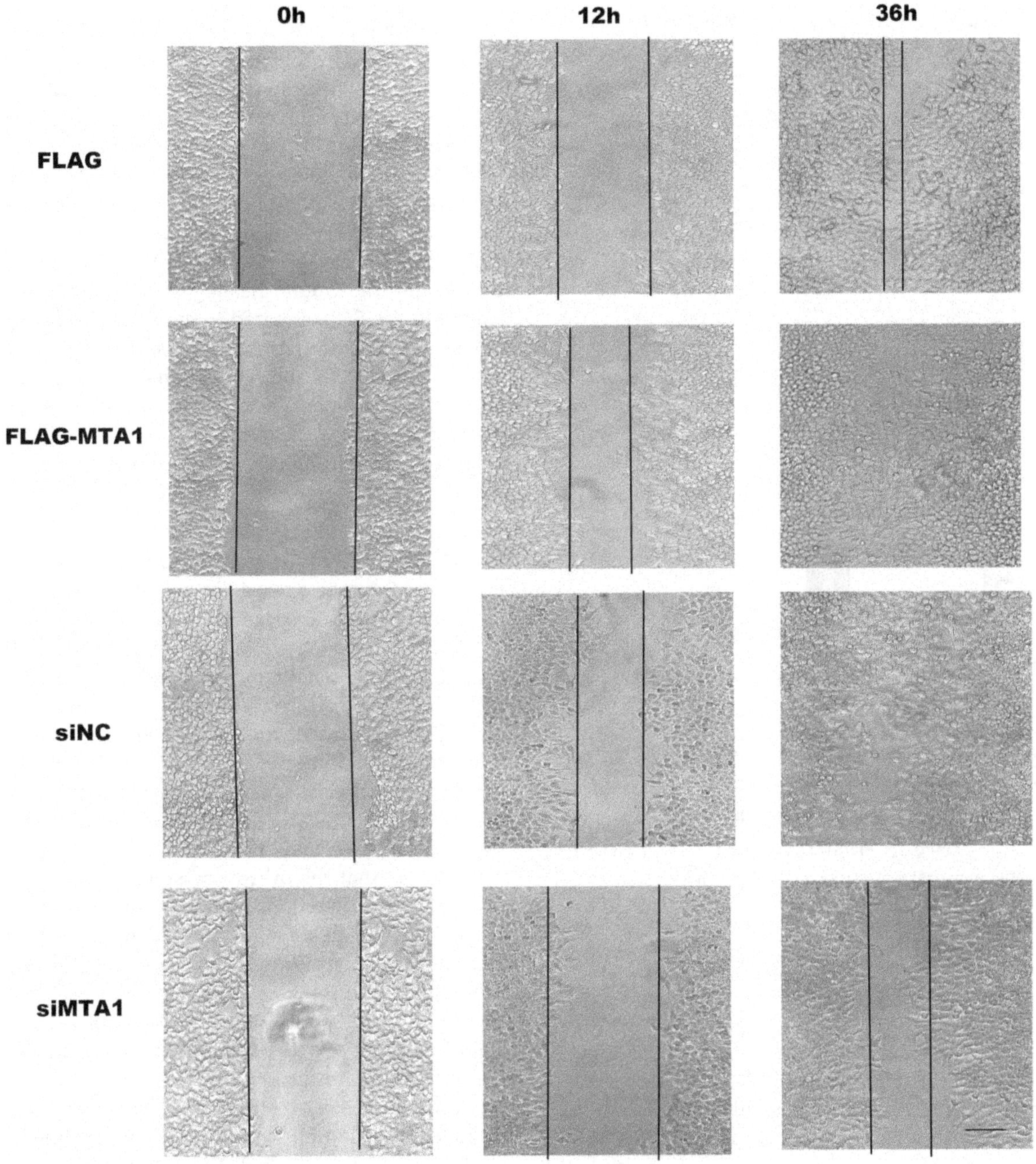

Fig. 2 MTA1 promotes A498 cell migration. A498 cells were transfected with pcDNA3.1-Flag, Flag-MTA1, siNC, and si-MTA1. After 24 h, cells in the four conditions were subjected to the wound healing assay. Macrographs were taken under ×100 magnification

knockdown of the MTA1 expression reduced the A498 cell invasion, compared to the siNC condition.

MTA1 regulates the NF-κB signaling pathway and MPP2/MMP9 as well as the E-cadherin gene expression

Metalloproteinase have been reported to stimulate tumor cell invasion and migration [11]. Furthermore, MTA1 was found to promote invasion by depressing the transcriptional expression of E-cadherin [17]. Thus, we verified the expression of E-cadherin, MPP2, and MPP9 in the MTA1 overexpressed and knocked-down A498 cells by qRT-PCR. The results showed that MTA1 could repress the expression of E-cadherin (Fig. 4a) and up-regulate the expression of MPP2 and MPP9 (Fig. 4b, c).

As is well known, the NF-κB pathway is involved with the regulation of MPP expression [18–20]. To further

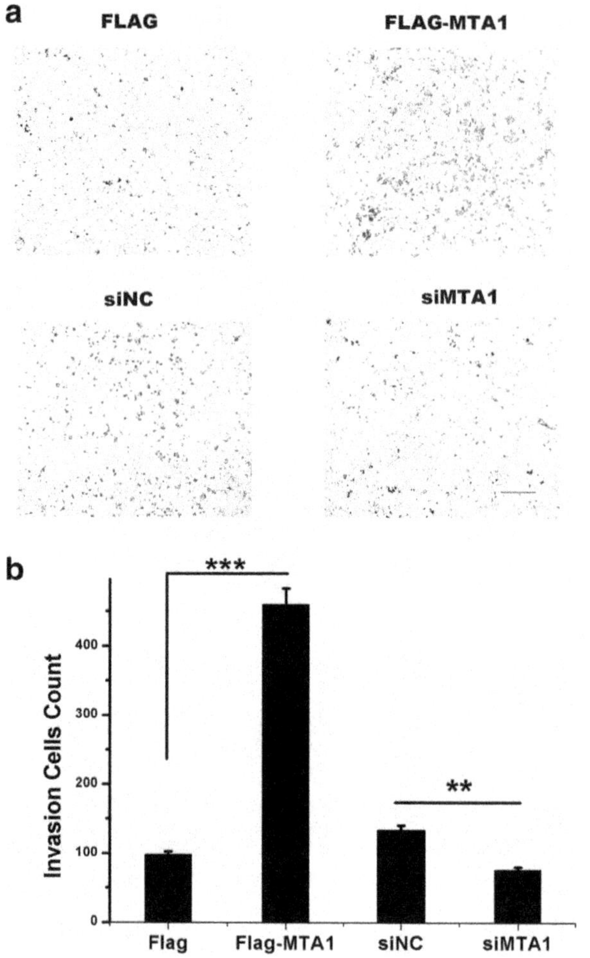

Fig. 3 MTA1 enhances the invasion of A498 cells. **a** A498 cells were transfected with pcDNA3.1-Flag, Flag-MTA1, siNC, and si-MTA1. After 24 h, the transwell cell invasion assay using A498 cells was performed, and macrographs were taken under ×40 magnification. Scale bar: 50 µm. **b** Image J was used to count the transmigrated cells and Student's *t* test to analyze differences. $^{**}p < 0.01$; $^{***}p < 0.001$

investigate the mechanism of MTA1-regulated expression of MPP2 and MPP9, western blotting analysis was used to test the NF-κB signaling pathway. As shown in Fig. 4d–f, MTA1 overexpression decreased the phosphorylation of p65 (p-p65), with no change in the levels of total p65. When we used the NF-κB inhibitor, PDTC (10 nM), to block the NF-κB signaling pathway, MTA1 had no effect on the expression of MPPs (Fig. 4b, c). These results suggested that MTA1 might regulate the expression of MPP2 and MPP9 through NF-κB.

We further studied the inhibitory role of PDTC treatment on migration and invasion of RCC cells. We transfected the A498 cells with pcDNA3.1-Flag, Flag-MTA1, and treated Flag-MTA1 with PDTC (10 nM), before performing the wound healing and transwell assays. As shown in Fig. 5a, compared to the Flag-MTA1 group, the invasion of Flag-MTA1 cells treated PDTC was lower. The transwell assay showed a similar result: PDTC treatment blocked the effect of MTA1 on invasion (Fig. 5b). These results suggested that MAT1 may affect invasion and migration through the NF-κB signaling pathway.

Discussion

MTA1 reportedly up-regulated and promoted the progression of tumor growth in many cancers, including lung, liver, breast, ovarian, gastric, and prostate cancers [7–9, 21, 22]. Nonetheless, the role of MTA1 in RCCs is still unclear. In renal cancers, ccRCC comprises nearly 80% of all RCCs. In this study, we selected 109 pairs of ccRCCs and adjacent normal tissues and demonstrated that the expression level of MTA1 was significantly up-regulated in ccRCC tissues, compared to the surrounding tissue (Fig. 1 and Table 1). Moreover, MTA1 was highly expressed in A498 and 768-O RCC cell lines (Fig. 1).

We found that the overexpression of MTA1 markedly promoted A498 cell migration and invasion in vitro (Figs. 2, 3), which strongly suggests that MTA1 was the key factor regulating the metastasis of RCCs. However, the clinical-pathological analysis revealed that positive MTA1 expression in RCCs was associated with the age of patients and T stage and grade but not with the lymph node metastasis (Table 2). This apparent contradiction could likely be attributed to the small number of cases with lymph node metastasis enrolled in this study, which did not lead to a statistically significant

(See figure on next page.)

Fig. 4 MTA1 regulated the expression of metastasis-related factors via the NFκB pathway. A498 cells were transfected with pcDNA3.1-Flag, Flag-MTA1, siNC, and si-MTA1. **a** Protein levels of MTA1; cells were collected for WB with MTA1 and GAPDH antibodies. The bands of over-expressed MTA1 were from Additional file 1: Fig. 2A and down-expressed MTA1 were from Additional file 1: Fig. 2B with arrow. **b** Cells were lysed and used in qRT-PCR assays to measure the E-cadherin mRNA expression. Statistical analysis was performed using Student's *t* test. **b, c** A498 cells were transfected with pcDNA3.1-Flag and Flag-MTA1. After 36 h, the Flag-MTA1 group was treated with 10 nM PDTC for 12 h. Then cells were harvested for qRT-PCR evaluation to measure the mRNA expression of MMP2 (**b**) and MMP9 (**c**). Statistical analysis was performed using ANOVA. **d** A498 cells were transfected with pcDNA3.1-Flag, Flag-MTA1, siNC, and si-MTA1. After 48 h, cells were subjected to western blotting analysis using antibodies targeting p-p65, p65 and ACTB. The bands of p-p65, p65 and ACTB were from Additional file 1: Fig. 3. **e, f** Image J was used to calculate the gray scanned bands of p-p65 (**b**) and p65 (C). $^{*}p < 0.05$; $^{**}p < 0.01$; $^{***}p < 0.001$, $^{****}p < 0.0001$; *NS* not significant

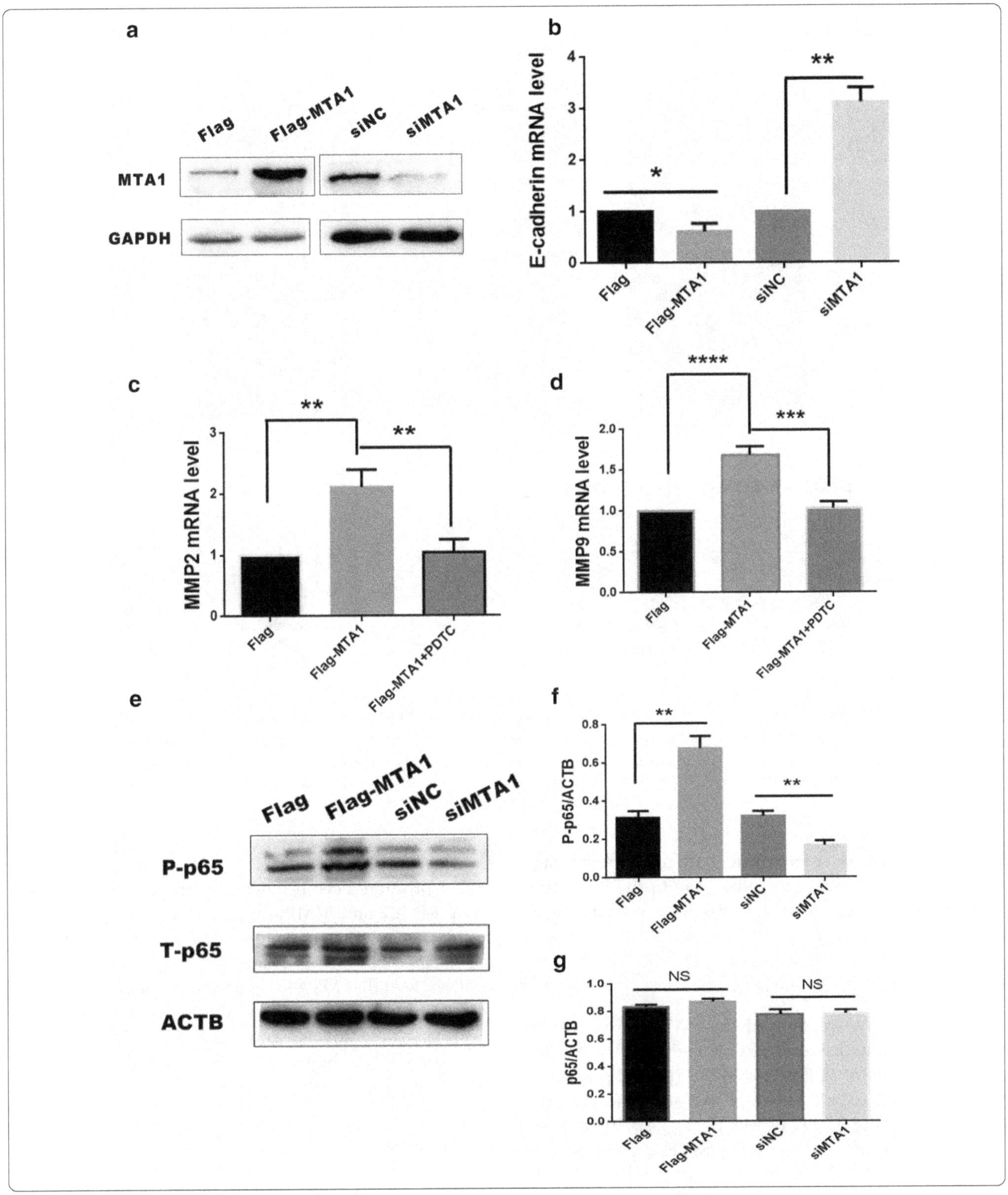

difference. Furthermore, Table 2 reports that 19 MTA1-positive cases were present, while only 4 MTA1-positive cases presenting lymph node metastasis were present. A similar result was shown in the no lymph node metastasis group, that is, MTA1-postive cases were more common than cases with negative MTA1. This trend is consistent with the results in our in vitro experiments. In addition, the enrolled cases were nearly

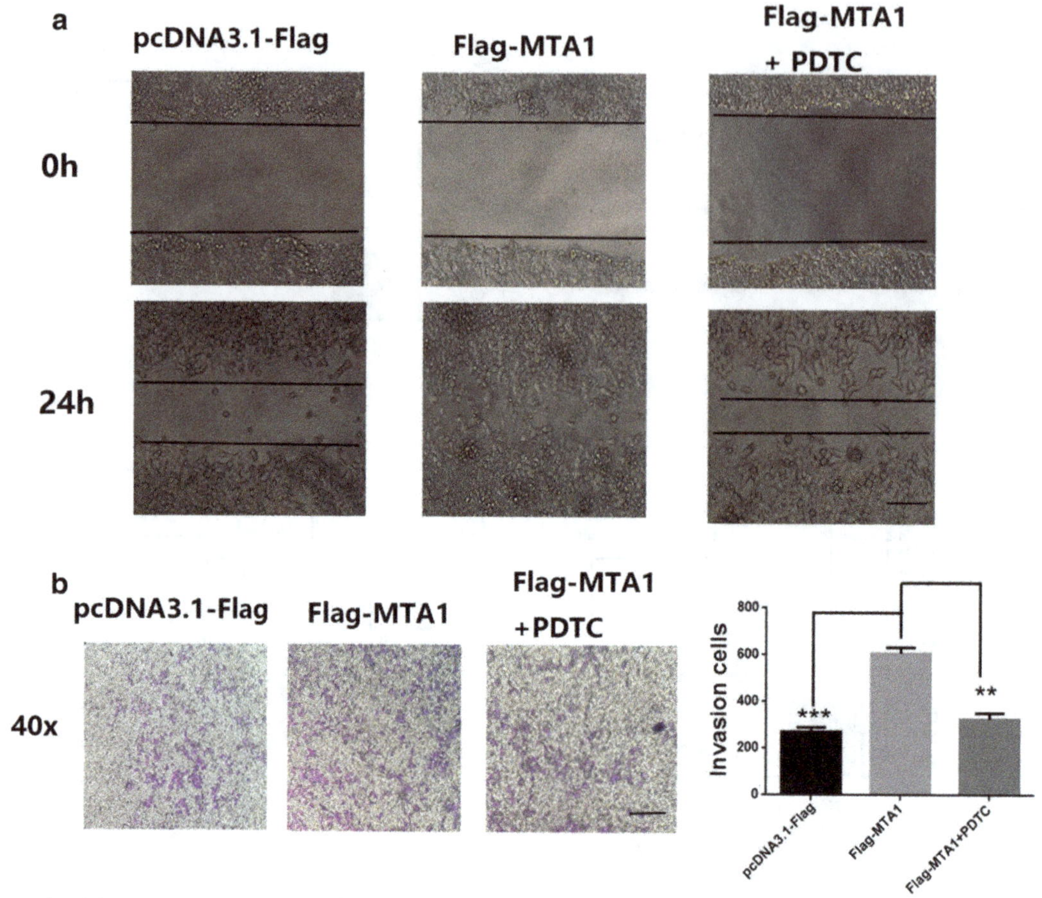

Fig. 5 MTA1 regulated the migration and invasion of RCC cells via NF-κB. A498 cells were transfected with pcDNA3.1-Flag, Flag-MTA1, and Flag-MTA1 + PDTC (10 nM). **a** In the wound healing assay, MTA1 improved the migration of RCC cells, while the addition of the inhibitor PDTC blocked the effect of MTA1 on migration. Scale bar: 100×. **b** In the transwell assay, MTA1 markedly induced invasion of A498 cells, but compared to the MTA1 group, the invasion of MTA1 + PDTC A498 cells was lower. $^{**}p < 0.01$; $^{***}p < 0.001$; Scale bar: ×40

early-stage; thus, over half of the patients in early-stage disease showed MTA1 positivity. Due to the limitation of the metastasis group sample size, future studies with a larger number of cases are needed to further examine the relationship between MTA1 and lymph node metastasis or distant metastasis.

Mechanistically, we showed that MTA1 was able to regulate the metastasis of RCCs by mediating the expression of E-cadherin, MPP2, and MPP9 (Fig. 4). Moreover, we used PDTC to inhibit the NF-κB signaling pathway, which limited the effects of MTA1 (Fig. 4). Further, the in vitro migration and invasion assays in the presence of PDTC treatment showed that NF-κB played a vital role in the MTA1-mediated migration and invasion (Fig. 5). Considering all the above evidence, we concluded that MTA1 mediated the migration and invasion of RCCs by targeting E-cadherin, MPP2, and MPP9 via the NF-κB pathway. Similar to our findings relative to the MTA1-mediated migration and invasion of RCCs by targeting E-cadherin, MPP2, and MPP9, Yao et al. reported that MTA1 promoted cell proliferation and invasion by regulating MMP2 and MMP9 in gastric cancers [13]. MTA1 could have an effect on some signaling pathways, including hedgehog, PI3K, HIF, and AKT [8, 12]. Bui-Nguyen et al. showed that MTA1 was a target gene of NF-κB [18]. In this study, we revealed that the NF-κB signaling pathway was a new downstream target for MTA1, although the mechanism of how MTA1 affects the NF-κB signaling pathway requires further study.

Conclusions

In summary, our study found that MTA1 is overexpressed in RCC cells and tissues. MTA1 mediated the tumor cell migration and invasion in cultured cells through the regulation of E-cadherin, MPP2, and MPP9 via the NF-κB pathway. These results suggested that MTA1 might play a vital role in the progression of RCC.

Abbreviations

MTA1: Metastasis-associated gene 1; RCC: Renal cell carcinoma; MMP2: Matrix metalloproteinase 2; MMP9: Matrix metalloproteinase 9.

Acknowledgments

None.

Authors' contributions

W. S., C.L., and S.S. conceived and designed the study. C.L completed most of experiments and analyses. Y.H., Q.L., and Z.L. performed some experiments and analyses. W. S., C.L., and S.S. drafted the manuscript. W. S and S.S. critically revised the manuscript. All authors read and approved the final manuscript.

Author details

[1] Department of Urology, Haikou Municipal Hospital, Haikou 570208, Hainan, China. [2] Department of Neurology, Haikou Municipal Hospital, Haikou 570208, Hainan, China. [3] Department of Urology, Danzhou People's Hospital, Danzhou 571799, Hainan, China. [4] Hubei Key Laboratory for Kidney Disease Pathogenesis and Intervention, Huangshi Central Hospital of Edong Healthcare Group, Hubei Polytechnic University School of Medicine, Huangshi, China.

References

1. Petejova N, Martinek A. Renal cell carcinoma: review of etiology, pathophysiology and risk factors. Biomed Pap Med Fac Univ Palacky Olomouc Czechoslovakia. 2016;160(2):183–94.
2. Shingarev R, Jaimes EA. Renal cell carcinoma: new insights and challenges for a clinician scientist. Am J Physiol Renal Physiol. 2017;313(2):F145–54.
3. Zhang ZL, Li YH, Xiong YH, Hou GL, Yao K, Dong P, Liu ZW, Han H, Qin ZK, Zhou FJ. Oncological outcome of surgical treatment in 336 patients with renal cell carcinoma. Chin J Cancer. 2010;29(12):995–9.
4. Prenen H, Gil T, Awada A. New therapeutic developments in renal cell cancer. Crit Rev Oncol Hematol. 2009;69(1):56–63.
5. Wang T, Li W, Huang H, Wang C. Metastasis-associated 1 (MTA1) gene expression promotes angiogenesis in mouse xenografts from human non-small cell lung cancer (NSCLC) cells. Med Sci Monit Int Med J Exp Clin Res. 2019;25:484–91.
6. Dannenmann C, Shabani N, Friese K, Jeschke U, Mylonas I, Brüning A. The metastasis-associated gene MTA1 is upregulated in advanced ovarian cancer, represses ERbeta, and enhances expression of oncogenic cytokine GRO. Cancer Biol Ther. 2008;7(9):1460–7.
7. Dhar S, Kumar A, Li K, Tzivion G, Levenson AS. Resveratrol regulates PTEN/Akt pathway through inhibition of MTA1/HDAC unit of the NuRD complex in prostate cancer. Biochem Biophys Acta. 2015;1853(2):265–75.
8. Hannafon BN, Gin AL, Xu YF, Bruns M, Calloway CL, Ding WQ. Metastasis-associated protein 1 (MTA1) is transferred by exosomes and contributes to the regulation of hypoxia and estrogen signaling in breast cancer cells. Cell Commun Signal CCS. 2019;17(1):13.
9. Lv ZY, Zhao ZS, Ye ZY, Wang YY, Wang HJ, Yang Q. Metastasis-associated protein 1 (MTA1) in gastric cancer tissues is positively associated with poorer prognosis. Pathol Res Pract. 2018;214(4):536–41.
10. Kumar R, Wang RA, Bagheri-Yarmand R. Emerging roles of MTA family members in human cancers. Semin Oncol. 2003;30(5):30–7.
11. Song Q, Wang B, Liu M, Ren Z, Fu Y, Zhang P, Yang M. MTA1 promotes the invasion and migration of oral squamous carcinoma by inducing epithelial-mesenchymal transition via the hedgehog signaling pathway. Exp Cell Res. 2019;382(1):111450.
12. Wang H, Fan L, Wei J, Weng Y, Zhou L, Shi Y, Zhou W, Ma D, Wang C. Akt mediates metastasis-associated gene 1 (MTA1) regulating the expression of E-cadherin and promoting the invasiveness of prostate cancer cells. PLoS ONE. 2012;7(12):e46888.
13. Yao Y, Feng S, Xiao M, Li Y, Yang L, Gong J. MTA1 promotes proliferation and invasion in human gastric cancer cells. Onco Targets Ther. 2015;8:1785–94.
14. Wang Z, Yuan C, Huang Y, Liu Z, Yu X, Lv C, Su Z. Decreased expression of apoptosis-inducing factor in renal cell carcinoma is associated with poor prognosis and reduced postoperative survival. Oncol Lett. 2019;18(3):2805–12.
15. Si W, Xie W, Deng W, Xiao Y, Karnik SS, Xu C, Chen Q, Wang QK. Angiotensin II increases angiogenesis by NF-kappaB-mediated transcriptional activation of angiogenic factor AGGF1. FASEB J. 2018;32(9):5051–62.
16. Zhou B, Si W, Su Z, Deng W, Tu X, Wang Q. Transcriptional activation of the Prox1 gene by HIF-1alpha and HIF-2alpha in response to hypoxia. FEBS Lett. 2013;587(6):724–31.
17. Kai L, Wang J, Ivanovic M, Chung YT, Laskin WB, Schulze-Hoepfner F, Mirochnik Y, Satcher RL Jr, Levenson AS. Targeting prostate cancer angiogenesis through metastasis-associated protein 1 (MTA1). Prostate. 2011;71(3):268–80.
18. Bui-Nguyen TM, Pakala SB, Sirigiri RD, Xia W, Hung MC, Sarin SK, Kumar V, Slagle BL, Kumar R. NF-kappaB signaling mediates the induction of MTA1 by hepatitis B virus transactivator protein HBx. Oncogene. 2010;29(8):1179–89.
19. Zhang JF, Wang P, Yan YJ, Li Y, Guan MW, Yu JJ, Wang XD. IL33 enhances glioma cell migration and invasion by upregulation of MMP2 and MMP9 via the ST2-NF-kappaB pathway. Oncol Rep. 2017;38(4):2033–42.
20. Zhang J, Zhang DL, Jiao XL, Dong Q. S100A4 regulates migration and invasion in hepatocellular carcinoma HepG2 cells via NF-kappaB-dependent MMP-9 signal. Eur Rev Med Pharmacol Sci. 2013;17(17):2372–82.
21. Li D, Qian J, Hong Z. Expression and clinical significance of MTA1 in non-small cell lung cancer. Chin J Lung Cancer. 2008;11(6):775–9.
22. Nair SS, Bommana A, Pakala SB, Ohshiro K, Lyon AJ, Suttiprapa S, Periago MV, Laha T, Hotez PJ, Bethony JM, et al. Inflammatory response to liver fluke *Opisthorchis viverrini* in mice depends on host master coregulator MTA1, a marker for parasite-induced cholangiocarcinoma in humans. Hepatology. 2011;54(4):1388–97.

5

8q24 clear cell renal cell carcinoma germline variant is associated with *VHL* mutation status and clinical aggressiveness

Jeanette E. Eckel-Passow[1*], Huihuang Yan[1], Matthew L. Kosel[1], Daniel Serie[2], Paul A. Decker[1], Robert B. Jenkins[3] Brian Costello[4], Bradley Leibovich[4], Thai H. Ho[5] and Alexander Parker[2]

Abstract

Background: The four most commonly-mutated genes in clear cell renal cell carcinoma (ccRCC) tumors are *BAP1*, *PBRM1*, *SETD2* and *VHL*. And, there are currently 14 known RCC germline variants that have been reproducibly shown to be associated with RCC risk. However, the association of germline genetics with tumor genetics and clinical aggressiveness are unknown.

Methods: We analyzed 420 ccRCC patients from The Cancer Genome Atlas. Molecular subtype was determined based on acquired mutations in *BAP1*, *PBRM1*, *SETD2* and *VHL*. Aggressive subtype was defined clinically using Mayo SSIGN score and molecularly using the ccA/ccB gene expression subtype. Publically-available Hi-C data were used to link germline risk variants with candidate target genes.

Results: The 8q24 variant rs35252396 was significantly associated with *VHL* mutation status (OR = 1.6, $p = 0.0037$) and SSIGN score (OR = 1.9, $p = 0.00094$), after adjusting for multiple comparisons. We observed that, while some germline variants have interactions with nearby genes, some variants demonstrate long-range interactions with target genes.

Conclusions: These data further demonstrate the link between rs35252396, *HIF* pathway and ccRCC clinical aggressiveness, providing a more comprehensive picture of how germline genetics and tumor genetics interact with respect to tumor development and progression.

Keywords: Kidney, GWAS, Subtype, Hi-C

Background

The majority (>90%) of kidney cancer is classified as renal cell carcinoma (RCC) and approximately 85% of RCCs are further classified as the clear cell subtype (ccRCC). The etiology of ccRCC has been extensively studied and smoking, obesity and hypertension are recognized environmental risk factors that increase the risk of developing ccRCC. Additionally, genome-wide association studies (GWAS) have to date identified 14 germline variants that are associated with risk of RCC [1–5]. The value of these germline genetic explorations notwithstanding, the functional impact of the germline variants associated with RCC and ccRCC specifically remains largely unknown. Furthermore, the association of germline genetics with tumor genetics and tumor aggressiveness are largely unknown. In some cancers investigators have reported that germline variants are associated with specific molecularly-defined tumor subtypes, and in some cases the association is large enough to suggest clinical relevance (e.g., rs55705857 has an odds ratio > 6 in *IDH*-mutated glioma) [6–8]. To date, similar

*Correspondence: eckelpassow.jeanette@mayo.edu
[1] Division of Biomedical Statistics and Informatics, Mayo Clinic, 200 First Street SW, Rochester, MN 55905, USA
Full list of author information is available at the end of the article

analyses linking germline variants with tumor subtypes have not been performed for RCC or ccRCC specifically. The value of identifying associations of genetic variants with specific molecular subtypes of a tumor centers on the ability to provide evidence of the involvement of specific developmental pathways that can help inform the biology of ccRCC tumor evolution, progression and novel prevention efforts. Related to this, we now have access to a catalog of acquired tumor alterations that are commonly present in ccRCC [9, 10]. Motivated by the opportunity to combine data on germline genetics associated with ccRCC risk with specific acquired molecular alterations found in ccRCC tumor tissue, we advance the field by evaluating for the first time the association of known ccRCC germline variants with these acquired alterations in order to better understand ccRCC development and progression. Moreover, we also evaluated the association of these known germline variants with well-known and validated clinical measures of ccRCC aggressiveness. Finally, we leverage Hi-C data to identify candidate target genes for the 14 germline variants that are the focus of this investigation.

Methods

The Cancer Genome Atlas (TCGA) data

Raw genotyping data from Affymetrix 6.0 array were obtained from germline DNA for 420 ccRCC patients, as well as corresponding clinical and pathological data. Somatic mutations of the four most frequently-mutated genes in ccRCC (*BAP1*, *PBRM1*, *SETD2* and *VHL*) were obtained from TCGA [9]. The clear cell A and clear cell B (ccA/ccB) gene expression subtype classification has been reproducibly shown to be associated with outcome [11, 12] and was obtained from [9]. The Mayo SSIGN score has also been reproducibly shown to be associated with outcome [13–16]. The Mayo SSIGN score is derived from an additive model that contains tumor stage, tumor size, tumor grade and presence of necrosis, and was calculated as described previously [17].

Statistical methods

Quality control was performed on the genotying data for the 420 ccRCC TCGA patients, including 95% call rate (zero germline variants failed), 95% sample call rate (zero samples failed), Hardy–Weinberg equilibrium (821 variants failed with $p < 0.000001$), minor allele frequency (MAF; 216,942 variants had MAF < 0.05), sex check (100% concordance) and population stratification (all Caucasian). Genotyping data were phased and imputed using the Michigan Imputation Server with the Haplotype Reference Consortium (release 1) as the reference population. The imputation quality for each of the 14 variants is provided in Additional file 1: Table S1. An additive logistic regression model was used to assess the association between each of the 14 variants and subtype, with genotype coded as having 0, 1, or 2 copies of the minor allele for observed data and dosage was modeled as continuous for imputed data. A general linear model was used to assess the association between age of diagnosis and each of the 14 variants. To account for multiple testing, p values < 0.004 were considered statistically significant (0.05/14 = 0.004).

Hi-C analysis

Associations between known RCC germline variants and genes within two-to-five megabase (Mb) were evaluated using Hi-C data via the HUGIn web browser [18]. Additional genetic information, limited to what was available in HUGIn, was included such as frequently interacting regions (FIREs), topologically associating domain (TAD) boundary regions, and occupancy of histone marks H3K27ac, H3K4me1 and H3K4me3. Because RCC is thought to originate from the renal tubular epithelium, and mesodermal stem cells form the tubule of the kidney, analyses were performed using mesendoderm cells. Mesenchymal stem cells were also analyzed [19]; results were similar across the two cell lines. We also used Hi-C data from ccRCC cell line (*VHL* mutant) Caki2 (GSM2827127 and GSM2827128) [20], (*VHL* wild-type) embryonic kidney cell lines HEK293T (GSM1081530 and GSM1081531) and HEK293T RAD21cv that was treated with tobacco etch mosaic virus protease (GSM1081526 and GSM1081527) [21]. RAD21 is a core subunit of cohesin complex, which is known to play a role in mediating chromosomal loops. In RAD21cv (a RAD21-EGFP variant) cells, RAD21cv replaced endogenous RAD21 and was incorporated into the cohesin complex. For Caki2 and HEK293 data, reads were mapped with Bowtie 2 [22] and alignments from two replicates were combined. Chromatin interaction was identified with HOMER (https://homer.ucsd.edu/homer/interactions/) at 20-kb resolution, which takes into account the dependence of interaction frequency and linear distance along each chromosome. For each risk locus, we combined the virtual 4C plot generated by the HUGIn web browser with the interaction plot generated from internally-analyzed Hi-C data.

Results

TCGA ccRCC cohort

Table 1 describes the 420 TCGA ccRCC patients that were analyzed. Of the 376 patients with available whole exome sequencing data, 150 (40%) had a *VHL* mutation, 34 (9%) *BAP1* mutation, 119 (32%) *PBRM1* mutation and 48 (13%) *SETD2* mutation. We also subtyped patients according to disease aggressiveness using pathological

Table 1 Description of 420 TCGA ccRCC patients

	N (%)
Sex	
Female	137 (32.6%)
Male	283 (67.4%)
Max tumor size	
N	376
Mean (SD)	6.5 (3.5)
Median	5.5
Q1, Q3	4.0, 8.5
Range	(1.1–25.0)
Stage	
Missing	44
Stage I	176 (46.8%)
Stage II	135 (35.9%)
Stage IV	65 (17.3%)
Grade	
Missing	44
G1	7 (1.9%)
G2	156 (41.5%)
G3	152 (40.4%)
G4	60 (16.0%)
GX	1 (0.3%)
Percent necrosis	
Missing	64
0	189 (53.1%)
2	4 (1.1%)
3	2 (0.6%)
5	42 (11.8%)
8	1 (0.3%)
10	23 (6.5%)
15	13 (3.7%)
20	6 (1.7%)
25	4 (1.1%)
30	72 (20.2%)
SSIGN group	
Missing	65
Low risk (0–3)	159 (44.8%)
Intermediate risk (4–7)	115 (32.4%)
High risk (8+)	81 (22.8%)
BAP1 mutated	
Missing	44
No	342 (91.0%)
Yes	34 (9.0%)
PBRM1 mutated	
Missing	44
No	257 (68.4%)
Yes	119 (31.6%)
SETD2 mutated	
Missing	44
No	328 (87.2%)
Yes	48 (12.8%)
VHL mutated	
Missing	44
No	226 (60.1%)
Yes	150 (39.9%)
ccA/ccB expression subtype	
Missing	68
ccB	168 (47.7%)
ccA	184 (52.3%)

indices defined by the Mayo SSIGN score [13] as well as molecularly according to the ccA/ccB gene expression subtype [11, 12]. Of the 355 patients that had available pathology data to calculate the Mayo SSIGN score, 81 (23%) were classified as aggressive (SSIGN score > 8). Using ccA/ccB to classify aggressiveness, of the 352 patients who had data, 168 (48%) were poor prognosis (ccB) subtype.

Association of RCC germline variants with frequently mutated genes

Using a case-case design, we evaluated the association of each of the 14 RCC germline variants with known ccRCC acquired alterations in *BAP1*, *PBRM1*, *SETD2* and *VHL* (Table 2). We observed a statistically significant association after adjusting for multiple comparisons between the 8q24 variant rs35252396 and *VHL* mutation (OR = 1.60, $p = 0.0037$). While not significant after adjusting for multiple testing, we also observed a candidate association between *EPAS1* variant rs7579899 and *SETD2* mutation (OR = 1.87, $p = 0.012$) (Table 2).

Association of RCC germline variants with aggressive ccRCC

We observed a statistically significant association between the 8q24 variant rs35252396 and Mayo SSIGN score (OR = 1.92, $p = 0.00094$) (Table 2). However, we did not observe a statistically-significant association between the known germline variants and ccA/ccB gene expression subtype.

Association of RCC germline variants with age at diagnosis

We did not observe a statistically-significant association between the known germline variants and age at diagnosis (Additional file 1: Table S2).

Table 2 Association of known RCC germline variants with RCC subtypes. Subtypes were defined molecularly based on individual acquired alterations, by mRNA molecular subtype (ccA/ccB) or clinically (Mayo SSIGN score).

RS ID	Chrom	REF	ALT	OR.bap1	P.bap1	OR.pbrm1	P.pbrm1	OR.setd2	P.setd2	OR.vhl	P.vhl	OR.ccAccB	P.ccAccB	OR.SSIGNcat	P.SSIGNcat
rs4381241	1	T	C	0.92	0.74	0.92	0.59	0.94	0.77	0.92	0.59	0.95	0.72	1.10	0.61
rs7579899	2	A	G	0.95	0.85	1.02	0.92	1.87	**0.012**	0.99	0.93	1.12	0.45	0.95	0.79
rs12105918	2	T	C	2.05	0.05	0.66	0.16	0.58	0.23	1.36	0.23	0.86	0.57	0.84	0.58
rs67311347	3	G	A	1.29	0.33	1.00	0.98	1.04	0.88	1.17	0.33	1.02	0.90	0.89	0.57
rs10936602	3	T	C	1.22	0.49	0.77	0.18	0.73	0.26	1.11	0.54	1.15	0.43	0.96	0.8
rs2241261	8	C	T	0.96	0.88	1.03	0.84	0.89	0.60	1.26	0.12	1.07	0.66	0.84	0.32
rs35252396[a]	8	A	C	1.17	0.57	0.95	0.77	0.97	0.89	1.60	*0.0037*	0.99	0.96	1.92	*0.00094*
rs35252396[a]	8	C	G	1.17	0.57	0.95	0.77	0.97	0.89	1.60	*0.0037*	0.99	0.96	1.92	*0.00094*
rs11813268	10	C	T	1.15	0.64	0.85	0.42	0.54	0.06	0.88	0.50	1.02	0.93	1.14	0.54
rs7105934	11	G	A	0.32	0.27	0.96	0.92	0.46	0.29	0.72	0.40	0.56	0.13	0.66	0.41
rs1800057	11	C	G	1.68	0.44	1.64	0.29	0.47	0.39	0.92	0.86	1.34	0.53	0.66	0.51
rs74911261	11	G	A	2.21	0.25	1.13	0.82	0.31	0.31	0.49	0.21	1.29	0.63	0.76	0.68
rs718314	12	A	G	1.05	0.86	0.93	0.67	0.89	0.65	1.11	0.55	0.94	0.72	1.07	0.74
rs4765623	12	C	T	1.13	0.65	0.99	0.94	0.64	0.07	1.08	0.63	0.92	0.60	0.95	0.77
rs4903064	14	T	C	1.35	0.25	0.90	0.55	1.19	0.45	1.06	0.72	1.04	0.83	0.96	0.82

Chrom denotes chromosome location, OR denotes odds ratio and p value is from a logistic regression model. Cells highlighted in italics denote associations that pass our multiple testing threshold (p value $< (0.05/14 = 0.004)$). Cells highlighted in bold denote candidate associations ($0.004 < p$ value < 0.05)

[a] rs35252396 is tri-allelic

Association of RCC germline variants with nearby genes

We evaluated the interaction of each of the known germline variants with putative target genes in mesendoderm cell lines and mesenchymal stem cells using publically-available Hi-C data. Hi-C identifies chromatin interactions to evaluate the three dimensional chromatin structures inside the nucleus, which may identify long-range interactions. Some germline variants demonstrated interactions with nearby genes: e.g., rs4381241 with *FAF1* (518.5 kb away), rs57579899 with *EPAS1* (16.8 kb away), rs12105918 with *ZEB2/ZEB2-AS1* (~70 kb away), rs1800057 with *ATM* (50.2 kb away) and rs4903064 with *DPF3* (81.4 kb away) (Fig. 1; Additional file 1: Figure S1). However, some of these variants showed additional long-range interactions that have not been reported previously: e.g., rs4381241 with *CDKN2C* and *TTC39A*, rs7579899 with *PRKCE*' rs12105918 with *ARHGAP15*, *GTDC1* and *TEX41*' rs1800057 with *CUL5*, *ACAT1*, *NPAT* and *EXPH5* and rs4903064 with *RGS6*. Other germline variants also demonstrated long-range interactions that have not been reported previously: e.g., rs10936602 with *SEC62* and *PHC3*, rs67311347 with *ENTPD3*, *CTNNB1* and *ULK4*, rs2241261 with *PEBP4* and *EGR3*, rs74911261 with *EXPH5*, rs718314 with *SSPN* and *ITPR2* and rs4765623 with *FAM101A* (Additional file 1: Figure S1). Additionally, rs35252396 demonstrated interactions with *PCAT1* and *PCAT2* in mesenchymal stem cells but not in mesendoderm cells (Fig. 2). Similarly, rs11813268 had interactions with *OBFC1* in mesenchymal stem cells but not in mesendoderm cells. Finally, we failed to identify genes within ± 1 Mb whose promoters interacted with rs7105934 in either mesenchymal stem cells or mesendoderm cells. All identified interactions were further evaluated in independent cell lines: *VHL*-mutant ccRCC cell line (Caki) and *VHL* wild-type embryonic kidney cell lines (HEK293 and HEK293 RAD21cv). A large proportion of the interactions were also identified in ccRCC or embryonic kidney cell lines. For example, rs10936602 interaction with *SEC62*, rs2241261 interactions with *PEBP4* and *EGR3*' rs1800057 and rs74911261 interactions with *EXPH5*, as well as rs718314 interaction with *SSPN* were confirmed in all three cell lines. Further, rs12105918 interaction with *GTDC1*, rs11813268 interaction with *OBFC1* and rs4765623 interaction with *FAM101A* were only identified in the ccRCC cell line, while rs7579899 interaction with *PRKCE*, rs35252396 interaction with *PCAT2*, and rs4903064 interaction with *DPF3* were only identified in the embryonic kidney cell lines.

Discussion

There are currently 14 known germline variants that are associated with risk of RCC; however, it remains unclear how germline genetics modify the risk of developing RCC or their association with tumor aggressiveness. To date, associations between germlines genetics and tumor genetics is largely unknown for RCC. With respect to tumor aggressiveness, previous investigators did not observe significant associations between a polygenic risk model that was derived from these 14 germline variants and age at onset or tumor stage [5]. However, the analyses were performed on overall RCC and not within relevant RCC subtypes. Herein, we not only evaluated ccRCC specifically, but also the association of these 14 variants with specific molecular (*BAP1*, *PBRM1*, *SETD2* and *VHL*) and clinically-aggressive subtypes of ccRCC. Using a case-case analysis, we observed that the 8q24 germline variant rs35252396 was significantly associated with tumor *VHL* mutation status as well as with the Mayo SSIGN score. Notably, the Mayo SSIGN score has been reproducibly shown to be associated with clinical outcome [13–16]. The 8q24 germline variant is located within *PVT1*, a candidate oncogene that is thought to regulate *MYC* to promote tumor formation. Of note, the 8q24 variant also overlaps a DNase I hypersensitive site and H3K4me1 peak from fetal kidney [23], indicating its location within a regulatory region. Through functional laboratory studies, investigators recently demonstrated that the 8q24 germline variant affects *HIF* binding to a *MYC* enhancer [24]. While the *EPAS1* (rs7579899) and *CCND1* (rs7105934) variants are also linked to the *HIF* pathway, we did not observe a statistically-significant association between these two variants and *VHL* mutation. Additionally, while it did not pass our multiple testing significance threshold, we also observed a candidate association between the *EPAS1* germline variant rs57579899 and *SETD2* tumor mutation ($p = 0.012$). We previously reported that loss of *SETD2* activity was associated with greater risk of ccRCC death [25].

While previous investigators did not observe a significant association between a RCC-derived polygenic risk model and tumor stage [5], we observed a significant association between the 8q24 germline variant and the Mayo SSIGN score. The difference could be due to the fact that the original analysis [5] was performed for overall RCC whereas our analyses were performed within a more homogeneous subtype of RCC, particularly, ccRCC. The Mayo SSIGN score is derived from an additive model that contains tumor stage, tumor size,

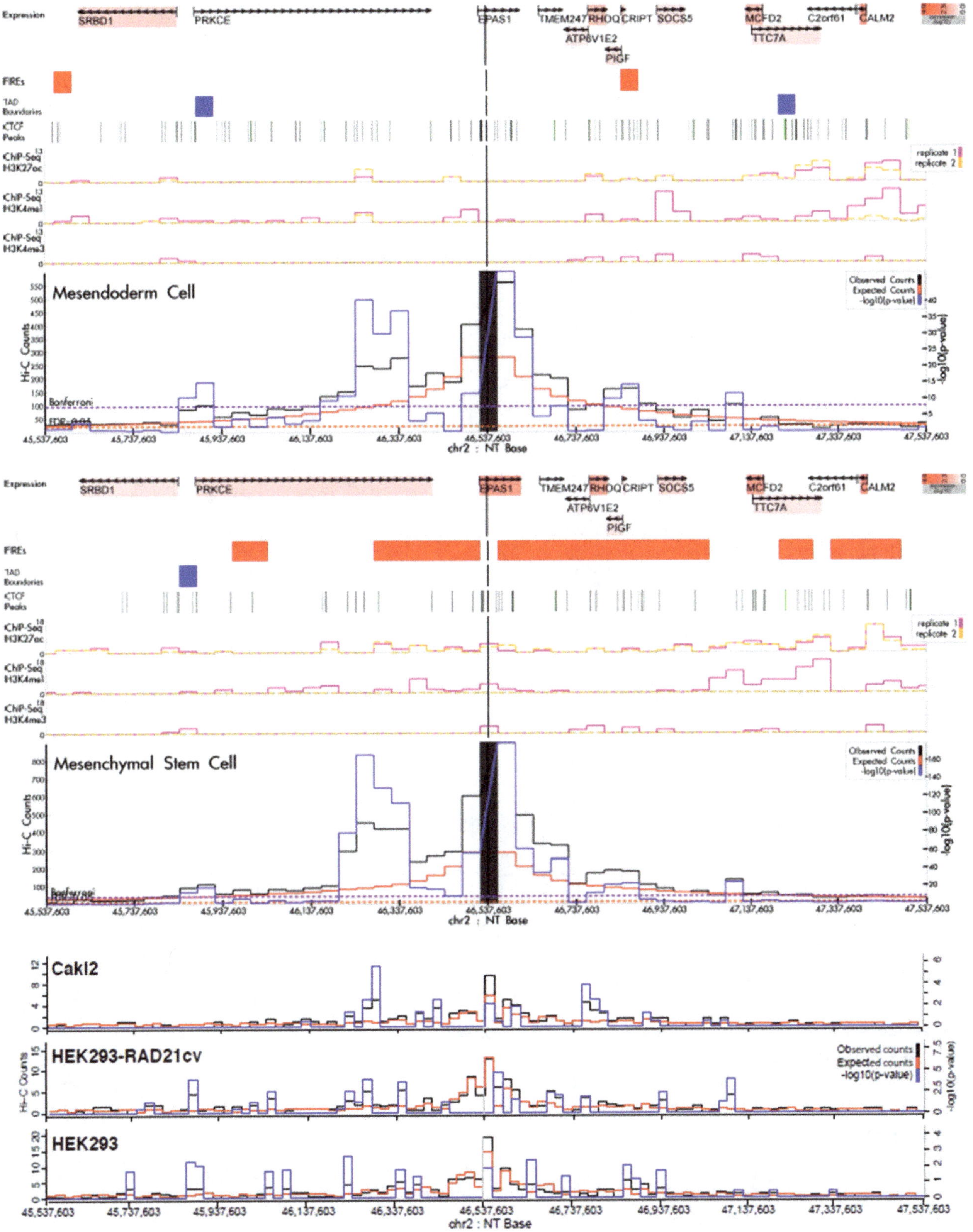

Fig. 1 Hi-C interactions for the *EPAS1* germline variant rs7579899. This variant was found to interact with *EPAS1* and *PRKCE*

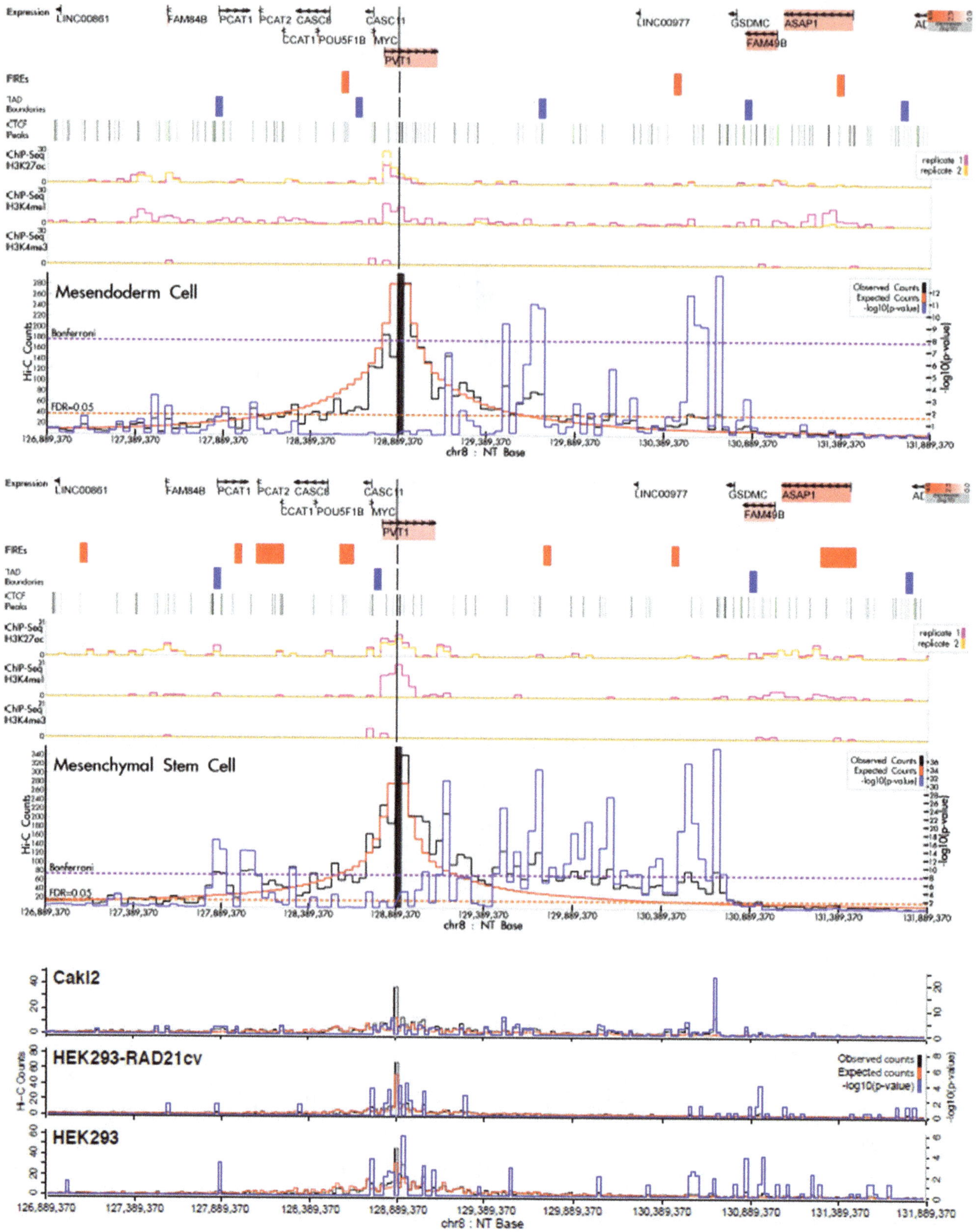

Fig. 2 Hi-C interactions for the 8q24 germline variant rs35252396. This variant showed interactions with *PCAT1* and *PCAT2*

tumor grade and presence of necrosis and the model has reproducibly been shown to be associated with outcome in ccRCC, with higher SSIGN score being associated with poorer prognosis [13–16]. While we observed a significant association of the 8q24 germline variant and the Mayo SSIGN score, we did not observe a significant association between any of the 14 variants and the molecularly-defined ccA/ccB expression subtype that has been linked to ccRCC aggressiveness [11, 12, 17].

Previous studies have performed expression quantitative trait loci (eQTL) analyses to evaluate function of the 14 RCC germline variants [2, 5]. Herein, we used Hi-C data to identify candidate target genes underlying the association of each of the 14 germline variants with ccRCC risk. While some variants demonstrated interactions with nearby genes, we observed additional long-range interactions. Laboratory studies are necessary to further understand these observations.

This study has limitations. We only analyzed associations of germline variants with somatic mutations, and no other acquired molecular alterations such as copy number variation. Additionally, because there are limited GWAS data available on patients who also have tumor molecular data, we did not validate the observed associations between the 8q24 germline variant and *VHL* tumor mutation nor the association between the *EPAS1* germline variant and *SETD2* tumor mutation. Similarly, Hi-C data are currently limited and thus we were not able to validate the Hi-C results. As such, the observed associations reported herein require validation in an external cohort.

Conclusion

We identified a significant association between the 8q24 germline variant and the presence of *VHL* somatic mutation. Additionally, we demonstrated for the first time an association between the 8q24 germline variant and ccRCC clinical aggressiveness as measured by the Mayo SSIGN score. Importantly, we additionally defined candidate target genes underlying the association between each of the 14 germline variants and risk of ccRCC. Together, these results further elucidate genes and pathways associated with ccRCC development. Specifically, these data further demonstrate the link between rs35252396 in the 8q24 region, *HIF* pathway and clinical aggressiveness, providing a more comprehensive biological understanding of the development of *VHL* mutated ccRCC tumors. Future work should evaluate how the rs35252396 germline variant and *VHL* mutation interact to affect treatment outcome and prognosis.

Supplementary information

Additional file 1: Supplementary Figure S1. Hi-C interactions for each of the 14 known RCC germline variants. Chromosome 1: rs4381241. **Supplementary Table S1**. Information on the 4 known RCC germline variants. R-square denotes the imputation quality and FRQ denotes the frequency of the variants for each of the aquired alterations that were evaluated. **Supplementary Table S2**. Association of known RCC germline variants with age of diagnosis.

Abbreviations

ccA: Clear cell A; ccB: Clear cell B; ccRCC: Clear cell renal cell carcinoma; eQTL: Expression quantitative trait loci; FIREs: Frequently interacting regions; GWAS: Genome wide association study; kb: Kilobase; MAF: Minor allele frequency; OR: Odds ratio; *p*: *p* Value; RCC: Renal cell carcinoma; SSIGN: Stage, sign, grade and necrosis; TAD: Topologically associating domain; TCGA: The Cancer Genome Atlas.

Acknowledgements

The results published here are in whole or part based upon data generated by the TCGA Research Network: https://cancergenome.nih.gov/.

Authors' contributions

The study was designed by JEEP and AP. Statistical and bioinformatics analyses were performed by HY, MK, DS and PD. Results were interpreted by JEEP, HY, RBJ, BC, BL, THH and AP. All authors contributed to the final version of the paper.

Author details

[1] Division of Biomedical Statistics and Informatics, Mayo Clinic, 200 First Street SW, Rochester, MN 55905, USA. [2] Department of Health Sciences Research, Mayo Clinic, Jacksonville, FL, USA. [3] Department of Laboratory Medicine and Pathology, Mayo Clinic, Rochester, MN, USA. [4] Department of Urology, Mayo Clinic, Rochester, MN, USA. [5] Division of Hematology and Medical Oncology, Mayo Clinic, Scottsdale, AZ, USA.

References

1. Gudmundsson J, Sulem P, Gudbjartsson DF, et al. A common variant at 8q24.21 is associated with renal cell cancer. Nat Commun. 2013;4:2776.
2. Henrion M, Frampton M, Scelo G, et al. Common variation at 2q22.3 (ZEB2) influences the risk of renal cancer. Hum Mol Genet. 2013;22:825–31.
3. Wu X, Scelo G, Purdue MP, et al. A genome-wide association study identifies a novel susceptibility locus for renal cell carcinoma on 12p11.23. Hum Mol Genet. 2012;21:456–62.
4. Purdue MP, Johansson M, Zelenika D, et al. Genome-wide association study of renal cell carcinoma identifies two susceptibility loci on 2p21 and 11q13.3. Nat Genet. 2011;43:60–5.
5. Scelo G, Purdue MP, Brown KM, et al. Genome-wide association study identifies multiple risk loci for renal cell carcinoma. Nat Commun. 2017;8:15724.
6. Eckel-Passow JE, Lachance DH, Molinaro AM, et al. Glioma groups based on 1p/19q, IDH, and TERT promoter mutations in tumors. N Engl J Med. 2015;372:2499–508.
7. Kuchenbaecker KB, McGuffog L, Barrowdale D, et al. Evaluation of polygenic risk scores for breast and ovarian cancer risk prediction in BRCA1 and BRCA2 mutation carriers. J Natl Cancer Inst. 2017;109:djw302.
8. Lecarpentier J, Silvestri V, Kuchenbaecker KB, et al. Prediction of breast and prostate cancer risks in male BRCA1 and BRCA2 mutation carriers using polygenic risk scores. J Clin Oncol. 2017;35:2240–50.

9. Tcga TCGA. Comprehensive molecular characterization of clear cell renal cell carcinoma. Nature. 2013;499:43–9.
10. Sato Y, Yoshizato T, Shiraishi Y, et al. Integrated molecular analysis of clear-cell renal cell carcinoma. Nat Genet. 2013;45:860–7.
11. Brannon AR, Reddy A, Seiler M, et al. Molecular stratification of clear cell renal cell carcinoma by consensus clustering reveals distinct subtypes and survival patterns. Genes Cancer. 2010;1:152–63.
12. Brooks SA, Brannon AR, Parker JS, et al. ClearCode34: a prognostic risk predictor for localized clear cell renal cell carcinoma. Eur Urol. 2014;66:77–84.
13. Frank I, Blute ML, Cheville JC, et al. An outcome prediction model for patients with clear cell renal cell carcinoma treated with radical nephrectomy based on tumor stage, size, grade and necrosis: the SSIGN score. J Urol. 2002;168:2395–400.
14. Zigeuner R, Hutterer G, Chromecki T, et al. External validation of the Mayo Clinic stage, size, grade, and necrosis (SSIGN) score for clear-cell renal cell carcinoma in a single European centre applying routine pathology. Eur Urol. 2010;57:102–9.
15. Ficarra V, Novara G, Galfano A, et al. The "Stage, Size, Grade and Necrosis" score is more accurate than the University of California Los Angeles Integrated Staging System for predicting cancer-specific survival in patients with clear cell renal cell carcinoma. BJU Int. 2009;103:165–70.
16. Parker WP, Cheville JC, Frank I, et al. Application of the Stage, Size, Grade, and Necrosis (SSIGN) Score for clear cell renal cell carcinoma in contemporary patients. Eur Urol. 2017;71:665–73.
17. Eckel-Passow JE, Igel DA, Serie DJ, et al. Assessing the clinical use of clear cell renal cell carcinoma molecular subtypes identified by RNA expression analysis. Urol Oncol. 2015;33(68):e17-23.
18. Schmitt AD, Hu M, Jung I, et al. A compendium of chromatin contact maps reveals spatially active regions in the human genome. Cell Rep. 2016;17:2042–59.
19. Myszczyszyn A, Czarnecka AM, Matak D, et al. The role of hypoxia and cancer stem cells in renal cell carcinoma pathogenesis. Stem Cell Rev. 2015;11:919–43.
20. ENCODE Project Consortium. An integrated encyclopedia of DNA elements in the human genome. Nature. 2012;489:57–74.
21. Zuin J, Dixon JR, van der Reijden MI, et al. Cohesin and CTCF differentially affect chromatin architecture and gene expression in human cells. Proc Natl Acad Sci USA. 2014;111:996–1001.
22. Langmead B, Salzberg SL. Fast gapped-read alignment with Bowtie 2. Nat Methods. 2012;9:357–9.
23. Kundaje A, Meuleman W, Ernst J, et al. Integrative analysis of 111 reference human epigenomes. Nature. 2015;518:317–30.
24. Grampp S, Platt JL, Lauer V, et al. Genetic variation at the 8q24.21 renal cancer susceptibility locus affects HIF binding to a MYC enhancer. Nat Commun. 2016;7:13183.
25. Ho TH, Kapur P, Joseph RW, et al. Loss of histone H3 lysine 36 trimethylation is associated with an increased risk of renal cell carcinoma-specific death. Mod Pathol. 2016;29:34–42.

6

Comparison of ultrasound-assisted and pure fluoroscopy-guided extracorporeal shockwave lithotripsy for renal stones

Tsung-Hsin Chang[1*], Wun-Rong Lin[1,2], Wei-Kung Tsai[1,2], Pai-Kai Chiang[1,2], Marcelo Chen[1,2,3], Jen-Shu Tseng[1*] and Allen W. Chiu[1,4]

Abstract

Background: In this study, we aimed to compare the efficacy and clinical outcomes of shock wave lithotripsy (SWL) for patients with renal stones using pure fluoroscopy (FS) or ultrasound-assisted (USa) localization with two lithotripters.

Methods: We retrospectively identified 425 patients with renal calculi who underwent SWL with either a LiteMed LM-9200 ELMA lithotripter (209 cases), which combined ultrasound and fluoroscopic stone targeting or a Medispec EM-1000 lithotripter machine (216 cases), which used fluoroscopy for stone localization and tracking. The patient demographic data, stone-free rates, stone disintegration rates, retreatment rates and complication rates were analyzed.

Results: The USa group had a significantly higher overall stone-free rate (43.6 vs. 28.2%, $p < 0.001$) and stone disintegration rate (85.6 vs. 64.3%, $p < 0.001$), as well as a significantly lower retreatment rate (14.8 vs. 35.6%, $p < 0.001$) and complication rate (1.9 vs. 5.5%, $p = 0.031$) compared with the FS group. This superiority remained significant in the stone size < 1 cm stratified group. In the stone size > 1 cm group, the stone-free rate (32.4 vs. 17.8%, $p = 0.028$), disintegration rate (89.2 vs. 54.8%, $p = 0.031$) and retreatment rate (21.6 vs. 53.4%, $p < 0.001$) were still significantly better in the USa group, however there was no significant difference in the complication rate. The most common complication was post-SWL-related flank pain.

Conclusion: SWL is a safe and non-invasive way of treating renal stones. This study compared two electromagnetic shock wave machines with different stone tracking systems. LiteMed LM-9200 ELMA lithotripter, which combined ultrasound and fluoroscopic stone targeting outperformed Medispec EM-1000 lithotripter, which used fluoroscopy for stone localization and tracking, with better stone-free rates and disintegration rates, as well as lower retreatment rates and complications with possible reduced radiation exposure.

Keywords: Shock wave lithotripsy, Nephrolithiasis, Kidney, Ultrasonography

Background

Extracorporeal shock wave lithotripsy (SWL) has been used as a non-invasive method of urolithiasis management since the 1980's [1]. It has been proven to be a safe, efficient way of treating non-infected upper urinary tract stones and remains one of the most commonly used treatment modality for renal stones worldwide today.

*Correspondence: KeithChang0910@gmail.com; urojst@gmail.com
[1] Department of Urology, MacKay Memorial Hospital, No. 92, Sec. 2, Zhongshan N. Rd., Taipei City 10449, Taiwan
Full list of author information is available at the end of the article

Contemporary studies have shown that the success rate of SWL for renal stones ranges from 47 to 92% [2–7]. This highly variable result is due to various crucial factors, including stone composition and size [8–11], skin to stone distance [12], lithotripter energy power [13] and frequency [14, 15], patient positioning [16], and patient tolerance and respiration [16, 17]. Less than half of the administered shockwaves may be accurately focused on the targeted calculus [18], and the excessive energy and shockwaves can cause damage to the parenchyma and adjacent organs. Chen et al. [19] demonstrated increased accuracy of stone targeting by using an electromagnetic lithotripter integrated with both ultrasound real-time tracking system and traditional fluoroscopy (LiteMed LM-9200 ELMA). Through the alternative use of ultrasound and fluoroscopy, the energy of the lithotripter may be more focused on the target stone during the whole session, thus increasing SWL efficiency. However, only a few studies have compared the efficacy of ultrasound-based lithotripters with fluoroscopy-based lithotripters. It is difficult to compare efficacy between different institutions due to variabilities in treatment protocols and operators. The current study compared the efficacy and clinical outcomes of two electromagnetic lithotripters using different stone localization methods (LiteMed LM-9200 ELMA lithotripter: combined ultrasound and fluoroscopic stone targeting; Medispec EM-1000 lithotripter: pure fluoroscopic stone targeting), in a single center with 2 hospital branches, using the same group of urologists and the same set of patients and surgical indications. The machines were operated by the same two experienced technicians, which minimizes operator and institutional related bias.

The aim of the current study was to compare the efficacy and clinical outcomes of these two different stone localization modalities in the treatment of renal stones in one single medical center.

Methods

The present study retrospectively reviewed the medical records of patients with radio-opaque kidney stones with stone size between 0.5 to 2.0 cm who underwent SWL in a single medical center with 2 hospital branches between January 2013 and March 2019. Exclusion criteria were patients with congenital anomalies or urinary diversion, pediatric patients or patients who received SWL as a combination therapy with other treatment modalities. Patients with radiolucent stones were also excluded as plain x-rays were used as the standard follow-up modality.

All patients underwent imaging and laboratory studies prior to SWL. Plain abdominal radiography of the kidneys, ureter and bladder (KUB), renal sonography, intravenous urography (IVU) and abdominal computed tomography (CT) were used to diagnose and identify the stones. The size of the stones were measured on the KUB using maximal stone diameters.

Patients underwent SWL at two branches of our medical center with either a LiteMed LM-9200 ELMA lithotripter or Medispec LTD EM-1000 lithotripter, depending on their location. The distance between the two branches of our medical center were about 10 km with about a 20 min driving time and both were located in the northern part of the city. There were no regional characteristics different between the patients of the two branches, such as water composition and eating habits. The energy source of both lithotripters was an electromagnetic shockwave source. The focal length was 145 mm for EM-1000 and 125 mm for LM-9200. All SWL treatments were performed on an ambulatory basis by the same group of urologists. Both machines were operated by the same two experienced technicians. The LiteMed LM-9200 ELMA lithotripter used ultrasonography and fluoroscopy for dual focusing of stone localization and tracking, while the EM1000 machine used only fluoroscopy for stone visualization, with an integrated computerized fluoroscopic X-ray (Visionspec™). The LiteMed LM-9200 machine has a auto-firing system, the shockwaves will only be fired when the stone is in the focal zone.

The same standardized SWL protocol was used for both machines except for the stone localization method. The patient was placed in a supine position without a restraint belt. The cushion size and lubricating jelly used were the same in both branch. and the stone was located by the fluoroscopy in both group. In the USa group, ultrasound was combined use for dual stone localization before initiating the SWL session and during the treatment for real time tracking of the stone. While in the FS group, only pure fluoroscopy was used throughout the whole session. During SWL, the initial energy level was set at 14KV and could gradually increased up to 19 kV if the stones did not show adequate fragmentation under low energy settings. The shock wave rate was set at 60 shocks per minute for both lithotripters. The maximum number of shockwaves delivered in one session was 3,000. Light intravenous propofol and dormicum were used as analgesics or for sedation if the patient suffered from pain or could not tolerate lying still in the supine position throughout the SWL session. The patient's position was adjusted throughout the SWL session for better stone visualization. If the patient's stone is still in focal zone, the position of the patient will not be changed to avoid constant de-coupling and re-coupling. In the FS group, the position was checked and adjusted after every 600 shocks or when the patient moved. While in the USa group, positioning was adjusted based on the ultrasound tracking of the stone location throughout the SWL session. All patient received SWL sessions on an ambulatory basis, analgesics with Diclofenac or Acetaminophen were prescribed for post-operative pain control.

Patients were evaluated at 4, 12 and 24 weeks after the SWL session by KUB. Stone-free status was defined as the absence of radiographic residual stones in the follow-up imaging, any residual fragments visible on KUB was considered as non-stone-free. The KUB x-ray. Stone disintegration was defined as the presence of stone destruction, fragmentation or a decrease in size in the post-session KUB compared with the pre-session KUB. Retreatment was defined as the need for further surgical intervention (repeat SWL, rigid ureteroscopic lithotripsy (URSL), retrograde intrarenal surgery (RIRS) or percutaneous nephrolithotomy (PCNL)) for symptomatic patients or patients with residual stone fragments > 0.5 cm. Complications were classified according to the Clavien-Dindo classification system. All data were analyzed and compared using t-tests and chi-squared tests with IBM SPSS statistics version 25.0 software. Statistical significance was set at $p < 0.05$.

The present study, including its research protocols and data collection, were approved by the Mackay Memorial Hospital Institutional Review Board. All personal information was de-identified prior to data analysis, thus ensuring patient data confidentiality.

Results

Of the 425 included patients, 209 were treated with USa SWL and 216 were treated with FS SWL. The mean age of patients was 53.3 ± 13.2 years in the USa group and 53.8 ± 12.4 years in the FS group ($p = 0.538$). Comparison of the two groups revealed that the FS group was significantly more male dominated ($p = 0.016$) and there were significantly larger stones in the USa group (1.03 ± 0.37 cm vs. 0.87 ± 0.33 cm, $p < 0.005$) (Table 1).

Table 1 Patient demographics and stone characteristics

Characteristic	USa	FS	p value
Number of patients	209	216	
Patient age (mean ± SD)	53.3 ± 13.2	53.8 ± 12.4	0.568
Patient gender			0.016
Male, n (%)	130 (62.2%)	158 (73.1%)	
Female, n (%)	79 (37.8%)	58 (26.8%)	
Stone size (cm)	1.03 ± 0.37	0.87 ± 0.33	0.008
> 1 cm (n)	111	73	
< 1 cm (n)	98	143	

Statistical analysis revealed better treatment outcomes in the USa group. The overall stone free rate was significantly better in the USa group compared with the FS group (USa 43.5% vs. FS 28.2%, $p < 0.001$), and the overall stone disintegration rates were significantly higher (USa 85.6% vs. FS 64.3%, $p < 0.001$). Significant lower retreatment (USa 14.8% vs. FS 35.6%, $p < 0.001$) and complication rates (USa 1.9% vs. FS 5.5%, $p = 0.031$) were noted in the USa group compared with the FS group (Table 2).

Patients were further stratified by stone size (< 1 cm and ≥ 1 cm), and the results were similar following stratification. In the group with renal stones < 1 cm the USa group had a significantly higher stone free rate (USa 56.1% vs. FS 33.5%, $p < 0.001$) and stone disintegration rate (USa 81.6% vs. FS 69.2%, $p = 0.031$) compared with the FS group. The USa group also had a significantly lower retreatment rate (USa 7.1% vs. FS 26.5%, $p < 0.001$) and complication rate (USa 1.0% vs. FS 6.9%, $p = 0.029$) (Table 3).

In the group with stones > 1 cm, the USa group still had a significantly better stone free rate (USa 32.4% vs. FS 17.8%, $p = 0.028$), stone disintegration rate (USa 89.2% vs. FS 54.8%, $p < 0.001$) and retreatment rate (USa 21.6% vs. FS 53.4%, $p < 0.001$) compared with the FS group. However, the complication rates were not statistically different between the two groups (US 2.7% vs. FS 4.1%, $p = 0.599$), but the USa group did still have a lower complication ratio (Table 4).

The most common complication was post-SWL-related flank pain (Clavien-Dindo grade I), which occurred in 1 (0.5%) USa group patient and 11 (5.1%) FS group patients, however no cases required hospitalization. In all

Table 2 Overall outcomes, stone free rate, complication, retreatment rate

	US (n = 209)	FS (n = 216)	p value
Stone free rate (%)	91 (43.5)	61 (28.2)	< 0.001
Disintegrate rate (%)	179 (85.6)	139 (64.3)	< 0.001
Retreatment rate (%)	31 (14.8)	77 (35.6)	< 0.001
Complication rate (%)	4 (1.9)	13 (6.0)	0.031

Table 3 Stone size < 1 cm, outcomes, stone free rate, complication, retreatment rate

	US (n = 98)	FS (n = 143)	p value
Stone free rate (%)	55 (56.1)	48 (33.5)	< 0.001
Disintegrate rate (%)	80 (81.6)	99 (69.2)	0.031
Retreatment rate (%)	7 (7.1)	38 (26.5)	< 0.001
Complication rate (%)	1 (1.0)	10 (6.9)	0.029

Table 4 Stone size>1 cm, outcomes, stone free rate, complication, retreatment rate

	US (n=111)	FS (n=73)	p value
Stone free rate (%)	36 (32.4)	13/ (17.8)	0.028
Disintegrate rate (%)	99 (89.2)	40 (54.8)	<0.001
Retreatment rate (%)	24 (21.6)	39 (53.4)	<0.001
Complication rate (%)	3 (2.7)	3 (4.1)	0.599

cases symptoms were controlled with intravenous/intramuscular or oral non-steroidal anti-inflammatory drugs (NSAIDs). In the USa group, 1 patient developed ureteral stone street after SWL; the patient had a 1.7 cm renal stone and required further RIRS for obstruction release and residual stone removal (grade 3). Another patient had a urinary tract infection and required hospitalization for intravenous antibiotics (grade 2). In the FS group, 2 patients developed post-SWL ureteral stone street, and one required URSL for stone removal (grade 3); the other patient had stone passage during follow up (grade 2).

Discussion

SWL has been the primary treatment option for renal and upper urinary calculi since its introduction in the early 1980's [20]. Two major international urological associations: the European association of urology and the American urological association both recommend SWL as the treatment of choice for small to intermediate renal stones. However, the treatment has certain limitations which may predict poor treatment efficacy, including steep and narrow infundibulum, long lower pole calyx, and shockwave-resistant stones [21, 22].

To maximize the efficacy and outcomes while minimizing complications of SWL, certain options regarding patient and stone characteristics have been proposed [16]. Obese patients and those with a higher body mass index (BMI) may have a larger skin to stone distance revealed during clinical examination, which could lead to unfavorable SWL success rates [12, 23]. Some studies highlighted the importance of anatomical location and the architecture of the stones as measured by CT Hounsfield units [8–11].

Other evidence showed that during SWL sessions, the energy and frequency emitted by the lithotripter notably contributed to stone disintegration. It is recommended that the treatment strategy starts from a low energy level and low frequency rate, and then gradually increases. Starting from a low energy level has been shown to pre-sensitize the kidney and cause renal vasoconstrictions [13, 24], thus reducing renal damage and improving patient tolerance. Low frequency shock wave rates have been proven to be associated with better stone fragmentation in many previous studies [14, 25–27]. Although there is no gold standard for optimal treatment frequency, it has been shown that frequency rates of 60 shocks per minute (1 Hz) and 90 shocks per minute (1.5 Hz) both had better outcomes compared with 120 shocks per minute (2 Hz) [14, 25–27]. Decreasing both the initial energy and shock wave frequency results in a reduced total number of shock waves and energy being delivered, thus reducing the possible damage to the kidney, and therefore decreasing the possibility of complications and improving patient comfort. The patient could be more easily adapted to this treatment, thus minimizing patient movement and the use of sedative agents. In this way, energy delivery could be more focused on the target and stone disruption could be improved. The training and experience of the technicians and operators performing the procedure also has an impact on the success of an SWL session, studies have shown that the stone free rate improves as the operator completes a learning curve [28, 29].

In the current study, the SWL session starts with a low energy (14KV) and low frequency setting (60 Hz) in order to maximize the treatment effect. All of the SWL sessions were performed by the same two technicians who have over 10 years of experience. The authors consider this to be a strength of the current study. Using the same low-frequency, low energy machine setup and having SWL sessions performed by the same two experienced operators, the SWL efficiency could be maximized while minimizing the inter-operator bias and learning curve bias.

Last but not least, the impact of the patient's stability during the SWL session must be considered. Patient movement and respiration during the SWL session can cause kidney movement [17], thus causing shock waves to be misdirected and focused away from the target. Excessive energy and inaccurate shockwaves may cause damage to the parenchyma and adjacent organs. Even when patients are under sedation or anesthesia during SWL, respiration related mistargeting remains inevitable. Constant tracking of the stone under a continuous fluoroscope could be the solution, however this may cause excessive ionizing radiation exposure. To overcome this problem, Chang et al. developed a real-time tracking ultrasound based system for renal stones [30]. In vitro and animal studies [31] showed the system to be efficient, and it could increase the accuracy of renal stone targeting and the efficiency of stone fragmentation.

The major advantage that ultrasound provides is real-time tracking of the stone without excessive radiation exposure to the patient. Although the dose of radiation during one SWL session may not be much and is not a worrisome dose compared to other invasive radiological procedures, the cumulative effect of ionizing radiation that needs to take into account includes the pre-treatment diagnostic imaging studies, such as CT or IVU, and possible repeat SWL treatment at a later date.

Chen et al. [19] reported on their clinical experience of renal stone treatment using an electromagnetic lithotripter integrated with an ultrasound-based real-time tracking system. Their results demonstrated increased accuracy of stone targeting with less shockwaves applied. Smith et al. [32] also compared the stone free rates between the USa localization technique and the traditional FS localization technique. The results revealed equivalent outcomes using the two different stone localization modalities but with the added benefit of no ionization exposure when using the USa technique. A randomized prospective study conducted by Van Besien et al. [33] demonstrated similar results, with the USa SWL stone-free rate not being inferior to the FS SWL, but with no need for ionizing radiation. This is probably most beneficial in pediatric patients, as children are 2–7 times more radiation-sensitive than adults [34]. In a study evaluating the outcomes and radiation exposure of children with cystine stones, Goren et al. [35] demonstrated that USa SWL was more effective and applied less ionizing radiation doses for pediatric patients. Also, in faintly radiopaque stones, such as cystine stones, USa-guided SWL has better visualization of the stones than a fluoroscope.

In the current study, the USa group had a larger baseline stone size. Despite this, the USa group had a significantly better stone-free rate, stone-disintegration rate and a lower retreatment rate; this was regardless of stone size stratification. This result indicates better stone localization and targeting with the assistance of real-time ultrasound, which causes better stone fragmentation and secondarily leads to better stone clearance and lower retreatment rates. As for safety, the USa group had a significantly lower complication rate for smaller stones, and a lower complication rate for larger stones, although this did not reach statistical significance. These results further indicate the theoretical benefit of ultrasound tracking, that is, better accuracy leads to less surrounding tissue damage, which would be more significant in smaller targets.

Previously reported stone-free rate of ESWL ranged around 47 to 92% [2–7]. In our study, the main reason of our relative lower stone-free rates is because that stone-free status was more strictly defined. Stone-free status was defined as the absence of radiographic residual stones in the follow-up imaging, any residual fragments visible on KUB was considered as non-stone-free, even the fragments were less than 2 mm or 4 mm, which was the most commonly used criteria in clinical practice and other studies.

Previous studies had certain limitations, such as small patient numbers or a lack of head to head comparisons [19, 32]. Despite its randomized prospective study design, Van Besein's study failed to show statistical significance between the different localization methods, this may be related to the small number of studied patients. A strength of the current study compared to others is that we have a large number of study patients, two similar energy source lithotripters using the same SWL protocol, and all procedures were performed by the same two experienced technicians, which provides strong head-to-head comparison while minimizing bias between different institutions and operators.

However, there were several limitations to the present study that need to be addressed. First, its retrospective study design limited the bias control, such as stone composition and anatomic parameters. Second, radiation exposure was not recorded besides self-reported preference by the two technicians. Third, CT was not routinely in every patient to assess factors that affect ESWL results, such as CT values, stone-to-skin distance and BMI. In addition, we compared two different electromagnetic lithotripters. Different lithotripters' acoustic output, efficiency, and collateral effects vary between models. Therefore, further strictly controlled studies are needed to support the conclusion. Lastly, SWL and localization techniques are very operator-dependent. The current study was conducted in one single center and only two technicians operated the machine, thus minimizing inter-operator and institutional bias. Further studies could be conducted in a larger set of patients who are prospectively randomized.

Conclusions

SWL is a safe and non-invasive way of treating renal stones. this study compared two electromagnetic shock wave machines with different stone tracking systems. LiteMed LM-9200 ELMA lithotripter, which combined ultrasound and fluoroscopic stone targeting outperformed Medispec EM-1000 lithotripter, which used fluoroscopy for stone localization and tracking, with better stone-free rates and disintegration rates, as well as lower retreatment rates and complications with possible reduced radiation exposure.

Abbreviations

CT: Computed tomography; SWL: Shock wave lithotripsy; KUB: Kidneys, ureter and bladder; IVU: Intravenous urography; URSL: Ureteroscopic lithotripsy; RIRS: Retrograde intrarenal surgery; PCNL: Percutaneous nephrolithotomy.

Acknowledgements

Not applicable.

Authors' contributions

THC: project development, data collection, data analysis, and manuscript writing. WRL: data collection and data analysis. WKT: data collection and data analysis. PKC: data collection and data analysis. MC: project development, data analysis, and manuscript editing. JST: project development, data analysis, and manuscript editing. AWC: manuscript editing. All authors have read and approved the manuscript.

Author details

[1] Department of Urology, MacKay Memorial Hospital, No. 92, Sec. 2, Zhongshan N. Rd., Taipei City 10449, Taiwan. [2] Mackay Medical College, No.46, Sec. 3, Zhongzheng Rd., Sanzhi Dist., New Taipei City 252, Taiwan. [3] Mackay Junior College of Medicine, Beitou District, Nursing, and Management, No.92, Shengjing Road, Taipei City 11272, Taiwan. [4] School of Medicine, National Yang-Ming University, No.145, Zhengzhou Rd., Datong Dist., Taipei City 10341, Taiwan.

References

1. Chaussy C, Brendel W, Schmiedt E. Extracorporeally induced destruction of kidney stones by shock waves. Lancet (London, England). 1980;2(8207):1265–8.
2. Fialkov JM, Hedican SP, Fallon B. Reassessing the efficacy of the Dornier MFL-5000 lithotriptor. J Urol. 2000;164(3 Pt 1):640–3.
3. Nafie S, Dyer JE, Minhas JS, Mills JA, Khan MA. Efficacy of a mobile lithotripsy service: a one-year review of 222 patients. Scand J Urol. 2014;48(3):324–7.
4. Chung VY, Turney BW. The success of shock wave lithotripsy (SWL) in treating moderate-sized (10–20 mm) renal stones. Urolithiasis. 2016;44(5):441–4.
5. Nielsen TK, Jensen JB. Efficacy of commercialised extracorporeal shock wave lithotripsy service: a review of 589 renal stones. BMC Urol. 2017;17(1):59.
6. Abdel-Khalek M, Sheir KZ, Mokhtar AA, Eraky I, Kenawy M, Bazeed M. Prediction of success rate after extracorporeal shock-wave lithotripsy of renal stones–a multivariate analysis model. Scand J Urol Nephrol. 2004;38(2):161–7.
7. Lee CC, Lin WR, Hsu JM, Chow YC, Tsai WK, Chiang PK, Chen M, Chiu AW. Comparison of electrohydraulic and electromagnetic extracorporeal shock wave lithotriptors for upper urinary tract stones in a single center. World J Urol. 2019;37(5):931–5.
8. El-Nahas AR, El-Assmy AM, Mansour O, Sheir KZ. A prospective multivariate analysis of factors predicting stone disintegration by extracorporeal shock wave lithotripsy: the value of high-resolution noncontrast computed tomography. Eur Urol. 2007;51(6):1688–93 (**discussion 1693–1684**).
9. Nakasato T, Morita J, Ogawa Y. Evaluation of Hounsfield Units as a predictive factor for the outcome of extracorporeal shock wave lithotripsy and stone composition. Urolithiasis. 2015;43(1):69–75.
10. Cui HW, Devlies W, Ravenscroft S, Heers H, Freidin AJ, Cleveland RO, Ganeshan B, Turney BW. CT Texture analysis of ex vivo renal stones predicts ease of fragmentation with shockwave lithotripsy. J Endourol. 2017;31(7):694–700.
11. Williams JC Jr, Paterson RF, Kopecky KK, Lingeman JE, McAteer JA. High resolution detection of internal structure of renal calculi by helical computerized tomography. J Urol. 2002;167(1):322–6.
12. Patel T, Kozakowski K, Hruby G, Gupta M. Skin to stone distance is an independent predictor of stone-free status following shockwave lithotripsy. J Endourol. 2009;23(9):1383–5.
13. Handa RK, McAteer JA, Connors BA, Liu Z, Lingeman JE, Evan AP. Optimising an escalating shockwave amplitude treatment strategy to protect the kidney from injury during shockwave lithotripsy. BJU Int. 2012;110(11 Pt C):E1041-1047.
14. Pace KT, Ghiculete D, Harju M, Honey RJ. Shock wave lithotripsy at 60 or 120 shocks per minute: a randomized, double-blind trial. J Urol. 2005;174(2):595–9.
15. Davenport K, Minervini A, Keoghane S, Parkin J, Keeley FX, Timoney AG. Does rate matter? The results of a randomized controlled trial of 60 versus 120 shocks per minute for shock wave lithotripsy of renal calculi. J Urol. 2006;176(5):2055–8 (**discussion 2058**).
16. Kroczak T, Scotland KB, Chew B, Pace KT. Shockwave lithotripsy: techniques for improving outcomes. World J Urol. 2017;35(9):1341–6.
17. Suramo I, Paivansalo M, Myllyla V. Cranio-caudal movements of the liver, pancreas and kidneys in respiration. Acta Radiol. 1984;25(2):129–31.
18. Kuwahara M, Kambe K, Taguchi K, Saito T, Shirai S, Orikasa S. Initial experience using a new type extracorporeal lithotripter with an anti-misshot control device. J Lithotr Stone Dis. 1991;3(2):141–6.
19. Chen CJ, Hsu HC, Chung WS, Yu HJ. Clinical experience with ultrasound-based real-time tracking lithotripsy in the single renal stone treatment. J Endourol. 2009;23(11):1811–5.
20. Chaussy C, Schmiedt E, Jocham D, Brendel W, Forssmann B, Walther V. First clinical experience with extracorporeally induced destruction of kidney stones by shock waves. J Urol. 1982;127(3):417–20.
21. Turk C, Petrik A, Sarica K, Seitz C, Skolarikos A, Straub M, Knoll T. EAU Guidelines on Interventional Treatment for Urolithiasis. Eur Urol. 2016;69(3):475–82.
22. Pradere B, Doizi S, Proietti S, Brachlow J, Traxer O. Evaluation of guidelines for surgical management of urolithiasis. J Urol. 2018;199(5):1267–71.
23. Wiesenthal JD, Ghiculete D, Ray AA, Honey RJ, Pace KT. A clinical nomogram to predict the successful shock wave lithotripsy of renal and ureteral calculi. J Urol. 2011;186(2):556–62.
24. Handa RK, Bailey MR, Paun M, Gao S, Connors BA, Willis LR, Evan AP. Pretreatment with low-energy shock waves induces renal vasoconstriction during standard shock wave lithotripsy (SWL): a treatment protocol known to reduce SWL-induced renal injury. BJU Int. 2009;103(9):1270–4.
25. Honey RJ, Schuler TD, Ghiculete D, Pace KT. A randomized, double-blind trial to compare shock wave frequencies of 60 and 120 shocks per minute for upper ureteral stones. J Urol. 2009;182(4):1418–23.
26. Li K, Lin T, Zhang C, Fan X, Xu K, Bi L, Han J, Huang H, Liu H, Dong W, et al. Optimal frequency of shock wave lithotripsy in urolithiasis treatment: a systematic review and meta-analysis of randomized controlled trials. J Urol. 2013;190(4):1260–7.
27. Yilmaz E, Batislam E, Basar M, Tuglu D, Mert C, Basar H. Optimal frequency in extracorporeal shock wave lithotripsy: prospective randomized study. Urology. 2005;66(6):1160–4.
28. Lee C, Best SL, Ugarte R, Monga M. Impact of learning curve on efficacy of shock wave lithotripsy. Radiol Technol. 2008;80(1):20–4.
29. Okada A, Yasui T, Taguchi K, Niimi K, Hirose Y, Hamamoto S, Ando R, Kubota Y, Umemoto Y, Tozawa K, et al. Impact of official technical training for urologists on the efficacy of shock wave lithotripsy. Urolithiasis. 2013;41(6):487–92.
30. Chang CC, Liang SM, Pu YR, Chen CH, Manousakas I, Chen TS, Kuo CL, Yu FM, Chu ZF. In vitro study of ultrasound based real-time tracking of renal stones for shock wave lithotripsy: part 1. J Urol. 2001;166(1):28–32.
31. Chang CC, Manousakas I, Pu YR, Liang SM, Chen CH, Chen TS, Yu FM, Yang WH, Tong YC, Kuo CL. In vitro study of ultrasound based real-time tracking for renal stones in shock wave lithotripsy: part II—a simulated animal experiment. J Urol. 2002;167(6):2594–7.
32. Smith HE, Bryant DA, KooNg J, Chapman RA, Lewis G. Extracorporeal shockwave lithotripsy without radiation: ultrasound localization is as effective as fluoroscopy. Urol Ann. 2016;8(4):454–7.
33. Van Besien J, Uvin P, Hermie I, Tailly T, Merckx L. Ultrasonography is not inferior to fluoroscopy to guide extracorporeal shock waves during treatment of renal and upper ureteric calculi: a randomized prospective study. Biomed Res Int. 2017;2017:7802672.
34. Richardson RB. Stem cell niches and other factors that influence the sensitivity of bone marrow to radiation-induced bone cancer and leukaemia in children and adults. Int J Radiat Biol. 2011;87(4):343–59.
35. Goren MR, Goren V, Ozer C. Ultrasound-guided shockwave lithotripsy reduces radiation exposure and has better outcomes for pediatric cystine stones. Urol Int. 2017;98(4):429–35.

7

Functional and oncologic outcomes of robot-assisted simple enucleation with and without renal arterial cold perfusion in complex renal tumors: A propensity score-matched analysis

Qun Lu[1†], Xiaozhi Zhao[1†], Changwei Ji[1], Suhan Guo[2], Xuefeng Qiu[1], Guangxiang Liu[1], Shiwei Zhang[1], Xiaogong Li[1], Gutian Zhang[1], Xuebin Zhang[3] and Hongqian Guo[1*]

Abstract

Background: To compare robot-assisted simple enucleation with renal arterial cold perfusion (RACP-RASE) and RASE alone in complex renal tumors with regard to perioperative, functional and oncologic outcomes by propensity score-matched analysis.

Methods: Data from 351 patients who underwent RACP-RASE or RASE for complex renal tumors were recorded between September 2014 and December 2017. Propensity score-matched analysis was performed on age, sex, BMI, ECOG score, tumor side and size, preoperative estimated glomerular filtration rate (eGFR), RENAL score and PADUA score.

Results: The study included 31 RACP-RASE and 320 RASE procedures. RENAL score and PADUA score were higher and tumor diameter was greater under RACP-RASE than RASE. After matching, the two groups were similar in estimated blood loss (208.3 vs 230.7 ml; $p=0.696$) and ischemic time (34.8 vs 32.8 min; $p=0.342$). The RACP-RASE group had significantly longer operative time than the RASE group (264.1 ± 55.7 vs 206.9 ± 64.0 min, $p=0.001$). There was no difference in the incidence of postoperative complications between the two groups (13.8% vs 24.1%; $p=0.315$), as was the overall incidence of positive surgical margins (3.4 vs 0%; $p=1.000$). The changes in eGFR significantly differed between the two groups at 3 months ($p=0.018$) and 12 months ($p=0.038$). More patients in the RASE group were CKD upstaged ($p=0.043$). At multivariable analysis, preoperative eGFR and the type of procedure were significant predictive factors for a change of more than 10% in eGFR at 3 months postoperatively. There was no local recurrence or distant metastasis during follow-up.

*Correspondence: dr.ghq@nju.edu.cn
†Qun Lu and Xiaozhi Zhao contributed equally to this work
[1] Department of Urology, Drum Tower Hospital, Medical School of Nanjing University, Institute of Urology, Nanjing University, 321 Zhongshan Rd., Nanjing 210008, Jiangsu, People's Republic of China
Full list of author information is available at the end of the article

Conclusions: RACP-RASE is an effective and safe technique for complex renal tumors that can provide appropriate temporary arterial occlusion and renal hypothermic perfusion. Renal arterial cold perfusion may be helpful in protecting renal function in RASE as compared with warm ischemia.

Keywords: Renal cell carcinoma, Enucleation, Robotic partial nephrectomy, Perfusion, Hypothermia

Background

An increasing number of patients with renal tumors have been detected at an early stage because of the widespread practice of health examination. Partial nephrectomy (PN) has become the standard therapy for treating localized renal tumors, and it provides desirable oncological and functional results not inferior to radical nephrectomy [1]. Traditionally, standard partial nephrectomy (SPN) includes removal of the tumor and a visible rim of healthy parenchyma [2, 3]. Simple enucleation (SE) is an alternative nephron-sparing technique that minimizes the thickness of normal parenchyma surrounding the tumor [4, 5]. About 82% of renal masses have a demonstrable pseudocapsule [6], providing an avascular plane to enucleate the mass. Several studies have revealed that SE can preserve more normal renal parenchyma than SPN [4, 7].

Renal ischemia during PN may result in postoperative kidney insufficiency due to ischemia/reperfusion injury. Although it is generally considered that temporary hilar control during PN won't affect the short-term renal function significantly [8, 9], decline in renal function averages about 20% in the operated kidney [10]. The risk factors like advanced age, hypertension, or the ischemia time exceeding 30 min further aggravate kidney injury. Some studies have reported that organ hypothermia has been applied to prolong the ischemia time and decrease the degree of kidney damage [11]. Lowering the renal temperature can decrease the renal metabolism and limit the hypoxia-induced injury pathways [12]. Several ways of hypothermic protection have been reported, such as surface cooling with ice slush, renal arterial cold perfusion using angiography, and retrograde transureteral perfusion.

With advanced characteristics such as magnified 3-D vision with high definition quality and precise control with articulating instruments, the da Vinci surgical system may overcome the disadvantages present in laparoscopic PN and significantly shorten the learning curve [13]. The surgical indications for robotic PN have expanded to more complex renal lesions, like completely endophytic or hilar tumors.

In this study, we present our initial experience with renal function protection technology combining robot-assisted simple enucleation (RASE) and renal arterial cold perfusion (RACP-RASE) for treating complex renal tumors. We describe the technique detailedly and present the results on perioperative, functional and oncologic outcomes comparing RACP-RASE and RASE alone.

Methods

Patients

The data of 351 patients who underwent RASE or RACP-RASE for clinical localized renal tumors were collected from September 2014 to December 2017. We detected the perioperative, functional and oncologic date. All the procedures were completed by one surgeon (Hongqian Guo). According to the tumor characteristics and our experience, we assessed the ischemia time during SE preoperatively. If the ischemia time may well exceed 30 min, we would perform RACP-RASE. The patients in RACP-RASE group were mostly with complex renal tumors, including endophytic, hilar, and renal tumors larger than 7 cm, which accounted for 77.4% of patients. The rest had a deep single lesion with renal sinus or collecting system contact in which prolonged ischemia time was anticipated. All patients in RACP-RASE group received a preoperative consultation of the Department of Radiology Intervention, and the interventional radiologist developed a proposal according to the three-dimensional reconstruction of renal artery. The study was approved by the local ethics committee, and all patients signed the informed consent.

Demographic data and perioperative outcomes of all patients were obtained. Level of functioning was classified by the Eastern Cooperative Oncology Group (ECOG) criteria [14]. The tumor presentation pattern was classified according to the Patard classification [15]. The score of renal tumors were determined by an experienced radiologist in conjunction with an urologist on the basis of the RENAL nephrometry score system and PADUA nephrometric classification [16, 17]. Postoperative complications were stratified according to the Clavien–Dindo grading system [18]. Estimated glomerular filtration rate (eGFR) calculated by the modification of diet renal disease formula was used to assess the kidney function [19]. Chronic kidney disease (CKD) was defined by the National Kidney Foundation Kidney Disease Outcome Quality Initiative classification. We counted the time of balloon catheterization into total operative time in RACP-RASE group.

(See figure on next page.)

Fig. 1 Intraoperative showing: incision of the renal parenchyma near the tumor edge until the tumor pseudocapsule is identified or the bleeding is interfering with the safe removal of the tumor (**A**). The renal artery is blocked by an inflating balloon, and cold ischemia is achieved by perfusion of chilled Ringers until the renal parenchyma becomes bleached (**B**). Removing the tumor with blunt dissection by using the natural cleavage plane between the tumor and normal parenchyma (**C–E**). The renal surface is examined to rule out tumor infiltration and hemorrhage in the tumor bed is controlled by bipolar coagulation without sutures conventionally (**F**). The single-layer renorrhaphy technique is performed for renal reconstruction (**G**). Deflating the balloon and inspecting the parenchymal defect (**H**)

Surgical technique

Before anesthesia the patient was first sent to the Radiology Intervention Department, and the renal artery balloon catheter was punctured through the femoral artery to achieve cold perfusion under the guidance of fluoroscopy. The interventional radiologist inserted a 5.5Fr balloon angiocatheter in the renal artery as distally as possible to avoid accidental shifting of the catheter. If the trunk of the renal artery was short, a 4Fr balloon catheter was placed in each of the two branches of the renal artery. The patient was then taken to the operative room in a horizontal position. After anesthesia the patient was placed in the lateral position. The Si da Vinci surgical system (Intuitive Surgical, Sunnyvale, CA, USA) was used for RASE. We employed two 8-mm ports for the instruments and one 12-mm port for the camera, and the transperitoneal approach was routinely used. The Fenestrated or Maryland grasper on the left arm and the monopolar scissor on the right arm were generally used in RASE.

The method of tumor enucleation was described in our previous study [20]. The enucleation began with a cold incision a few millimeters around the lesion without ischemia. When the tumor capsule was seen or hemorrhage blurred the surgical field, the renal artery was blocked by inflating 0.5–1.0 ml saline solution into the catheter balloon. Cold ischemia was achieved by perfusion of chilled Ringers lactate through the catheter at the rate of 20 ml/min, and the enucleation wound contributed to the outflow of the perfusion fluid. The surgeon then enucleated the tumor without visible normal parenchyma around it by blunt dissection. After the tumor was removed, the tumor bed was easily detected to rule out possible tumor infiltration because the renal parenchyma became bleached. Hemostasis was controlled by bipolar coagulation, and the collecting system fracture was ligated using a single suture. The cortical defect was usually closed with horizontal and interrupted sutures. Then the perfusion was stopped and the balloon was deflated. Finally, the parenchyma defect was detected to rule out bleeding, and additional sutures was employed if necessary (Fig. 1).

Pathology

Tumors pathology were staged according to the TNM classification [21]. The histological subtypes of tumor were classified by the 2004 version of WHO classification. The nuclear grade was classified by the 2016 WHO/ISUP grading [22]. All specimens were grossly analyzed for surgical margin evaluation.

Statistical analysis

We used the Mann–Whitney U-test or the Pearson chi-square test to compare the variables. A propensity score-matched analysis was used to minimize the selection bias of treatment. The propensity score was derived from a multivariable logistic model including the variables of age, sex, BMI, ECOG score, tumor side and size, preoperative eGFR, RENAL score and PADUA score. According to the propensity score, the RACP-RASE patients were matched 1:1 without replacement to the RASE patients by using nearest-neighbour matching within a caliper set at 0.05. A 2-sided p value < 0.05 was considered statistically significant and the analysis was performed using SPSS 17.0 (SPSS Inc., Chicago, IL).

Results

The characteristics of the patients before and after the propensity score matching were shown in Table 1. This study included 31 patients who underwent RACP-RASE and 320 who underwent RASE. The two groups were comparative in age, sex, BMI, ECOG score, symptoms and preoperative eGFR. Anatomical complexity scores (RENAL score and PADUA score) were higher and tumor diameter was greater for patients with RACP-RASE than RASE.

Within the propensity score matched cohort, a total of 58 patients were matched, with 29 patients in each group. Complex tumor features after matching were shown in Table 2. In the RACP-RASE group, 5 patients had tumors larger than 7 cm, 6 patients had completely intrarenal tumors, 12 patients had hilar tumors, and 1 patient had multiple tumors. The rest had a deep single lesion with renal sinus or collecting system contact. The RACP-RASE group had more hilar tumors than RASE group (41.4 vs 13.8%, $p = 0.019$).

Surgical, pathological and functional results before and after matching were shown in Table 3. After matching, the RACP-RASE and RASE groups were similar in ischemic time (34.8 ± 9.4 vs 32.8 ± 7.2 min) and estimated blood loss (208.3 ± 93.8 vs 230.7 ± 135.7 ml). The operative

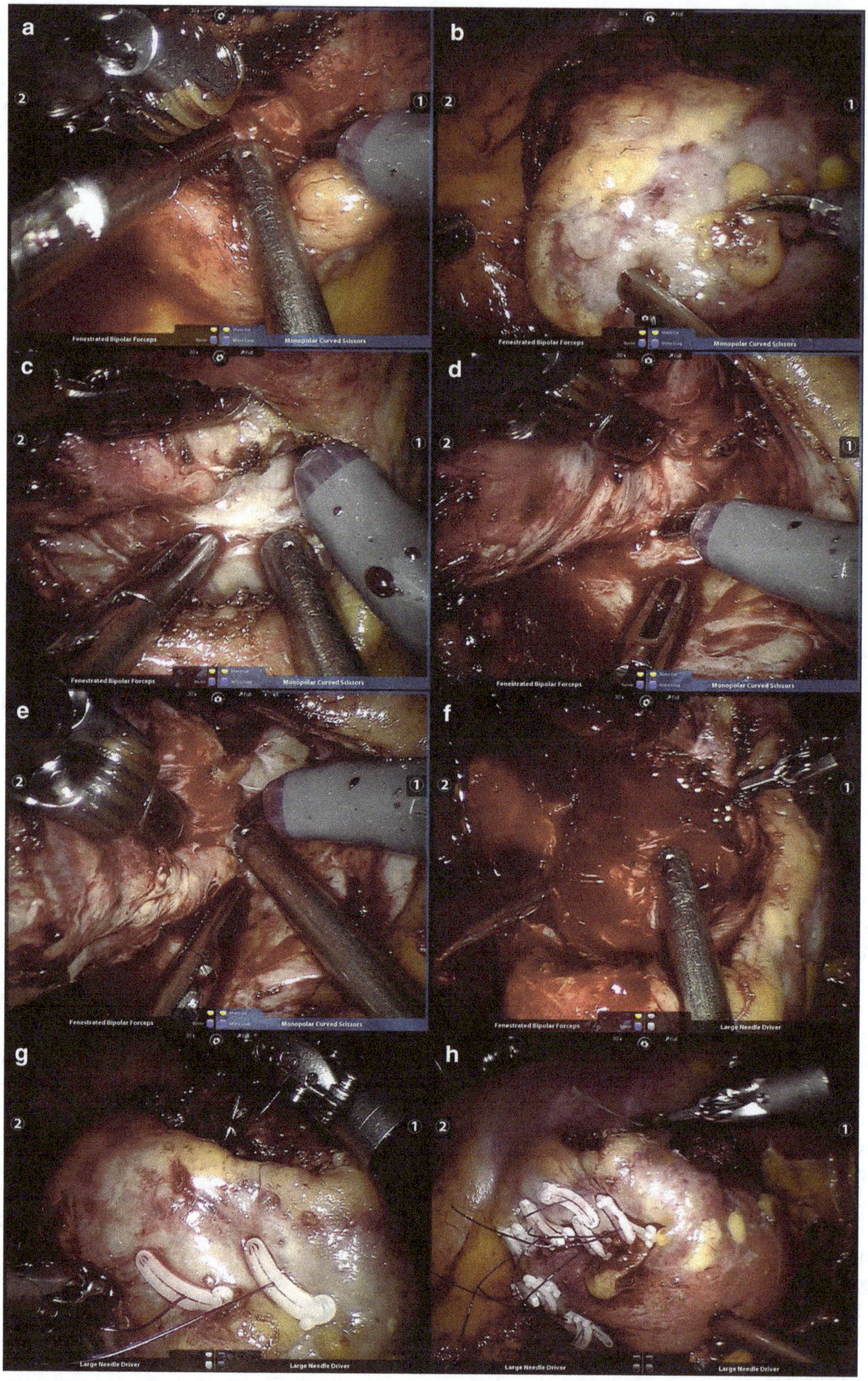
a
b
c
d
e
f
g
h
Fenestrated Bipolar Forceps
Monopolar Curved Scissors
Large Needle Driver

Table 1 Preoperative patient data and tumor characteristics before and after propensity-score matching

	Pre-matching			Post-matching		
	RACP-RASE, n = 31	RASE, n = 320	*p* value	RACP-RASE, n = 29	RASE, n = 29	*p* value
Age, years, mean ± SD	52.9 ± 12.9	53.7 ± 13.6	0.695	52.5 ± 13.2	54.4 ± 14.3	0.460
Sex (n, %)			0.810			0.780
Male	19 (61.3%)	189 (59.1%)		19 (65.5%)	20 (69.0%)	
Female	12 (38.7%)	131 (40.9%)		10 (34.5%)	9 (31.0%)	
BMI, mean ± SD	24.6 ± 3.4	24.2 ± 3.1	0.714	24.3 ± 3.1	24.1 ± 3.2	0.646
ECOG (n, %)			0.547			0.368
0	21 (67.7%)	233 (72.8%)		20 (69.0%)	23 (79.3%)	
≥ 1	10 (32.3%)	87 (27.2%)		9 (31.0%)	6 (20.7%)	
Side (n, %)			0.645			0.421
Left	18 (58.1%)	172 (53.8%)		16 (55.2%)	19 (65.5%)	
Right	13 (41.9%)	148 (46.2%)		13 (44.8%)	10 (34.5%)	
Symptoms at diagnosis (n, %)			0.706			0.389
Asymptomatic	27 (87.1%)	291 (90.9%)		25 (86.2%)	27 (93.1%)	
Symptomatic	4 (12.9%)	29 (9.1%)		4 (13.8%)	2 (6.9%)	
Preoperative eGFR, ml/min/1.73m^2, median (IQR)	101 (80–111)	97 (80–116)	0.960	98 (79–109)	91 (76–110)	0.539
Clinical tumor size, cm, mean ± SD	5.1 ± 1.3	3.9 ± 1.6	**0.000**	5.0 ± 1.7	4.9 ± 1.8	0.870
RENAL score, median (IQR)	10 (10–11)	8 (6–9)	**0.000**	10 (10–11)	10 (10–11)	0.709
PADUA score, median (IQR)	11 (11–12)	9 (7–10)	**0.000**	11 (11–12)	11 (11–12)	0.683

Bold indicated that the *p* value was statistically significant

RACP-RASE robot-assisted simple enucleation with renal arterial cold perfusion, *RASE* robot-assisted simple enucleation, *BMI* body mass index, *ECOG* Eastern Cooperative Oncology Group, *eGFR* estimated glomerular filtration rate, *IQR* interquartile range

Table 2 Complex tumor features after propensity-score matching

	Post-matching		
	RACP-RASE, n = 29	RASE, n = 29	*p* value
Larger than 7 cm	5 (17.2%)	3 (10.3%)	0.703
Completely intrarenal tumor	6 (20.7%)	4 (13.8%)	0.487
Hilar tumor	12 (41.4%)	4 (13.8%)	**0.019**
Multiple tumors	1 (3.4%)	0 (0.0%)	1.000

Bold indicated that the *p* value was statistically significant

time of RACP-RASE group was significantly longer than the RASE group (264.1 ± 55.7 vs 206.9 ± 64.0 min, $p = 0.001$). The rate of renal sinus entry was comparable (58.6% vs 48.3%). The RACP-RASE group had 1 conversion (3.4%) to radical nephrectomy for oncological reasons, and the RASE group had 1 conversion (3.4%) to radical nephrectomy for significant hemorrhage. The 2 groups did not differ in the incidence of postoperative complications (13.8% vs 24.1%, $p = 0.315$). The complications were mainly Clavien–Dindo grade 1 or 2 complications. Clavien–Dindo grade 3 complications occurred in no RACP-RASE patients and in 1 RASE patient. Overall, 89.7% of RACP-RASE patients and 82.8% RASE patients had malignant tumors, and clear cell carcinoma was the most common histotype. There was no difference in the rate of positive surgical margins between 2 groups (3.4 vs 0%, $p = 1.000$). The only 1 patient with positive margin in RASE group showed no local recurrence to date.

Regarding the renal functional outcomes after matching, the median eGFR 3 months postoperatively was 93 and 84 ml/min per 1.73 m^2 ($p = 0.287$) for the RACP-RASE and RASE groups, with a median -6.3 and -12.0 percentage change, respectively ($p = 0.018$). Only 1 patient in the RASE group had acute renal injury. The median eGFR 12 months postoperatively was 88 and 80 ml/min per 1.73 m^2, respectively ($p = 0.186$), with a median − 5.8 and − 11.7 percentage change ($p = 0.038$). The changes in eGFR significantly differed between the two groups. A total of 17.2% of patients in the RACP-RASE group and 41.4% in the RASE group were CKD upstaged ($p = 0.043$). No patient required temporary or permanent dialysis. At multivariable analysis, preoperative eGFR and the type of procedure were significant predictive factors for a change of more than 10% in eGFR at 3 months postoperatively (Table 4).

The median follow-up with RACP-RASE and RASE was 22 months (range 15–30) and 28 months (range

Table 3 Surgical, pathological and functional outcomes for RACP-RASE and RASE before and after propensity-score matching

	Pre-matching			Post-matching		
	RACP-RASE, n = 31	RASE, n = 320	*p* Value	RACP-RASE, n = 29	RASE, n = 29	*p* Value
Operative time, min, mean ± SD	262.6 ± 57.1	175.6 ± 45.5	**0.000**	264.1 ± 55.7	206.9 ± 64.0	**0.001**
Ischemic time, min, mean ± SD	35.9 ± 10.8	22.8 ± 7.3	**0.000**	34.8 ± 9.4	32.8 ± 7.2	0.342
Estimated blood loss, ml, mean ± SD	212.6 ± 94.2	179.1 ± 123.6	**0.005**	208.3 ± 93.8	230.7 ± 135.7	0.696
Entry into sinus (n, %)	19 (61.3%)	63 (19.7%)	**0.000**	17 (58.6%)	14 (48.3%)	0.430
Conversions (n, %)						
Open conversion	0 (0.0%)	2 (0.6%)	1.000	0 (0.0%)	0 (0.0%)	–
Radical conversion	1 (3.2%)	6 (1.9%)	1.000	1 (3.4%)	1 (3.4%)	1.000
Length of stay, d, mean ± SD	7.9 ± 1.4	7.9 ± 2.0	0.429	7.8 ± 1.4	8.6 ± 2.3	0.370
Postoperative complications (n, %)	4 (12.9%)	35 (10.9%)	0.973	4 (13.8%)	7 (24.1%)	0.315
Clavien 1–2	4 (12.9%)	31 (9.7%)		4 (13.8%)	6 (20.7%)	
Clavien 3–4	0 (0.0%)	4 (1.3%)		0 (0.0%)	1 (3.4%)	
Tumor histology (n, %)			1.000			0.703
Malignant	28 (90.3%)	286 (89.4%)		26 (89.7%)	24 (82.8%)	
Benign	3 (9.7%)	34 (10.6%)		3 (10.3%)	5 (17.2%)	
Positive margins (n, %)	1 (3.2%)	5 (1.6%)	1.000	1 (3.4%)	0 (0.0%)	1.000
Postoperative eGFR, ml/min/1.73m^2, median (IQR)						
3 months	93 (73–108)	92 (79–110)	0.670	93 (74–107)	84 (60–105)	0.287
12 months	88 (73–114)	93 (81–112)	0.453	88 (77–108)	80 (61–98)	0.186
Acute renal injury (n, %)	1 (3.2%)	3 (0.9%)	0.795	0 (0.0%)	1 (3.4%)	1.000
Postoperative change in eGFR, %, median (IQR)						
3 months	− 6.3 (− 11.3 to − 2.4)	− 3.2 (− 19.4 to − 2.3)	0.849	− 6.3 (− 10.3 to − 2.4)	− 12.0 (− 17.5 to − 6.7)	**0.018**
12 months	− 5.8 (− 15.5 to 1.9)	− 2.0 (− 17.4 to 10.0)	0.551	− 5.8 (− 12.7 to 0.1)	− 11.7 (− 18.9 to − 4.0)	**0.038**
CKD upstaging n (%)	6 (19.4%)	68 (21.3%)	0.805	5 (17.2%)	12 (41.4%)	**0.043**

Bold indicated that the *p* value was statistically significant

Table 4 Multivariate analysis for a change of more than 10% in eGFR at 3 months postoperatively

Variable	OR	CI	*p* value
Age	0.955	0.894–1.019	0.163
ECOG	1.308	0.305–5.602	0.717
Clinical tumor size	1.196	0.684–2.093	0.530
PADUA score	1.952	0.668–5.707	0.222
Preoperative eGFR	0.968	0.941–0.997	**0.029**
RASE vs RACP-RASE	0.090	0.020–0.408	**0.002**

Bold indicated that the *p* value was statistically significant

14–45). No local recurrence or distant metastasis occurred during follow-up.

Discussion

Here we compared the perioperative, functional and oncologic outcomes of RACP-RASE and RASE alone by propensity score-matched analysis. After matching, the two groups were similar in estimated blood loss and ischemic time. Operative time was longer in RACP-RASE group than RASE group. The main reason was that we counted the time of balloon catheterization into total operative time in RACP-RASE group. It also took minutes to transport patients from the Radiology Intervention Department to the operative room. The total incidence of postoperative complications was comparable between two groups, as was the incidence of positive surgical margins. The changes in eGFR significantly differed between the two groups at 3 months and 12 months. RACP-RASE is a safe and acceptable technique for complex renal tumors that can achieve temporary control of renal artery and provide hypothermic perfusion for the kidney. Renal arterial cold perfusion was helpful in protecting renal function in RASE as compared with warm ischemia.

Nephron-sparing surgeries, including SE and SPN, offer perioperative outcomes similar to those of radical nephrectomy with the advantage of renal function preservation [23, 24]. Minimally invasive surgery especially robotic surgery has the potential benefits for postoperative rapid recovery. In previous studies various techniques of renal cooling in PN have been reported. Gill et al. described an ice slush technique in an open approach with good functional outcomes [25]. Cold ureteral perfusion was also used in laparoscopic PN but without an outcome study [26].

Renal arterial cold perfusion is the most common physiological form of renal hypothermia, and the method has been applied in clinical practice for many years [27, 28]. It replaces the residual blood of kidney and cools the renal parenchyma quickly. Moreover, it prevents intravascular coagulation and makes the surgical visibility clearer. Cold perfusion is also used in kidney transplantation for the organ preservation and in vivo PN through open or laparoscopic approaches [29, 30]. To our knowledge, this is the first study to combine the technology of renal arterial cold perfusion and RASE.

The balloon catheters have the advantage of providing renal hypothermia and renal artery block in RASE for larger tumors or completely intrarenal tumors. The patients should be detailly evaluated, and the catheter should be placed as distally as possible in the renal artery, because of the easy shifting or insufficient occlusion of the balloon. Moreover, any major movement of the body should also be avoided.

Tumor enucleation has been demonstrated in several previous studies. It basically means of enucleate the tumor by blunt dissection along the pseudocapsule as anatomical landmark, without visible normal parenchyma [31]. Therefore the SE technique could maximumly preserve normal renal parenchyma theoretically [5, 32], and it could avoid influencing the renal function by reducing the ischemia time. Moreover, the single-layer renorrhaphy could avoided compressing the deep vessels and reduced the suture time, thereby reducing the ischemic necrosis of the sutured parenchyma.

We observed a median of − 6.3 and − 12.0 percentage change at 3 months, and a median of − 5.8 and − 11.7 percentage change at 12 months in the RACP-RASE and RASE groups, respectively. The changes in eGFR significantly differed between the two groups. More cases in the RASE group were CKD upstaged compared with RACP-RASE group. No postoperative acute renal failure or renal replacement therapy occurred. Multivariable analysis revealed that preoperative eGFR and the procedure type were significant predictive factors for a more than 10% change in eGFR at 3 months postoperatively. A major restriction of RASE technique is time because kidney injury is expected if the ischemia time exceeds 30 min. Lowering the renal temperature can decrease the renal metabolism and limit the hypoxia-induced injury pathways. Therefore, RACP-RASE may be applied to decrease the degree of kidney damage and prolong the ischemia time.

There are several limitations to this study. First, this is a retrospective and small sample study. Second, this study lacks of randomization. Third, this study lacks a standardized manner of the procedure choice which was mainly based on the tumor complexity, and this leads to selection bias.

Conclusions

Our initial experience with RACP-RASE technique revealed that renal arterial cold perfusion can provide appropriate temporary arterial occlusion and renal hypothermic perfusion during RASE. Renal arterial cold perfusion may be helpful in protecting renal function in RASE as compared with warm ischemia. RACP-RASE is an effective and safe technique with complex tumors such as completely intrarenal and hilar tumors. Long-term study with large patient sample is needed.

Abbreviations

PN: Partial nephrectomy; SPN: Standard partial nephrectomy; SE: Simple enucleation; RASE: Robot-assisted simple enucleation; RACP-RASE: Robot-assisted simple enucleation with renal arterial cold perfusion; ECOG: Eastern Cooperative Oncology Group; BMI: Body mass index.

Acknowledgements

None.

Authors' contributions

HG and QL participated in the design of this study. QL and XZ contributed to data collection, data analysis and manuscript writing. CJ, SG and XQ took part in data collection and management. GL, SZ and XL involved in manuscript editing. GZ and XZ contributed to project development and manuscript writing. All authors read and approved the final manuscript.

Author details

[1] Department of Urology, Drum Tower Hospital, Medical School of Nanjing University, Institute of Urology, Nanjing University, 321 Zhongshan Rd., Nanjing 210008, Jiangsu, People's Republic of China. [2] School of Public Health, Nanjing Medical University, Nanjing 210029, Jiangsu, People's Republic of China. [3] Department of Radiology, Drum Tower Hospital, Medical School of Nanjing University, Nanjing 210008, Jiangsu, People's Republic of China.

References

1. Ljungberg B, Bensalah K, Canfield S, et al. EAU guidelines on renal cell carcinoma: 2014 update. Eur Urol. 2015;67(5):913–24.
2. Kaouk JH, Khalifeh A, Hillyer S, et al. Robot-assisted laparoscopic partial nephrectomy: step-by-step contemporary technique and surgical outcomes at a single high-volume institution. Eur Urol. 2012;62(3):553–61.

3. Blair BM, Lehman EB, Jafri SM, et al. Predicted versus observed 30-day perioperative outcomes using the ACS NSQIP surgical risk calculator in patients undergoing partial nephrectomy for renal cell carcinoma. Int Urol Nephrol. 2018;50(7):1249–56.
4. Blackwell RH, Li B, Kozel Z, et al. Functional implications of renal tumor enucleation relative to standard partial nephrectomy. Urology. 2017;99:162–8.
5. Minervini A, Serni S, Tuccio A, et al. Simple enucleation versus radical nephrectomy in the treatment of pT1a and pT1b renal cell carcinoma. Ann Surg Oncol. 2012;19(2):694–700.
6. Azhar RA, de Castro Abreu AL, Broxham E, et al. Histological analysis of the kidney tumor-parenchyma interface. J Urol. 2015;193(2):415–22.
7. Lu Q, Zhao X, Ji C, et al. Modified laparoscopic simple enucleation with single-layer suture technique versus standard laparoscopic partial nephrectomy for treating localized renal cell carcinoma. Int Urol Nephrol. 2017;49(2):239–45.
8. Shekarriz B, Shah G, Upadhyay J. Impact of temporary hilar clamping during laparoscopic partial nephrectomy on postoperative renal function: a prospective study. J Urol. 2004;172(1):54–7.
9. Larcher A, Meskawi M, Valdivieso R, et al. Comparison of renal function detriments after local tumor ablation or partial nephrectomy for renal cell carcinoma. World J Urol. 2016;34(3):383–9.
10. Mir MC, Ercole C, Takagi T, et al. Decline in renal function after partial nephrectomy: etiology and prevention. J Urol. 2015;193(6):1889–98.
11. Steffens J, Humke U, Ziegler M, et al. Partial nephrectomy with perfusion cooling for imperative indications: a 24-year experience. BJU Int. 2005;96(4):608–11.
12. Maathuis MH, Leuvenink HG, Ploeg RJ. Perspectives in organ preservation. Transplantation. 2007;83(10):1289–98.
13. Mottrie A, De Naeyer G, Schatteman P, et al. Impact of the learning curve on perioperative outcomes in patients who underwent robotic partial nephrectomy for parenchymal renal tumours. Eur Urol. 2010;58(1):127–32.
14. Oken MM, Creech RH, Tormey DC, et al. Toxicity and response criteria of the Eastern Cooperative Oncology Group. Am J Clin Oncol. 1982;5(6):649–55.
15. Patard JJ, Leray E, Cindolo L, et al. Multi-institutional validation of a symptom based classification for renal cell carcinoma. J Urol. 2004;172(3):858–62.
16. Ficarra V, Novara G, Secco S, et al. Preoperative aspects and dimensions used for an anatomical (PADUA) classification of renal tumours in patients who are candidates for nephron-sparing surgery. Eur Urol. 2009;56(5):786–93.
17. Kutikov A, Uzzo RG. The R.E.N.A.L. nephrometry score: a comprehensive standardized system for quantitating renal tumor size, location and depth. J Urol. 2009;182(3):844–53.
18. Dindo D, Demartines N, Clavien PA. Classification of surgical complications: a new proposal with evaluation in a cohort of 6336 patients and results of a survey. Ann Surg. 2004;240(2):205–13.
19. Levey AS, Bosch JP, Lewis JB, et al. A more accurate method to estimate glomerular filtration rate from serum creatinine: a new prediction equation. Ann Intern Med. 1999;130(6):461–70.
20. Zhao X, Lu Q, Campi R, et al. Endoscopic Robot-Assisted Simple Enucleation versus laparoscopic simple enucleation with single-layer renorrhaphy in localized renal tumors: a propensity score-matched analysis from a high-volume centre. Urology. 2018;121:97–103.
21. Edge SB, Compton CC. The American Joint Committee on Cancer: the 7th edition of the AJCC cancer staging manual and the future of TNM. Ann Surg Oncol. 2010;17(6):1471–4.
22. Moch H. The WHO/ISUP grading system for renal carcinoma. Pathologe. 2016;37(4):355–60.
23. Huang WC, Levey AS, Serio AM, et al. Chronic kidney disease after nephrectomy in patients with renal cortical tumours: a retrospective cohort study. Lancet Oncol. 2006;7(9):735–40.
24. Mari A, Tellini R, Di Maida F, et al. Predictors of early postoperative and mid-term functional outcomes in patients treated with Endoscopic Robot-Assisted Simple Enucleation (ERASE): results from a tertiary referral center. Minerva Urol Nefrol. 2020;72(4):490–7.
25. Gill IS, Abreu SC, Desai MM, et al. Laparoscopic ice slush renal hypothermia for partial nephrectomy: the initial experience. J Urol. 2003;170(1):52–6.
26. Weld KJ, Venkatesh R, Huang J, et al. (2006) Evolution of surgical technique and patient outcomes for laparoscopic partial nephrectomy. Urology. 2006;67(3):502–6 **(discussion 506–7)**.
27. Marberger M, Georgi M, Guenther R, et al. Simultaneous balloon occlusion of the renal artery and hypothermic perfusion in in situ surgery of the kidney. J Urol. 1978;119(4):463–7.
28. Liu F, Yuan H, Li X, et al. Application of hypothermic perfusion via a renal artery balloon catheter during robot-assisted partial nephrectomy and effect on renal function. Acad Radiol. 2019;26(8):e196–201.
29. Janetschek G, Abdelmaksoud A, Bagheri F, et al. Laparoscopic partial nephrectomy in cold ischemia: renal artery perfusion. J Urol. 2004;171(1):68–71.
30. Beri A, Lattouf JB, Deambros O, et al. Partial nephrectomy using renal artery perfusion for cold ischemia: functional and oncologic outcomes. J Endourol. 2008;22(6):1285–90.
31. Mari A, Di Maida F, Tellini R, et al. Oncologic outcomes in patients treated with Endoscopic Robot Assisted Simple Enucleation (ERASE) for renal cell carcinoma: results from a tertiary referral center. Eur J Surg Oncol. 2019;45(10):1977–82.
32. Puppo P, Introini C, Calvi P, et al. Long term results of excision of small renal cancer surrounded by a minimal layer of grossly normal parenchyma: review of 94 cases. Eur Urol. 2004;46(4):477–81.

8

Preoperative anaemi and thrombocytosis predict adverse prognosis in non-metastatic renal cell carcinoma with tumour thrombus

Ruotao Xiao[1,2], Chuxiao Xu[1,2], Wei He[1,2], Lei Liu[1], Hongxian Zhang[1], Cheng Liu[2] and Lulin Ma[2*]

Abstract

Background : This study aimed to determine the prognostic value of preoperative blood parameters in renal cell carcinoma (RCC) and tumour thrombus (TT) patients that were surgically treated.

Method: We retrospectively analysed clinicopathological data and blood parameters of 146 RCC and TT patients that were surgically treated. Univariate or multivariate Cox regression analyses were performed to determine the risk factors associated with progression-free survival (PFS) and overall survival (OS). Kaplan-Meier analysis and logistic regression were performed to study the risk factors. Receiver operating characteristic curves were applied to test improvements in the predictive accuracy of the established prognosis score.

Results: On univariate and multivariate analysis, anaemia (HR 2.873, P = 0.008) and lymph node metastasis (HR 4.811, P = 0.015) were independent prognostic factors linked to OS. Besides, thrombocytosis (HR 2.324, P = 0.011), histologic subtype (HR 2.835, P = 0.004), nuclear grade (HR 2.069, P = 0.033), and lymph node metastasis (HR 5.739, P = 0.001) were independent prognostic factors associated with PFS. Kaplan–Meier curves revealed that patients with anaemia exhibited worse OS than those without it (P = 0.0033). Likewise, patients with thrombocytosis showed worse PFS than those without it (P < 0.0001). Adding the anaemia and thrombocytosis to the SSIGN score improved its predictive accuracy related to OS and PFS. Preoperative anaemia was linked to more symptom at presentation (OR 3.348, P = 0.006), longer surgical time (OR 1.005, P = 0.001), more blood loss (OR 1.000, P = 0.018), more transfusion (OR 2.734, P = 0.004), higher thrombus level (OR 4.750, P = 0.004) and higher nuclear grade (OR 3.449, P = 0.001) while thrombocytosis was associated with more symptom at presentation (OR 7.784, P = 0.007).

Conclusions: Preoperative anaemia and thrombocytosis were adverse prognostic factors in non-metastatic RCC patients with TT. Also, both preoperative anaemia and thrombocytosis can be clinically used for risk stratification of non-metastatic RCC and TT patients.

Keywords: Anaemia, Thrombocytosis, Renal cell carcinoma, Tumour thrombus, Prognosis

Background

Renal cell carcinoma (RCC) accounts for 3% of all malignant tumours worldwide [1]. With the advancement of surgical procedures and adjuvant therapy, the long-term prognostic outcome of RCC has become favourable with a 5-year survival rate of 80–90% in most histological subtypes[2]. Based on pathological data, RCC subtype, tumour grade, sarcomatoid and rhabdoid features, and TNM stage are commonly used prognostic factors of RCC [3]. Combining these factors, several prognostic models have established to predict survival among the RCC patients and validated their usefulness externally[3].

*Correspondence: malulin@bjmu.edu.cn

[2] Department of Urology, Peking University Third Hospital, No.49 North Garden Road, Haidian District, 100191 Beijing, People's Republic of China

Full list of author information is available at the end of the article

Notably, preoperative blood parameters can be used to reflect the inflammatory status and health conditions of patients in an economic and convenient manner. The inflammation status has been well associated with genesis, progression, and metastasis of tumours [4]. Preoperative inflammation indicators such as neutrophils, lymphocytes, platelets, neutrophil-lymphocyte ratio (NLR), and the platelet lymphocyte ratio (PLR) have been reported for prognostic value in urologic malignancies such as prostate and bladder cancers [5, 6]. Previously, in RCC too, elevated neutrophils, platelets, NLR, PLR, and decreased lymphocytes were linked to poor survival rates [7–9]. Moreover, other preoperative blood parameters such as haemoglobin, AST/ALT, albumin have been suggested to hold prognostic values predicting survival in RCC [10]. Recently, a novel prognostic system incorporating preoperative blood parameters has also been designed to improve prognostic accuracy to predict metastatic RCC [11].

Intriguingly, 4–10% of RCC patients exhibit thrombus either in the renal vein or inferior vena cava [12]. Due to the complexity of the inflammatory status and rarity of data, the prognostic significance of preoperative blood parameters has not been extensively studied yet. Therefore, this study was aimed to determine the prognostic value of preoperative blood parameters in RCC and TT patients that were surgically treated.

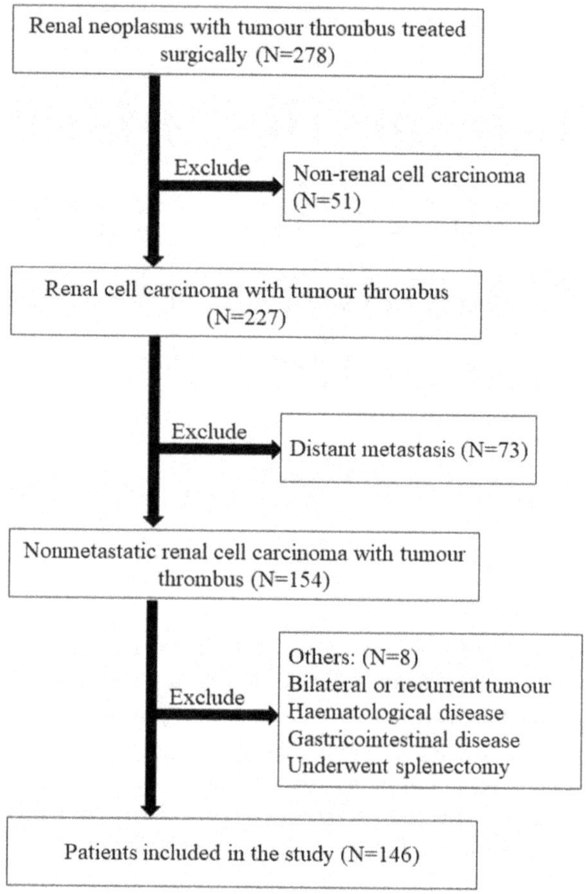

Fig. 1 Flow chart showing the inclusion/exclusion criteria of the patients

Methods

Patient population

After approval from the Peking University Third Hospital Medical Science Research Ethics Committee, we retrospectively analysed the clinicopathological data of 278 patients. These were diagnosed with renal neoplasms and tumour thrombus receiving nephrectomy and thrombectomy at our institute between Jan 2014 and Dec 2019. The excluding criteria were as follows: (1) non-renal cell carcinoma, (2) preoperative suspicious distant metastasis, (3) bilateral or recurrent tumour, (4) combined with hematological disease or gastrointestinal disease, (5) a past-history of splenectomy. The flow chart describing the inclusion criteria of patients is shown in Fig. 1. Finally, data belonging to 146 patients were used for further research. The corresponding clinicopathological data and blood parameters were obtained using the patients' medical and pathological records.

Clinical and pathologic evaluation

The clinicopathological variables included age, sex, body mass index (BMI), symptoms at presentation, American Society of Anesthesiologists (ASA) score, surgical data (approach, time, blood loss, segmental resection of vena cava, and transfusion), tumour thrombus level (TT), tumour size and side, and tumour pathology (histologic subtype, nuclear grade, lymph node status, necrosis, and invasion of venous wall). Tumour thrombus levels were defined according to the Mayo classification using the preoperative images [13]. Nuclear grade was defined according to Fuhrman grade before 2016 and WHO/IUSP classification after 2016 [14]. SSIGN score was used to stratify the study cohort in low-risk (score 2–4), intermediate-risk (score 5–7), and high-risk (score 8–11) groups [15]. Patients' routine laboratory examinations were analysed for a period of one week before the surgery. The corresponding blood parameters including neutrophil count (NEU), platelet count (PLT), lymphocyte count (LYM), haemoglobin level (HGB), albumin level (ABL), serum creatine (SCR), plasma AST and ALT, serum calcium (SCa) and alkaline phosphatase (ALP) levels were obtained. NLR and PLR were calculated using the neutrophil and platelet counts. $PLT \geq 300 \times 10^9/L$ was defined as thrombocytosis. $HGB \leq 120$ g/L for males and $HGB \leq 115$ g/L for females were defined as anaemia.

Follow up

After surgery, all patients were followed up and prognostic data were obtained through a clinic visit or by telephone until July 2020. Patients were recommended to a follow up for every 3 months in the first year, every 6 months in the next 2 years, and yearly thereafter. At each visit, laboratory examinations, X-ray, ultrasonic scan, or abdominal CT were performed. Patients who had recurrence or metastasis during follow-up were recommended to receive tyrosine kinase inhibitors (TKIs) as adjuvant therapy. Overall survival (OS) was calculated from the date of surgery to death and progression-free survival (PFS) was calculated from the date of surgery to tumour recurrence or metastasis.

Statistical analysis

The prognostic value (OS and PFS) of preoperative blood parameters and clinicopathologic data were assessed using the univariate and multivariate Cox proportional hazards regression model. Potential predictors with a significance of $P<0.10$ in the univariable Cox regression analysis or with clinic value were included in the subsequent multivariable regression analysis (with forward stepwise likelihood ratio method). The OS and PFS were estimated using the Kaplan–Meier curves and survival differences were compared using the log-rank test. Association among risk factors and clinicopathological characteristics was analysed using the logistic regression model. Time-dependent receiver operating characteristic (ROC) curves were performed to analyse the improvement of the modified model compared to the conventional model [16]. All statistical analyses were performed with SPSS Statistics 22.0 (IBM Corp, Armonk, NY, USA) and R software (Version 4.0.3). All comparisons were subjected to Two-tailed tests, and $P<0.05$ was considered statistically significant.

Results

The baseline clinical and pathological variables of 146 RCC and TT patients that were treated surgically are shown in Table 1. Among these, the majority (n = 113, 77.4%) of patients were male. The patients' median age was 60 year (IQR 54–66.25). Of these, the majority of patients had TT levels classified to Mayo 0–II (n = 118, 80.8%) than Mayo III–IV (n = 28, 19.2%). According to SSIGN score, patients in the low-risk (score2–4), intermediate-risk (score 5–7), and high-risk (score 8–11) groups were 49 (33.5%), 76 (52.1%), and 21 (13.4%) respectively. At the last follow-up, 139 (95.2%) patients were followed up for a median of 19 months (IQR 8–32). Twenty-eight (19.2%) patients died with the mean OS of 46.82 months (median OS was not reached). The 1-year and 3-year cumulative OS rates were 90.3% and 73.4% respectively. Fifty-two (35.6%) patients had disease progression with the median PFS of 37 months (IQR 22–60). The 1-year and 3-year cumulative PFS rates were 87.2% and 50.7% respectively.

Table 1 Univariate Cox regression analysis of prognostic factors correlated with overall survival and progression-free survival

Characteristics	All cohort (n = 146)
Age, y, median. (IQR)	60 (54–66.25)
Sex, no. (%)	
Male	113 (77.4)
Female	33 (22.6)
BMI, kg/m^2, median. (IQR)	23.87 (21.44–26.65)
Symptom at presentation, no. (%)	
Absent	38 (26)
Present	108 (74)
ASA score, no. (%)	
I–II	129 (88.3)
III	17 (11.7)
Surgical approach, no. (%)	
Open	59 (40.4)
Laparoscopic	87 (59.6)
Surgical time, min, median. (IQR)	305.5 (224.25–400)
Blood loss, ml, median. (IQR)	600 (200–1650)
Transfusion, no. (%)	61 (41.8)
Segmental resection of vena cava, no. (%)	27 (18.5)
Tumour side, no. (%)	
Left	52 (35.6)
Right	94 (64.4)
Tumour size, cm, median. (IQR)	8.25 (6.48–10)
Tumour thrombus level, no. (%)	
0–II	118 (80.8)
III–IV	28 (19.2)
Invasion of venous wall, no. (%)	53 (41.4)
Histology subtype, no. (%)	
Clear cell	124 (84.9)
Non-CCRCC	22 (15.1)
Nuclear grade, no. (%)	
I–II	61 (41.7)
III–IV	85 (58.3)
lymph node metastasis, no. (%)	9 (5.9)
Necrosis, no. (%)	66 (45.8)
SSIGN score	
Low-risk (score 2–4)	49 (33.5)
Intermediate-risk (score 5–7)	76 (52.1)
High-risk (score 8–11)	21 (13.4)

IQR interquartile range, *BMI* body mass index, *ASA* American Society of Anesthesiologists, *CCRCC* clear cell renal cell carcinoma

Table 2 Preoperative blood parameters of patients with renal cell carcinoma and tumour thrombus treated surgically

Blood parameters (unit)	Median (IQR)
NEU (× 10^9/L)	4.31 (3.53–5.04)
LYM(× 10^9/L)	1.29 (1–1.62)
PLT (× 10^9/L)	235 (185.25–299)
HGB (g/L)	123 (111–139)
ALB (g/L)	40 (35.55–43.05)
SCR (umol/L)	89.5 (80–108.5)
ALT (u/L)	16 (11.75–26.25)
AST(u/L)	18 (15–24)
SCa (mmol/L)	2.28 (2.18–2.38)
ALP (u/L)	80 (65–101)
NLR	3.43 (2.39–4.49)
PLR	184.81 (118.89–273.57)
AST/ALT	1.13 (0.83–1.45)

NEU neutrophil count, *LYM* lymphocyte count, *PLT* platelet count, *HGB* hemoglobin, *ALB* albumin, *SCR* serum creatinine, *SCa* serum calcium, *ALP* alkaline phosphatase

The baseline preoperative blood parameters of the study cohort are shown in Table 2. Univariate analysis revealed that anaemia, SSIGN score, and lymph node metastasis were substantial predictors of OS. Besides, thrombocytosis, anaemia, histologic subtype, nuclear grade, lymph node metastasis, SSIGN score were significant predictors of PFS (Table 3). Stepwise multivariable analysis revealed that anemia (HR 2.873, P=0.008) and lymph node metastasis (HR 4.811, P=0.015) were independent prognostic factors associated with OS. Besides, thrombocytosis (HR 2.324, P=0.011), histologic subtype (HR 2.835, P=0.004), nuclear grade (HR 2.069, P=0.033), lymph node metastasis (HR 5.739, P=0.001) were independent predictors of PFS. Furthermore, anaemia and thrombocytosis were significant prognostic factors independent of the SSIGN scores to predict OS and PFS respectively (Table 4). Using the Kaplan–Meier survival analysis we found that patients with preoperative anaemia exhibited a significantly increased mortality risk than those without it. Besides, preoperative thrombocytosis was also significantly associated with an increased risk of earlier recurrence or metastasis than those without it (Fig. 2).

To investigate the improvement in predictive ability by adding anaemia and thrombocytosis to SSIGN score, we performed time-dependent ROC curves and compared the AUCs of the modified SSIGN model to the conventional SSIGN model. Figure 3 illustrates the modified SSIGN score exhibited better predictive accuracy than the conventional SSIGN in predicting 2-year (AUCs: 702 vs. 0.657), 3-year (AUCs: 721 vs. 0.627), and 4-year (AUCs: 0.750 vs. 0.716) OS. Likewise, the modified SSIGN score exhibited better predictive accuracy than the conventional SSIGN in predicting 2-year (AUCs: 0.711 vs. 0.640), 3-year (AUCs: 0.691 vs. 0.594), and 4-year (AUCs: 0.723 vs. 0.688) PFS.

Furthermore, the association between preoperative anaemia and thrombocytosis with clinicopathological characteristics is shown in Table 5. Preoperative anaemia was related to more symptom at presentation (OR 3.348, P=0.006), longer surgical time (OR 1.005, P=0.001), more blood loss (OR 1.000, P=0.018), more transfusion (OR:2.734, P=0.004), higher thrombus level (OR 4.750, P=0.001) and higher nuclear grade (OR 3.449, P=0.001). Moreover, patients with thrombocytosis were associated with more symptoms at presentation (OR 7.784, P=0.007).

Discussion

In this study, from a high-volume centre, we examined the data related to 146 RCC and TT patients who underwent surgical treatment. We found that patients with preoperative anaemia had significantly adverse OS than those without it. Likewise, thrombocytosis was linked to poor PFS. In multivariable analysis, we found that preoperative anaemia and thrombocytosis were the independent worse prognostic factors even after adjusting for the other known pathologic prognostic factors and SSIGN scores. Furthermore, adding anaemia and thrombocytosis to the SSIGN score improved its predictive accuracy related to OS and PFS. To the best of our knowledge, this is the first study analysing preoperative blood parameters that specifically focused on the RCC population with TT.

Previously, anaemia has been suggested as a prognostic factor in RCC. Kim et al. retrospectively analysed data of 4260 patients that had non-metastatic RCC and found anaemia was highly associated with worse recurrence-free survival (RFS), cancer-specific survival (CSS), and overall survival (OS) [17]. *Jiwei Huang et al.* analysed the data of 352 papillary RCC patients and found that patients with preoperative anaemia had significantly worse RFS, CSS, and OS than those without it ($P < 0.001$). Multivariable analysis revealed that anaemia was an independent prognostic factor in terms of RFS, CSS, and OS ($P < 0.001$) [18]. Xia et al. conducted a meta-analysis and found preoperative anaemia was associated with increased all-cause mortality, cancer-specific mortality, and disease recurrence [19]. Our study found that preoperative anaemia was a predictor of worse OS and PFS. However, after controlling for pathologic features, preoperative anaemia was only independently associated with OS but not with PFS. To our knowledge, preoperative anaemia represented worse nutrition status of patients either due to long term poor consumption or blood loss,

Table 3 Univariate Cox regression analysis of prognostic factors correlated with overall survival and progression-free survival

Variable	Overall survival			Progression-free survival		
	HR	95%CL	P-value	HR	95%CL	P-value
Age*	0.980	0.943–1.018	0.289	0.976	0.950–1.003	0.086
Sex (male vs. female)						
Male	Ref			Ref		
Female	0.874	0.330–2.315	0.787	0.801	0.390–1.645	0.545
ASA score						
I+II	Ref			Ref		
III	1.511	0.518–4.412	0.450	1.110	0.471–2.613	0.812
Symptom at presentation	1.858	0.745–4.629	0.184	1.878	0.978–3.603	0.058
Histologic subtype						
CCRCC	Ref			Ref		
Non-CCRCC	2.279	0.909–5.716	0.079	3.007	1.620–5.845	0.001
Tumour thrombus level						
0–II	Ref			Ref		
III–IV	1.259	0.525–3.022	0.606	1.149	0.609–2.167	0.669
Tumour size*	1.032	0.910–1.170	0.626	1.015	0.926–1.113	0.749
Invasion of venous wall	1.455	0.681–3.112	0.333	1.450	0.824–2.551	0.198
Nuclear grade						
I–II	Ref			Ref		
III–IV	2.283	0.955–5.456	0.063	2.368	1.255–4.468	0.008
Lymph node metastasis	5.622	1.872–16.888	0.002	3.871	1.504–9.962	0.005
Necrosis	1.889	0.850–4.198	0.119	1.709	0.946–3.028	0.066
SSIGN score						
Low-risk (score 2–4)	Ref			Ref		
Intermediate-risk (score 5–7)	2.158	0.771–6.039	0.143	2.311	1.125–4.749	0.023
High-risk (score 8–11)	5.653	1.808–17.677	0.003	3.799	1.598–9.033	0.003
Blood parameters						
NLR*	1.090	0.959–1.239	0.189	1.019	0.905–1.148	0.750
PLR*	1.001	0.998–1.004	0.377	1.002	1.000–1.004	0.084
AST/ALT*	1.117	0.553–2.256	0.758	1.212	0.983–1.765	0.238
Thrombocytosis	2.288	0.946–5.532	0.066	3.307	1.819–6.009	<0.001
Anaemia	2.991	1.384–6.467	0.005	2.065	1.196–3.566	0.009
ALB*	0.959	0.902–1.021	0.191	0.979	0.935–1.026	0.384
SCR*	1.003	0.987–1.019	0.714	0.994	0.981–1.007	0.376
SCa*	0.666	0.064–6.885	0.733	3.740	0.769–18.205	0.102
ALP*	1.006	0.998–1.013	0.150	1.001	0.995–1.008	0.638

*As continuous variable

thus it could independently affect OS. In our study, anaemia exhibited a higher level of TT, higher nuclear grade, and more symptoms at presentation. We speculate that it is advanced tumour biology rather than anaemia that had a more significant impact on PFS, although this hypothesis needs to be verified externally.

Interestingly, thrombocytosis had been established as a worse prognostic predictor in various cancers, including nasopharyngeal carcinoma [20], gynecologic malignancies [21], melanoma [22], and colorectal cancer [23]. In RCC too, thrombocytosis could be regarded as a potential prognostic indicator. Several studies have shown that patients with preoperative thrombocytosis had worse survival than those without it [24–26]. Although none of the studies linked thrombocytosis to worse prognosis in RCC population with TT, a study found that bland thrombus in RCC with TT is linked to adverse survival [27]. Data from our study suggest that

Table 4 Multivariate Cox regression analysis of blood parameter with clinicopathologic characteristics and SSIGN prognostic model

Variable	Overall survival			Progression-free survival		
	HR	95%CL	P	HR	95%CL	P
Model 1						
Age[1,2]	/	/	NS	/	/	NS
Symptom at presentation[1,2]	/	/	NS	/	/	NS
Histologic subtype[1,2]						
CCRCC	Ref			Ref		
Non-CCRCC	/	/	NS	2.835	1.403–5.728	0.004
Nuclear grade[1,2]						
I–II	Ref			Ref		
III–IV	/	/	NS	2.069	1.059–4.039	0.033
Lymph node metastasis[1,2]	4.811	1.365–16.961	0.015	5.739	2.136–15.420	0.001
Necrosis[2]	/	/	/	/	/	NS
Blood parameters						
PLR[2]	/	/	/	/	/	NS
Thrombocytosis[1,2]	/	/	NS	2.324	1.215–4.446	0.011
Anaemia[1,2]	2.873	1.310–6.299	0.008	/	/	NS
Model 2						
SSIGN score						
Low-risk (score 2–4)	Ref			Ref		
Intermediate-risk (score 5–7)	1.447	0.499–4.193	0.496	1.833	0.871–3.858	0.111
High-risk (score 8–11)	5.847	1.838–18.603	0.003	3.025	1.230–7.436	0.016
Blood parameters						
PLR[2]	/	/	/	/	/	NS
Thrombocytosis[1,2]	/	/	NS	2.375	1.245–4.469	0.008
Anaemia[1,2]	3.453	1.495–7.978	0.004	/	/	NS

NS not statistically significant

[1] The variable that was selected into the multivariate model correlated with overall survival

[2] The variable that was selected into the multivariate model correlated with progression-free survival

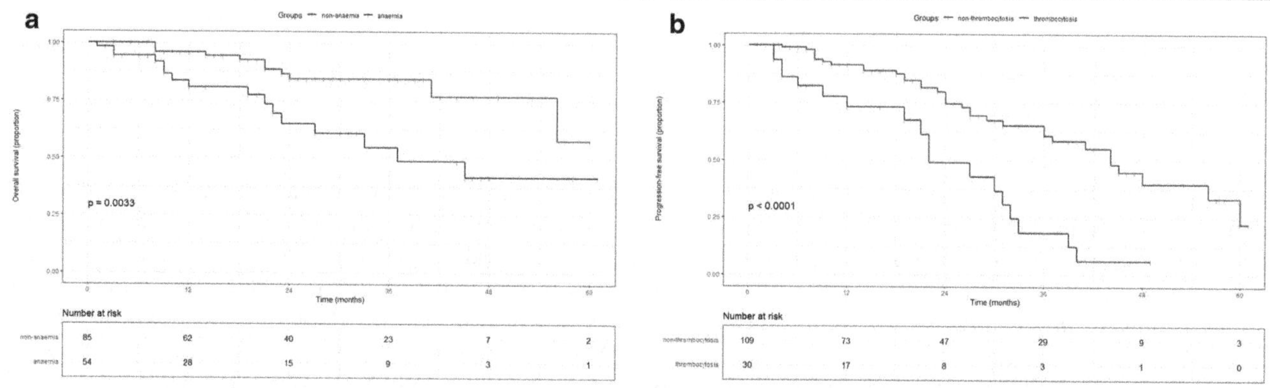

Fig. 2 Kaplan-Meier curves showing the cumulative survival of patients with renal cell carcinoma and tumour thrombus categorized by anaemia and thrombocytosis. **a** The overall survival curve for anaemic and non-anaemic patients; **b** the progression-free survival curve for thrombocytosis and non-thrombocytosis patients

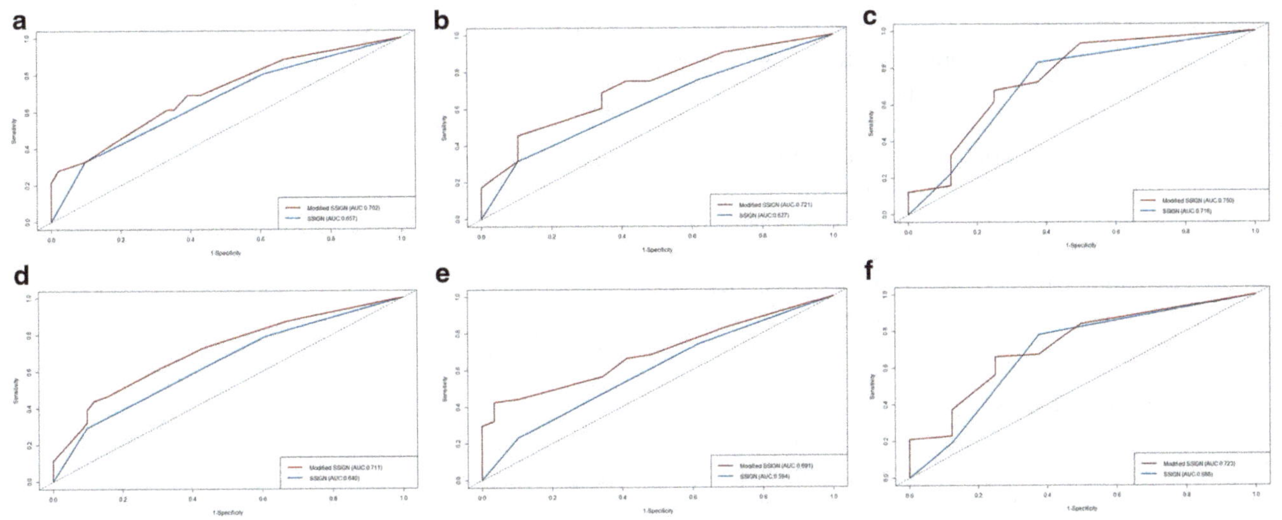

Fig. 3 Time-dependent ROC curves for modified SSIGN score and SSIGN score relate to overall survival (OS) and progression-free survival (PFS). **a** 2-year OS; **b** 3-year OS; **c** 4-year OS; **d** 2-year PFS; **e** 3-year PFS; **f** 4-year PFS

Table 5 Odds ratios and 95% confidence interval for the association of anaemia and thrombocytosis with clinicopathological characteristics

Variable	Anaemia			Thrombocytosis		
	OR	95%CL	P-value	OR	95%CL	P-value
Age, yr	0.998	0.966–1.031	0.893	1.008	0.970–1.047	0.679
ASA score (III vs. I–II)	1.791	0.648–4.952	0.262	0.396	0.086–1.826	0.235
Symptom at presentation	3.348	1.405–7.977	0.006	7.784	1.767–34.298	0.007
Surgical time, min	1.005	1.002–1.008	0.001	1.000	0.997–1.003	0.880
Blood loss, ml	1.000	1.000–1.001	0.018	1.000	0.999–1.000	0.137
Transfusion	2.734	1.374–5.441	0.004	1.284	0.593–2.782	0.526
Segmental resection of vena cava	0.465	0.199–1.084	0.076	0.857	0.327–2.244	0.754
Tumour thrombosis level (III–IV vs. 0–II)	4.750	1.910–11.814	0.001	1.474	0.579–3.750	0.416
Tumour size, cm	0.988	0.883–1.107	0.840	1.135	0.996–1.294	0.057
Invasion of venous wall	1.381	0.670–2.846	0.382	0.973	0.409–2.311	0.950
Histologic subtype (non-CCRCC vs. CCRCC)	2.449	0.971–6.175	0.058	1.677	0.621–4.527	0.308
Nuclear grade (III–IV vs. I–II)	3.449	1.653–7.196	0.001	2.315	0.990–5.412	0.053
lymph node metastasis	0.884	0.203–3.850	0.869	0.446	0.053–3.758	0.458
Necrosis	1.488	0.762–2.908	0.245	1.245	0.576–2.689	0.577

patients with thrombocytosis had an increased risk of recurrence or metastasis than those without it. Also, we found that thrombocytosis is an independent prognostic factor of PFS. Notably, the previous notion that platelets were mainly involved in limiting blood loss and promoting wound healing has been changed with recent preclinical and clinical findings. Studies now show that platelets can also promote tumorigenesis and metastasis through a crosstalk with cancer cells[28]. This rationalize preoperative thrombocytosis link to post-surgery higher risk of recurrence or metastasis. Therefore, we suggest that in cases of preoperative thrombocytosis, a follow-up plan should be closely monitored in populations with RCC and TT.

Nowadays many established prognostic models have been established to predict prognosis in patients with RCC [3]. Several clinicopathological features such as symptom at presentation, TNM stage, Fuhrman grade, and necrosis were regarded as prognostic factors in the current model [15]. To our knowledge, anaemia and thrombocytosis have already been added to the IMDC model to predict prognosis in patients with metastatic RCC [29]. Concerning nonmetastatic RCC, none of the models have included blood parameters. Since our study found that preoperative anaemia and thrombocytosis could serve as potential biomarkers predicting prognosis in patients with RCC and TT, we added these two factors to the SSIGN score and improved its predictive accuracy related to 2-year, 3-year, and 4-year OS and PFS. Thus, we propose that both anaemia and thrombocytosis should not be ignored as prognostic factors of worse survival in these patients.

Several factors such as NLR, PLR, AST/ALT, and ALB have shown their prognostic value in local and metastatic RCC [8–10, 30]. However, these blood parameters were not associated with prognosis in our study cohort. Previous studies demonstrated that these parameters reflected personal inflammatory conditions. To our knowledge, in patients with RCC and TT, the tumour thrombus was directly in contact with circulating blood. Thus, we speculated that the inflammatory condition was more complex in these unique populations and could not thoroughly be revealed by these inflammatory indices. Notably, Peyton et al. [9] also found that in patients with metastatic RCC and TT, NLR>4 was associated with worse survival. We think that an insufficient number of patients included in our study could be another reason to not find any statistical differences in these factors.

Nevertheless, this retrospective study had several limitations. Firstly, as mentioned above, the insufficient number of patients, short follow-up time, and insufficient outcome events could have limited the study of several blood parameters. Therefore, future studies are needed to externally validate the proposed risk factors in a large prospective cohort. Secondly, we did not have access to data related to concomitant drugs, which could have influenced blood counts (e.g., steroids). Thirdly, our research is a single-institutional retrospective review, which inherently had missing data and confounding bias that were beyond our control. Despite these limitations, these findings are significant as this is the only study to date that specifically focused on the impact of preoperative blood parameters in RCC patients with TT.

Conclusions

Both preoperative anaemia and thrombocytosis are the important independent prognostic factors in RCC patients with TT. We found that anaemia is associated with an increased risk of mortality while thrombocytosis is linked to a higher risk of earlier recurrence or metastasis. Furthermore, both preoperative anaemia and thrombocytosis could be clinically useful for risk stratifying patients undergoing surgery for non-metastatic RCC with TT.

Abbreviations

RCC: Renal cell carcinoma; TT: Tumour thrombus; SCR: Serum creatinine; ALB: Albumin; HGB: Haemoglobin; NLR: Neutrophil-lymphocyte ratio; PLR: Platelet lymphocyte ratio; NEU: Neutrophil count; PLT: Platelet count; LYM: Lymphocyte count; SCa: Serum calcium; ALP: Alkaline phosphatase; BMI: Body mass index; ASA: American Society of Anesthesiologists score; OS: Overall survival; PFS: Progression-free survival.

Acknowledgements

Not applicable.

Authors' contributions

RX collected and analysed the data and wrote the manuscript. CX, WH, LL, HZ made substantial contributions planning this work. LM and CL substantially revised the work and manuscript. All authors have read and approved the manuscript.

Author details

[1] Peking University Health Science Centre, 100191 Beijing, People's Republic of China. [2] Department of Urology, Peking University Third Hospital, No.49 North Garden Road, Haidian District, 100191 Beijing, People's Republic of China.

References

1. Ferlay J, Colombet M, Soerjomataram I, Dyba T, Randi G, Bettio M, Gavin A, Visser O, Bray F. Cancer incidence and mortality patterns in Europe: estimates for 40 countries and 25 major cancers in 2018. Eur J Cancer. 2018;103:356–87.
2. Keegan KA, Schupp CW, Chamie K, Hellenthal NJ, Evans CP, Koppie TM. Histopathology of surgically treated renal cell carcinoma: survival differences by subtype and stage. J Urol. 2012;188(2):391–7.
3. Sun M, Shariat SF, Cheng C, Ficarra V, Murai M, Oudard S, Pantuck AJ, Zigeuner R, Karakiewicz PI. Prognostic factors and predictive models in renal cell carcinoma: a contemporary review. Eur Urol. 2011;60(4):644–61.
4. Greten FR, Grivennikov SI. Inflammation and cancer: triggers, mechanisms, and consequences. Immunity. 2019;51(1):27–41.
5. Bahig H, Taussky D, Delouya G, Nadiri A, Gagnon-Jacques A, Bodson-Clermont P, Soulieres D. Neutrophil count is associated with survival in localized prostate cancer. BMC Cancer. 2015;15:594.
6. Zhang J, Zhou X, Ding H, Wang L, Liu S, Liu Y, Chen Z. The prognostic value of routine preoperative blood parameters in muscle-invasive bladder cancer. BMC Urol. 2020;20(1):31.
7. Huszno J, Kolosza Z, Mrochem-Kwarciak J, Rutkowski T, Skladowski K. The role of neutrophil-lymphocyte ratio, platelet-lymphocyte ratio, and platelets in the prognosis of metastatic renal cell carcinoma. Oncology. 2019;97(1):7–17.
8. Hu H, Yao X, Xie X, Wu X, Zheng C, Xia W, Ma S. Prognostic value of preoperative NLR, dNLR, PLR and CRP in surgical renal cell carcinoma patients. World J Urol. 2017;35(2):261–70.
9. Peyton CC, Abel EJ, Chipollini J, Boulware DC, Azizi M, Karam JA, Margulis V, Master VA, Matin SF, Raman JD, et al. The value of neutrophil to lymphocyte ratio in patients undergoing cytoreductive nephrectomy with thrombectomy. Eur Urol Focus. 2020;6(1):104–11.
10. Bezan A, Mrsic E, Krieger D, Stojakovic T, Pummer K, Zigeuner R, Hutterer GC, Pichler M. The preoperative AST/ALT (De Ritis) ratio represents a poor prognostic factor in a cohort of patients with nonmetastatic renal cell carcinoma. J Urol. 2015;194(1):30–5.
11. Chrom P, Stec R, Bodnar L, Szczylik C. Incorporating neutrophil-to-lymphocyte ratio and platelet-to-lymphocyte ratio in place of neutrophil

count and platelet count improves prognostic accuracy of the international metastatic renal cell carcinoma database consortium model. Cancer Res Treat. 2018;50(1):103–10.
12. Lardas M, Stewart F, Scrimgeour D, Hofmann F, Marconi L, Dabestani S, Bex A, Volpe A, Canfield SE, Staehler M, et al. Systematic review of surgical management of nonmetastatic renal cell carcinoma with vena caval thrombus. Eur Urol. 2016;70(2):265–80.
13. Blute ML, Leibovich BC, Lohse CM, Cheville JC, Zincke H. The Mayo Clinic experience with surgical management, complications and outcome for patients with renal cell carcinoma and venous tumour thrombus. BJU Int. 2004;94(1):33–41.
14. Moch H, Cubilla AL, Humphrey PA, Reuter VE, Ulbright TM. The 2016 WHO classification of tumours of the urinary system and male genital organs-part A: renal, penile, and testicular tumours. Eur Urol. 2016;70(1):93–105.
15. Frank I, Blute ML, Cheville JC, Lohse CM, Weaver AL, Zincke H. An outcome prediction model for patients with clear cell renal cell carcinoma treated with radical nephrectomy based on tumor stage, size, grade and necrosis: the SSIGN score. J Urol. 2002;168(6):2395–400.
16. Heagerty PJ, Lumley T, Pepe MS. Time-dependent ROC curves for censored survival data and a diagnostic marker. Biometrics. 2000;56(2):337–44.
17. Kim SH, Park B, Hwang EC, Hong SH, Jeong CW, Kwak C, Byun SS, Chung J. Retrospective multicenter long-term follow-up analysis of prognostic risk factors for recurrence-free, metastasis-free, cancer-specific, and overall survival after curative nephrectomy in non-metastatic renal cell carcinoma. Front Oncol. 2019;9:859.
18. Huang J, Feldman AS, Dong L, Cornejo K, Liu Q, Dahl DM, Wu S, Blute ML, Huang Y, Wu CL. Preoperative anemia as an independent prognostic indicator of papillary renal cell carcinoma. Clin Genitourin Cancer. 2015;13(5):e353–60.
19. Xia L, Hu G, Guzzo TJ. Prognostic significance of preoperative anemia in patients undergoing surgery for renal cell carcinoma: a meta-analysis. Anticancer Res. 2017;37(6):3175–81.
20. Chen YP, Zhao BC, Chen C, Shen LJ, Gao J, Mai ZY, Chen MK, Chen G, Yan F, Liu S, et al. Pretreatment platelet count improves the prognostic performance of the TNM staging system and aids in planning therapeutic regimens for nasopharyngeal carcinoma: a single-institutional study of 2,626 patients. Chin J Cancer. 2015;34(3):137–46.
21. Menczer J. Preoperative elevated platelet count and thrombocytosis in gynecologic malignancies. Arch Gynecol Obstet. 2017;295(1):9–15.
22. Rachidi S, Md P, Kaur MM, Lautenschlaeger TM, Li Z, Md P. Platelet count correlates with stage and predicts survival in melanoma. Platelets. 2019;30(8):1042–6.
23. Zhu X, Cao Y, Lu P, Kang Y, Lin Z, Hao T, Song Y. Evaluation of platelet indices as diagnostic biomarkers for colorectal cancer. Sci Rep. 2018;8(1):11814.
24. Życzkowski M, Prokopowicz G, Taborowski P, Nowakowski K, Rajwa P, Stelmach P, Paradysz A. Basic parameters of blood count, serum sodium, and creatinine as prognostic factors for renal cell carcinoma at five-year follow-up. Med Sci Monit Int Med J Exp Clin Res. 2018;24:3895–902.
25. Choi JY, Ko YH, Song PH. Clinical significance of preoperative thrombocytosis in patients who underwent radical nephrectomy for nonmetastatic renal cell carcinoma. Investig Clin Urol. 2016;57(5):324–9.
26. Hutterer GC, Krieger D, Mrsic E, Pohlmann K, Bezan A, Stojakovic T, Pummer K, Zigeuner R, Pichler M. Preoperative leucocytosis, thrombocytosis and anemia as potential prognostic factors in non-metastatic renal cell carcinoma. Anticancer Res. 2015;35(6):3463–9.
27. Hutchinson R, Rew C, Chen G, Woldu S, Krabbe LM, Meissner M, Sheth K, Singla N, Shakir N, Master VA, et al. The adverse survival implications of bland thrombus in renal cell carcinoma with venous tumor thrombus. Urology. 2018;115:119–24.
28. Haemmerle M, Stone RL, Menter DG, Afshar-Kharghan V, Sood AK. The platelet lifeline to cancer: challenges and opportunities. Cancer Cell. 2018;33(6):965–83.
29. Heng DY, Xie W, Regan MM, Harshman LC, Bjarnason GA, Vaishampayan UN, Mackenzie M, Wood L, Donskov F, Tan MH, et al. External validation and comparison with other models of the International Metastatic Renal-Cell Carcinoma Database Consortium prognostic model: a population-based study. Lancet Oncol. 2013;14(2):141–8.
30. Peng D, Zhang CJ, Tang Q, Zhang L, Yang KW, Yu XT, Gong Y, Li XS, He ZS, Zhou LQ. Prognostic significance of the combination of preoperative hemoglobin and albumin levels and lymphocyte and platelet counts (HALP) in patients with renal cell carcinoma after nephrectomy. BMC Urol. 2018;18(1):20.

9

Prognostic significance of preoperative neutrophil-to-lymphocyte ratio in papillary renal cell carcinoma patients after receiving curative surgery based on a retrospective cohort

Zhilei Zhang[1,2], Yongbo Yu[1,2], Jilu Zheng[1,2], Mingxin Zhang[1] and Haitao Niu[1*]

Abstract

Background: Inflammatory response biomarkers have been studied as promising prognostic factors in renal cell carcinoma, but few studies have focused on papillary renal cell carcinoma (PRCC). This study was performed to evaluate the prognostic value of the preoperative neutrophil-to-lymphocyte ratio (NLR) in PRCC patients.

Methods: In total, 122 postoperative PRCC patients selected from 366 non-clear cell renal cell carcinoma patients were enrolled from our institution between 2012 and 2020. The optimal cutoff value of the NLR was assessed by receiver operating characteristic (ROC) curve analysis, and the Kaplan–Meier method and Cox's proportional hazards regression models were performed to analyze the association of the NLR with overall survival (OS). In addition, the potential of tumor-node-metastasis (TNM) stage, the NLR and an NLR-TNM system to predict survival were compared with ROC curves, and clinical usefulness of the predicting models were assessed by decision curve analysis.

Results: A threshold value of 2.39 for the NLR for OS analysis was determined by ROC curve analysis. An NLR $\geq$ 2.39 was associated with a more advanced TNM stage ($P<0.01$) and larger tumors ($P<0.05$) than a low NLR, as well as pathological subtype II ($P<0.05$), and the patients with a high NLR also exhibited significantly worse overall survival outcomes ($P<0.05$). The NLR was determined to be a significant independent prognostic indicator by univariable and multivariable analyses (HR = 5.56, $P<0.05$). Furthermore, TNM stage and the NLR were integrated, and the area under the curve (AUC) of for the NLR-TNM system was larger than that of for the TNM system when predicting overall survival (0.84 vs 0.73, $P=0.04$). Decision curve analysis also demonstrated a better clinical value for the NLR-TNM model to predict the prognosis.

Conclusion: A high preoperative NLR was associated with poor clinical and pathologic parameters in patients with PRCC; moreover, the NLR was also an independent prognostic factor for the OS of patients with PRCC. The NLR-TNM system, which was a model that integrated the NLR with TNM staging, could improve the ability to predict overall survival.

Keywords: Papillary renal cell carcinoma (PRCC), Neutrophil-to-lymphocyte ratio (NLR), Overall survival (OS)

*Correspondence: niuht0532@126.com
[1] Department of Urology, The Affiliated Hospital of Qingdao University, Qingdao, China
Full list of author information is available at the end of the article

Background

Renal cell carcinoma (RCC) is a common malignant tumor of the urinary system. In 2018, approximately

175,000 RCC patients died worldwide, and approximately 400,000 new cases were diagnosed [1]. Widespread use of abdominal ultrasound and computed tomography (CT) has increased the number of incidentally detected RCCs [2]. Histologically, RCC can be divided into clear cell renal cell carcinoma (ccRCC), and non-clear cell carcinoma. Papillary renal cell carcinoma (PRCC) is a common subtype of non-clear cell carcinoma, accounting for 15–20% of RCC [3]. The 5-year overall survival rate of PRCC is reported to be significantly higher than that of clear cell carcinoma (80.5% vs 71.3%) [4]. Surgery is still the main treatment of PRCC, and recurrence after surgery often occurs in the advanced stage of PRCC, which may threaten survival and quality of life to a certain extent. Substantial evidence shows that inflammatory cells can induce tumor cell proliferation and metastasis through systemic inflammatory activation; therefore, inflammatory cells may be used to predict tumor prognosis [5–7]. Several indicators of systemic inflammation, such as c-reactive protein (CRP), the neutrophil-to-lymphocyte count ratio (NLR) and the platelet-to-lymphocyte count ratio (PLR), have been studied to predict the prognosis of various tumors [8, 9]. Among these indicators, the NLR is considered a valuable indicator for predicting tumor prognosis, such as that of lung cancer, liver cancer, esophageal cancer and ovarian cancer [10–12]. At present, there are few studies focusing on the prognosis of renal papillary cell carcinoma domestically or globally. Therefore, we used this background to analyze the value of the NLR in evaluating the prognosis of patients with renal papillary cell carcinoma following surgery.

Methods

Patients

A total of 366 patients with non-clear cell renal cell carcinoma (nccRCC) who underwent surgical treatment in the department of urology in our hospital from January 2012 to April 2020 were collected.

Inclusion criteria: (1) the medical records were complete. (2) No adjuvant treatment was performed before the operation. (3) The results of blood samplings were obtained within 1 week after admission. (4) The surgical method was partial nephrectomy or radical nephrectomy, and pathological results of specimens were confirmed by more than 2 pathologists as nccRCC with clean cutting edge and no residual.

Exclusion criteria: (1) patients with recent infectious diseases or a history of autoimmune diseases and infectious diseases; (2) patients with a history of primary tumor in other organs; (3) patients with preoperative radiotherapy or chemotherapy; (4) incomplete laboratory and pathological data.

After screening, a total of 122 patients diagnosed as papillary renal cell carcinoma (PRCC) were included in this study. This study was approved by the ethics committee of The Affiliated Hospital of Qingdao University.

Data collection

During the first week after admission, blood samples were obtained from all the patients. According to the results of peripheral blood test, neutrophil count ($\times 10^9$/L)/lymphocyte count ($\times 10^9$/L) was used to calculate the value of NLR. The optimal cutoff value of NLR was identified by an ROC analysis with OS as the primary endpoint, 2.39 was defined as the best cutoff value due to the maximum youden index value (sensitivity: 78.6%; specificity: 70.4%; youden index: 0.49). The cutoff value of CHOL (4.90) were defined by ROC with OS as the endpoint as well.

Follow up strategy: All patients after surgery were considered to be healthy, the first follow-up time in the first 2 years after the operation was every 3 months after operation, for the next 2 years, the follow up time was every 6 months and then annually for the last years, the follow-up included medical history, physical examination, laboratory blood tests and image information, information of death obtained by telephone interview was recorded. The follow-up period was up to 2020-11-01.

Statistics

Association with NLR between groups was analyzed by Chi-square test and Mann–Whitney U test, and the optimal threshold value of NLR was determined by the receiver operating characteristic (ROC) curve with OS as the primary endpoint. Kaplan–Meier method was utilized to estimate the survival rate of OS, and the survival estimate between groups divided by each cutoff value was compared by log-rank test. Univariable and multivariable COX regression analysis were used to determine the independent prognostic factors of OS. The abilities of different factors to predict OS were compared by the comparisons of the area under curve (AUC) of each parameter, and decision curve analysis was used to assess the clinical usefulness of the predicting models. SPSS ver. 22.0 (SPSS Inc., Chicago, IL, USA), R 4.0.3 (formerly AT&T, now Lucent Technologies), Graphpad Prism 8 (GraphPad Software Inc., La Jolla, CA, USA) and Medcalc v19.1.3 were used to analyze all the statistics. $P < 0.05$ of two sides was considered statistically significant.

Results

Patient characteristics

The patient clinicopathological characteristics were listed on Table 1, 122 PRCC patients with 88 (72.1%) males and 34 (27.9%) females aged from 7 to 81 (the

Table 1 Patient clinical characteristics

Characteristic	No. of patients (%)
Age/years	
<60	61 (50%)
≥60	61 (50%)
Gender	
Male	88 (72.1%)
Female	34 (27.9%)
BMI	
≥25	54 (44.3%)
<25	68 (55.7%)
Diabetes/hyperglycemia, n (%)	
Yes	20 (16.4%)
No	102 (83.6%)
TNM stage (AJCC8th)	
I	101 (82.7%)
II	10 (8.2%)
III	8 (6.6%)
IV	3 (2.5%)
Surgical type	
RN	64 (52.5%)
PN	58 (47.5%)
Tumor size(cm)	
<7	98 (80.3%)
≥7	24 (19.7%)
Subtype, n (%)	
I	64 (55.6%)
II	58 (44.4%)
Serum album(g/l)	
≥40	70 (57.4%)
<40	52 (42.6%)
NLR	
<2.39	78 (63.9%)
≥2.39	44 (36.1%)
CHOL	
<4.90	65 (53.3%)
≥4.90	57 (46.7%)
BUN/Cr	
<20	87 (57.8%)
≥20	35 (42.2%)

TNM tumor-node-metastasis, *CHOL* cholesterol, *NLR* neutrophil-to-lymphocyte ratio, *PN* partial nephrectomy, *RN* radical nephrectomy

mean age was 57.7). According to the histology, these patients were divided into two subtypes 64 (52.5%) I and 58 (47.5%) II, respectively. All patients were underwent curative surgery including radical nephrectomy 64 (52%) and partial nephrectomy 58 (47.5%). Based on the 8th TNM classification of AJCC guideline, 101 (82.7%), 10 (8.2%), 8 (6.6%) and 3 (2.5%) were distributed into I, II, III and IV stage. The median follow up time was 33 months (interquartile range, 16.75–52.5 months), 14 patients were died during the follow-up, and the survival rate of 1 year, 3 years and 5 years were 99.2%, 97.1% and 81.2% in our present study.

Associations between NLR and clinicopathological characteristics of the patients

ROC curve was used to identify the best cut-off value of NLR based on OS (overall survival) as the endpoint. The median preoperative NLR was 1.96 (IQR 1.42–2.82), and the optimal cut-off value of NLR was 2.39 in our study (83.3% sensitivity and 71.8% specificity) by ROC curves analysis, then 78 patients were categorized into the high NLR (≥2.39) group and 44 patients were identified into the low NLR (<2.39) group. Table 2 showed the association between different levels of NLR and clinicopathological characteristics, there were no significant differences between two groups with regard to the age, gender, BMI, surgical type and other clinical characteristics, patients with high NLR tend to have a more advanced TNM stage ($P<0.01$) and larger tumors ($P<0.05$) than a low NLR, as well as pathological subtype II ($P<0.05$).

Survival analysis

The 1 year, 3 year and 5 year survival rates were 100%, 98%and 84%in low NLR group, while the 1 year, 3 year and 5 year survival rates of high NLR group were 97.7%, 80.6% and 56.1%, respectively. The OS time of the high NLR group was shorter than the low NLR group ($P<0.01$), Fig. 1 showed the Kaplan–Meier survival curves for OS of patients with PRCC according to NLR levels, TNM stage and Tumor size levels, which were all significant predictors for OS ($P<0.05$) by the univariable analysis (Table 3), Patients with advanced TNM stage and larger tumor size were associated with worse OS.

In the univariable analysis the significant variables ($P<0.05$) were included into the following multivariate analysis, as shown in Table 3, NLR (HR=5.56, 95% CI 1.06–29.15, $P=0.04$) and TNM stage (HR=4.86, 95% CI 1.52–15.58, $P=0.01$) was the independent prognostic factors of OS, which demonstrated that patients with a NLR≥2.39 and advanced TNM stage were correlated with a shorter survival time.

Comparison of the predictive prognostic value of TNM stage, NLR and NLR-TNM model

To evaluate the ability of predicting OS in patients with PRCC, we further drew ROC curves for each parameter to calculated AUC of TNM stage, NLR and NLR-TNM (Fig. 2). The AUC of NLR-TNM system integrated NLR with TNM stage in predicting OS time were relatively higher than that of TNM and NLR alone (0.73 vs 0.78 vs 0.84 for TNM, NLR and NLR-TNM, respectively),

Table 2 Associations between NLR and clinicopathologic characteristics

Variables	NLR < 2.39 (n = 78)	NLR ≥ 2.39 (n = 44)	*P* value
Age/years			0.451
< 60	37 (47.4%)	24 (54.5%)	
≥ 60	41 (52.6%)	20 (45.5%)	
Gender			0.596
Male	55 (70.5%)	33 (75%)	
Female	23 (29.5%)	11 (25%)	
BMI			0.187
≥ 25	38 (48.7%)	16 (36.4%)	
< 25	40 (51.3%)	28 (63.6%)	
Diabetes/hyperglycemia, n (%)			0.363
No	67 (85.9%)	35 (79.5%)	
Yes	11 (14.1%)	9 (250.5%)	
TNM stage (AJCC 8th)			0.001[a]
I	71 (91%)	30 (68.2%)	
II	4 (5.1%)	6 (13.5%)	
III	3 (3.9%)	5 (11.5%)	
IV	0	3 (6.8%)	
Surgical type			0.063
RN	36 (46.2%)	28 (63.6%)	
PN	42 (53.8%)	16 (36.4%)	
Tumor size (cm)			0.011
< 7	68 (87.2%)	30 (68.2%)	
≥ 7	10 (12.8%)	14 (31.8%)	
Subtype, n (%)	0.022		
I	47 (60.3%)	17 (38.6%)	
II	31 (39.7%)	27 (61.4%)	
Serum album (g/l)			0.925
≥ 40	45 (57.7%)	25 (56.8%)	
< 40	33 (42.3%)	19 (43.2%)	
CHOL			0.085
< 4.90	37 (47.4%)	28 (63.6%)	
≥ 4.90	41 (52.6%)	16 (36.4%)	
BUN/Cr			0.274
< 20	53 (67.9%)	34 (77.3%)	
≥ 20	25 (32.1%)	10 (22.7%)	

TNM tumor-node-metastasis, *CHOL* cholesterol, *NLR* neutrophil-to-lymphocyte ratio, *PN* partial nephrectomy, *RN* radical nephrectomy

[a] Mann–Whitney U

which revealed that the predictive ability of NLR was higher than traditional TNM stage, after integrated NLR with TNM stage system, the NLR-TNM showed the better ability in predicting OS time ($P < 0.05$) (Table 4).

Figure 3 showed the decision curves of the predicted models of NLR, TNM stage and NLR-TNM, and a positive net benefit was compared among them, which demonstrated that using this NLR-TNM model in the current study to predict OS added more benefits than the other two models.

Discussion

In our study, we respectively analyzed 122 PRCC patients who underwent curative surgical treatment. An NLR ≥ 2.39 was closely correlated with a relatively advanced pathological stage and large tumor volume. In addition, the results demonstrated that a high preoperative NLR was an independent prognostic factor associated with shortened OS. These results were in line with other previous studies [13–15], which implies that the NLR is relevant for predicting poor clinical characteristics. Furthermore, the NLR-TNM system was relatively

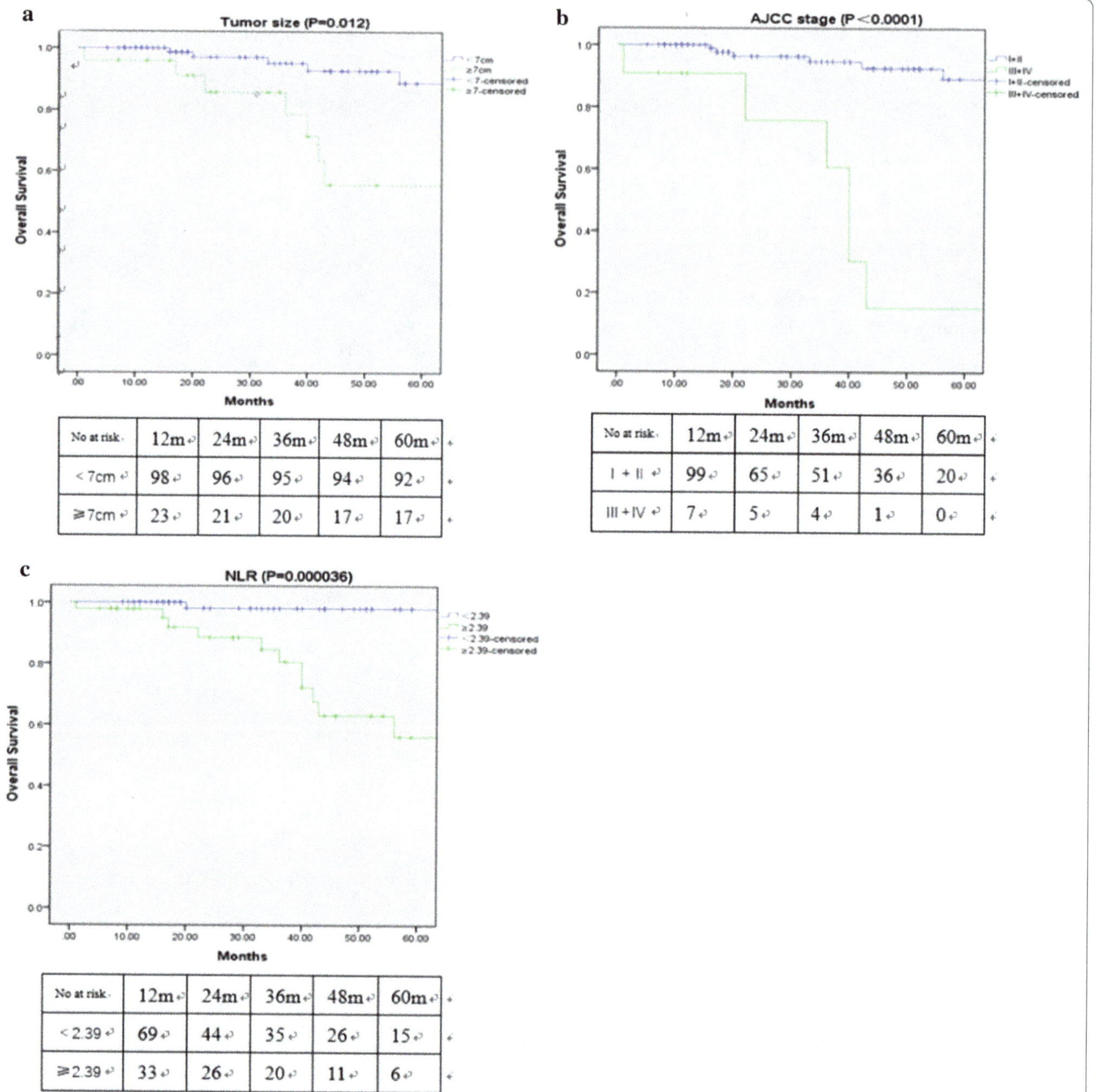

No at risk	12m	24m	36m	48m	60m
<7cm	98	96	95	94	92
≥7cm	23	21	20	17	17

No at risk	12m	24m	36m	48m	60m
I + II	99	65	51	36	20
III + IV	7	5	4	1	0

No at risk	12m	24m	36m	48m	60m
<2.39	69	44	35	26	15
≥2.39	33	26	20	11	6

Fig. 1 Kaplan–Meier survival curves for OS of patients with PRCC (papillary renal cell carcinoma) according to tumor size (**a**), TNM (AJCC) stage (**b**) and NLR levels (**c**). Patients with larger tumor size, advanced TNM stage and higher NLR were associated with worse OS

more accurate in predicting overall survival than the TNM stage or NLR alone.

Several immunohistochemical biomarkers and nomograms have been confirmed to be independent prognostic factors for the survival of RCC patients [16, 17]. The NLR is a tumor marker easily obtained from the peripheral blood. Previous research has reported that the NLR has been used to evaluate the tumor prognosis of localized renal cell carcinoma [18, 19], but most studies have focused on clear cell renal cell carcinoma, and there is a lack of studies on predictive models for pathological subtypes of papillary renal cell carcinoma. Huang et al. first reported that the NLR was associated with the RFS (recurrence-free survival) of non-metastatic papillary cell carcinoma patients [20], which revealed that an NLR≥3.6 was an independent predictor of RFS. This was similar to the conclusion of our study. Most different cutoff levels for the NLR with prognostic value for RCC range from 3

Table 3 Univariable and multivariable analyses of factors in relation to overall survival

Variables	Univariable		Multivariable	
	HR (95% CI)	*P* value	HR (95% CI)	*P* value
Age/years				
≥60 versus <60	1.072 (0.376–3.063)	0.896		
Gender				
(M vs F)	1.149 (0.351–3.7571)	0.818		
BMI				
≥25 versus <25	1.055 (0.365–3.051)	0.921		
Diabetes/hyperglycemia, n (%)				
Yes versus no	1.182 (0.328–4.258)	0.798		
TNM stage (AJCC 8th)				
III+IV versus I+II	12.845 (4.417–37.353)	0.001	4.859 (1.515–15.584)	0.008
Surgical type				
RN versus PN	2.67 (0.744–9.583)	0.132		
Tumor size (cm)				
≥7 versus <7	3.557 (1.24–10.205)	0.018	1.819 (0.60–5.51)	0.290
Subtype, n (%)				
I versus II	0.342 (0.106–1.098)	0.071		
Serum album (g/l)				
<40 versus ≥40	0.641 (0.214–1.92)	0.427		
CHOL				
<4.9 versus ≥4.9	0.988 (0.344–2.838)	0.983		
NLR				
≥2.39 versus <2.39	12.007 (2.675–53.886)	0.001	5.557 (1.059–29.149)	0.043
BUN/Cr				
≥20 versus <20	0.373 (0.082–1.706)	0.203		

TNM tumor-node-metastasis, *CHOL* cholesterol, *NLR* neutrophil-to-lymphocyte ratio, *PN* partial nephrectomy, *RN* radical nephrectomy

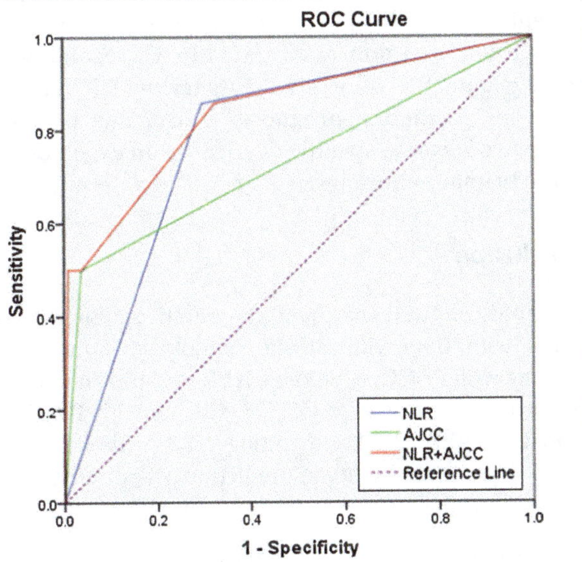

Fig. 2 Comparisons of TNM, NLR and NLR-TNM in prognosis prediction of 122 PRCC patients in present study using receiver operating characteristic curves. The AUC of TNM, NLR and NLR-TNM were 0.731 ($P=0.005$), 0.780 ($P=0.001$) and 0.839 ($P<0.0001$), respectively. *TNM* tumor-node-metastasis, *NLR* neutrophil-to-lymphocyte ratio

Table 4 Comparisons of the value of TNM, NLR and NLR-TNM systems in predicting prognosis of overall survival among the patients in present study

Model	AUC (95%CI)	*P*
TNM versus NLR-TNM	0.731 (0.644–0.808) versus 0.839 (0.761–0.899)	0.036
NLR versus NLR-TNM	0.780 (0.696–0.850) versus 0.839 (0.761–0.899)	0.034
NLR versus TNM	0.780 (0.696–0.850) versus 0.731 (0.644–0.808)	0.489

TNM tumor-node-metastasis, *NLR* neutrophil-to-lymphocyte ratio

to 5 [21], which was not consistent with our study, Most of the patients with PRCC in our study were staged early, and PRCC is a tumor with relatively low malignancy, which may contribute to this difference. Our study also found that a high preoperative NLR was related to poor overall survival in PRCC, indicating that the NLR could be used as an independent prognostic factor to predict prognosis.

The inflammatory response is an important factor in the occurrence of malignant tumors, and tumor cells

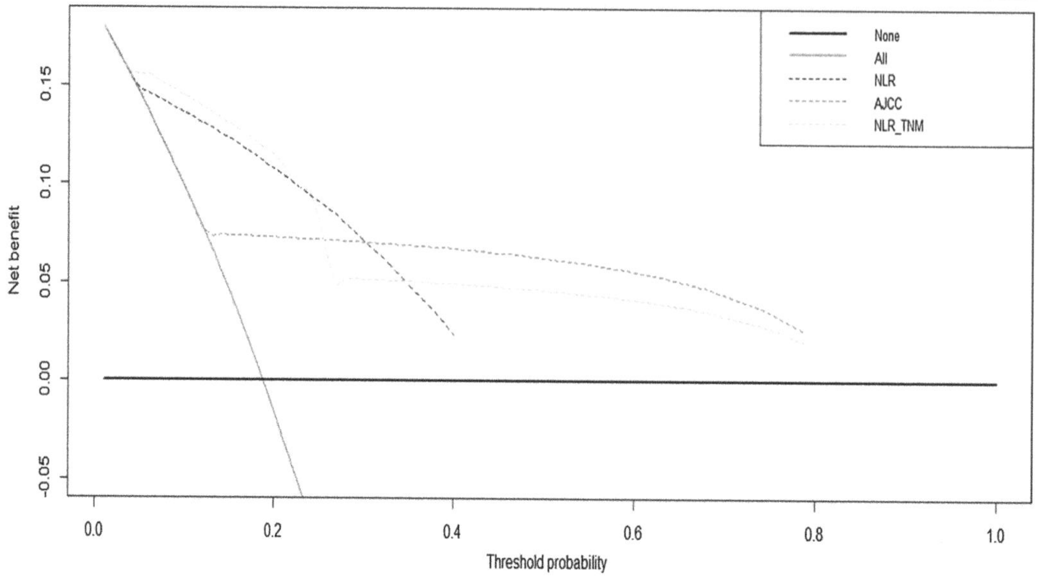

Fig. 3 Decision curve analysis for the TNM, NLR and NLR-TNM model. Notes: The y-axis measures the net benefit. The dotted line represents the model of TNM, NLR and NLR-TNM. The thin solid line represents the assumption that all patients are intervened. Thin thick solid line represents the assumption that no patients are intervened. The decision curve of NLR-TNM model showed the most benefit than the other two models

release a large number of inflammatory factors to change the tumor microenvironment, which can help tumor cells escape the host immune response. This escape leads to the proliferation and distant metastasis of tumor cells [22] and promotes the transformation of normal cells into tumor cells. Recent studies have shown that neutrophils can produce and release active cellular factors, such as IL6-1, IL-6 and VEGF, which changes the balance of inflammatory and anti-inflammatory in the tumor microenvironment [23]. Lymphocytes are important immune cells that contribute to tumor immune surveillance, which can inhibit tumor invasion. The NLR is a more accurate indicator of the inflammatory response level than either single factor composing the NLR. Therefore, a large number of studies have shown that a high NLR is associated with an advanced stage and a poor prognosis [24, 25], which was also supported by our study.

Since 2015, targeted therapy and immune checkpoint inhibitors have gradually become the main treatments for advanced metastatic renal carcinoma [26]. Vascular endothelial growth factor (VEGF) and vascular endothelial growth factor receptor (VEGFR) have become crucial targets of anticancer therapy because of their antiangiogenic functions. VEGF is a cellular activity factor produced by neutrophils, and whether the NLR can be used as a potential marker for the effect of targeted therapy remains to be determined. One study showed that the NLR was reduced by adjuvant sunitinib therapy for 4 weeks, with one endpoint of RFS improved [27]. Moreover, the NLR has been reported to be lower after the immunotherapy in metastatic RCC, with improved survival outcomes [28]. The systematic inflammatory response will be a very interesting focus of further research after neoadjuvant or adjuvant therapy in advanced RCC and PRCC.

Our study also had several limitations. First, our study was a respective study with a single-center, and the low incidence of PRCC led to the small sample of patients, so we did not divide the patients into metastatic PRCC and non-metastatic PRCC. Second, we did not evaluate the NLR after surgery, which limits the value for predicting prognosis. Third, due to a small number of disease specific deaths, we analyzed only OS as the primary endpoint.

Conclusion

This study showed that high preoperative NLR was associated with poor clinical and pathologic parameters of patients with PRCC. Moreover, NLR was also an independent prognostic factor of OS for patients with PRCC. The model of NLR-TNM integrating NLR with TNM stage could improve the ability of predicting overall survival.

Abbreviations

PRCC: Papillary renal cell carcinoma; NLR: Neutrophil-to-lymphocyte ratio; TNM: Tumor-node-metastasis; ROC: Receiver operating curve.

Acknowledgements

Not applicable.

Authors' contributions

All authors have read and approved the manuscript. All authors have agreed both to be personally accountable for the own contributions and to ensure that questions related to the accuracy or integrity of any part of the work. ZZ: Data Collection, Manuscript writing; YY, JZ: Data collection: MZ and HN: made supervision and helped reviewing the manuscript. All authors read and approved the final manuscript.

Author details

[1] Department of Urology, The Affiliated Hospital of Qingdao University, Qingdao, China. [2] Department of Clinical Medicine, Qingdao University, Qingdao, China.

References

1. Bray F, Ferlay J, Soerjomataram I, Siegel RL, Torre LA, Jemal A. Global cancer statistics 2018: GLOBOCAN estimates of incidence and mortality worldwide for 36 cancers in 185 countries. CA Cancer J Clin. 2018;68(6):394–424.
2. Pichler M, Hutterer GC, Chromecki TF, et al. Renal cell carcinoma stage migration in a single European centre over 25 years: effects on 5- and 10-year metastasis-free survival. Int Urol Nephrol. 2012;44(4):997–1004.
3. Humphrey PA, Moch H, Cubilla AL, Ulbright TM, Reuter VE. The 2016 WHO classification of tumours of the urinary system and male genital organs—part B: prostate and bladder tumours. Lyon: IARC Press; 2004.
4. Steffens S, Janssen M, Roos FC, et al. Incidence and long-term prognosis of papillary compared to clear cell renal cell carcinoma—a multicentre study. Eur J Cancer. 2012;48(15):2347–52.
5. Gores GJ. Inflammatory cytokines induce DNA damage and inhibit DNA repair in cholangiocarcinoma cells by a nitric oxide-dependent mechanism. Cancer Res. 2000;60(1):184–90.
6. Hainaut P, Plymoth A. Targeting the hallmarks of cancer: towards a rational approach to next-generation cancer therapy. Curr Opin Oncol. 2013;25(1):50.
7. Grebien F, Hantschel O, Wojcik J, et al. & Weinberg, Robert A. Hallmarks of Cancer: The Next Generation. 2011.
8. Szkandera J, Stotz M, Absenger G, et al. Validation of C-reactive protein levels as a prognostic indicator for survival in a large cohort of pancreatic cancer patients. Br J Cancer. 2014;110(1):183–8.
9. Kazuya N, Kuniya T. The modified Glasgow prognostic score as a predictor of survival after hepatectomy for colorectal liver metastases. Ann Surg Oncol. 2014;21(5):1711–8.
10. Cho HB, Hur HW, Sang WK, et al. Pre-treatment neutrophil to lymphocyte ratio is elevated in epithelial ovarian cancer and predicts survival after treatment. Cancer Immunol Immunother. 2009;58(1):15–23.
11. Aliustaoglu M, Bilici A, Ustaalioglu BB, et al. The effect of peripheral blood values on prognosis of patients with locally advanced gastric cancer before treatment. Med Oncol. 2010;27(4):1060–5.
12. Templeton AJ, Ace O, Mcnamara MG, et al. Prognostic role of neutrophil-to-lymphocyte ratio in solid tumors: a systematic review and meta-analysis. Breast Cancer Res. 2017;19(1):2.
13. Viers BR, Houston Thompson R, Boorjian SA, Lohse CM, Leibovich BC, Tollefson MK. Preoperative neutrophil-lymphocyte ratio predicts death among patients with localized clear cell renal carcinoma undergoing nephrectomy. Urol Oncol. 2014;32(8):1277–84.
14. Huang J, Dahl DM, Dong L, et al. Preoperative neutrophil-to-lymphocyte ratio and neutrophilia are independent predictors of recurrence in patients with localized papillary renal cell carcinoma. Biomed Res Int. 2015;2015:891045.
15. Wen RM, Zhang YJ, Ma S, Xu YL, Zheng JN. Preoperative neutrophil to lymphocyte ratio as a prognostic factor in patients with non-metastatic renal cell carcinoma. Asian Pac J Cancer Prev APJCP. 2015;16(9):3703–8.
16. Cindolo L, Patard J, Chiodini P, et al. Comparison of predictive accuracy of four prognostic models for nonmetastatic renal cell carcinoma after nephrectomy: a multicenter European study. Cancer. 2010;104(7):1362–71.
17. Karakiewicz PI, et al. Multi-institutional validation of a new renal cancer-specific survival nomogram. J Clin Oncol. 2007;25(11):1316–22.
18. Frank I, Blute ML, Cheville JC, Lohse CM, Weaver AL, Zincke H. An outcome prediction model for patients with clear cell renal cell carcinoma treated with radical nephrectomy based on tumor stage, size, grade and necrosis: the SSIGN score. J Urol. 2002;168(6):2395–400.
19. Viers BR, Boorjian SA, Frank I, et al. Pretreatment neutrophil-to-lymphocyte ratio is associated with advanced pathologic tumor stage and increased cancer-specific mortality among patients with urothelial carcinoma of the bladder undergoing radical cystectomy. Eur Urol. 2014;66(6):1157–64.
20. Huang J, Dahl DM, Liang D, et al. Preoperative neutrophil-to-lymphocyte ratio and neutrophilia are independent predictors of recurrence in patients with localized papillary renal cell carcinoma. Biomed Res Int. 2015;2015:1–9.
21. Byun SS, Hwang EC, Kang SH, et al. Prognostic significance of preoperative neutrophil-to-lymphocyte ratio in nonmetastatic renal cell carcinoma: a large. Multicenter Cohort Analysis Biomed Res Int. 2016;2016:5634148.
22. Byong S, Oh J, Won J. Prognostic value of C-reactive protein and neutrophil-to-lymphocyte ratio in patients with hepatocellular carcinoma. BMC Cancer. 2013;13:78.
23. Ingrid M, Markus M, Pascale K, Maria HG. Polymorphonuclear neutrophils and T lymphocytes: strange bedfellows or brothers in arms. Trends Immunol. 2009;30(11):522–30.
24. Hsu JT, Liao CK, Le PH, et al. Prognostic value of the preoperative neutrophil to lymphocyte ratio in resectable gastric cancer. Medicine (Abingdon). 2015;94(39):e1589.
25. Gu XB, Tian T, Tian XJ, Zhang XJ. Prognostic significance of neutrophil-to-lymphocyte ratio in non-small cell lung cancer: a meta-analysis. Sci Rep. 2015;5:12493.
26. Soerensen AV, Donskov F, Hermann GG, et al. Improved overall survival after implementation of targeted therapy for patients with metastatic renal cell carcinoma: results from the Danish Renal Cancer Group (DARENCA) study-2. Eur J Cancer. 2014;50(3):553–62.
27. Patel A, Ravaud A, Motzer RJ, Pantuck AJ, George DJ. Neutrophil-to-lymphocyte ratio as a potential prognostic factor of disease-free survival in high-risk renal cell carcinoma: analysis of the S-TRAC trial. J Clin Oncol. 2018;36(15_suppl):4562–4562.
28. Lalani AA, Xie W, Martini DJ, et al. Change in Neutrophil-to-lymphocyte ratio (NLR) in response to immune checkpoint blockade for metastatic renal cell carcinoma. J Immunother Cancer. 2018;6(1):5.

10

Hyperprogressive disease after radiotherapy combined with anti-PD-1 therapy in renal cell carcinoma

Chao Liu[1†], Jingjing Piao[2†] and Zhiyang Shang[1*]

Abstract

Background: Studies have shown that immune checkpoint inhibitors (ICIs) have limited efficacy and can even increase tumour burden in short time periods. This is usually called hyperprogressive disease (HPD). To date, there are few reports regarding HPD; fewer have analysed the relationship between HPD and radiotherapy combined with ICIs, and their conclusions are controversial.

Case presentation: A 42-year-old woman was diagnosed with stage IV renal clear cell carcinoma. The patient had previously received sorafenib and pazopanib as first- and second-line therapies, respectively. She received radiotherapy combined with nivolumab. Eighteen days after administration of the third dose of nivolumab, the patient's general condition deteriorated; this was associated with immune-related adverse events. Computed tomography showed that the diameter of left lung metastases had sharply increased. A biopsy of the lung metastasis showed no infiltration of lymphocytes. The patient's general condition worsened and she died of the disease on the 70th day after administration of the third dose of nivolumab.

Conclusions: This report describes the development of HPD following the administration of radiotherapy combined with ICIs in a case of advanced renal cell carcinoma. The case indicates that radiotherapy may show bidirectional regulation effects on anti-tumour immune response. If the immunosuppressive function of radiotherapy is dominant, combined with ICIs, it could result in HPD.

Keywords: Hyperprogressive disease, Radiotherapy, Immunotherapy, Renal clear cell carcinoma, Case report

Background

Immune checkpoint inhibitors (ICIs), especially antibodies against programmed death 1/programmed death-ligand 1 (PD-1/PD-L1) and cytotoxic T lymphocyte antigen-4 (CTLA-4), represent one of the most significant breakthroughs in the treatment of advanced malignancies; they have been approved to treat several solid tumours. However, despite the usefulness of these drugs, a significant number of patients do not respond to them. Therefore, improving the effectiveness of immunotherapy is a major goal of clinical research. Researchers have found that radiotherapy can promote the presentation of tumour antigens and induce immune-mediated anti-tumour responses, indicating that the combination of radiotherapy and ICIs may enhance the anti-tumour immune response [1, 2]. A secondary analysis of the KEYNOTE-001 phase 1 trial found that the overall survival

*Correspondence: shangzhiyang85@163.com
†Chao Liu and Jingjing Piao have contributed equally to this work
[1] Department of Oncology, Zhuozhou Hospital, No.129, Fanyang Road, Zhuozhou City, Hebei Province, China
Full list of author information is available at the end of the article

(OS) was significantly longer in patients who received pembrolizumab and radiotherapy than in patients who had not previously received radiotherapy [3]. Moreover, the PACIFIC study showed that compared with placebo, durvalumab significantly prolonged progression-free survival (PFS) and OS among patients with stage III unresectable non-small-cell lung cancer (NSCLC) who did not have disease progression after concurrent chemoradiotherapy [4].

Recently, the number of active clinical trials testing ICIs combined with radiotherapy has seen a dramatic increase [5], and some reports have found that locally applied radiotherapy can improve the curative effect of ICIs [6–8]. However, studies have also shown that ICI therapy has limited efficacy, and can even accelerate tumour growth rate and increase tumour burden in short time periods. This is usually called hyperprogressive disease (HPD) [9]. HPD generally defined as > twofold increase in progression pace, > 50% increase in tumor burden and time to treatment failure < 2 months [10]. The median OS was significantly shortened in patients with HPD compared to those without the disease.

Until now, very few studies have analysed the relationship between HPD and radiotherapy combined with ICIs. Here, we present the case of a patient with advanced renal cell carcinoma who developed HPD following the administration of radiotherapy combined with nivolumab, and we review the literature on HPD associated with this treatment modality. This article hopes to provide new perspectives for researchers to explore the mechanisms underlying HPD.

Case presentation

A 42-year-old woman was admitted to our hospital in March 2019 with a diagnosis of stage IV renal clear cell carcinoma (with multiple lung metastases). Her Eastern Cooperative Oncology Group (ECOG) and Royal Marsden Hospital (RMH) prognostic scores were 2 and 1 (albumin < 3.5 g/dL), respectively. The patient had previously received sorafenib and pazopanib as first- and second-line therapies, respectively, but these could not stop the progress of the disease. She had no history of autoimmune diseases, and her whole exome sequencing showed that the tumour mutation burden (TMB) was 127 mu/mb and no MDM2/4 amplification. The patient then received radiotherapy combined with nivolumab (180 mg, 3 mg/kg). The first dose of nivolumab was administered on 27 March 2019. After six days, she underwent radiotherapy. To induce systemic immune response and improve local tumour control, a suitable radiotherapy strategy was designed, including stereotactic body radiation therapy (SBRT) (24 Gy in 3 fractions) followed by the conventional 59.5 Gy in 17 fractions to the right kidney lesion (Fig. 1).

The diameter of the left lung metastases increased from 0.7 cm at baseline to 1.5 cm during radiotherapy, and showed no changes after completion of radiotherapy (Fig. 2a–c). After 14th days of radiotherapy, the patient was treated with the second and third doses of nivolumab (3 mg/kg every 2 weeks). Eighteen days after administration of the third dose of nivolumab, the patient's general condition deteriorated; this was associated with an immune-related adverse event, namely, inflammatory arthritis, which presented as severe pain and deformed joints in the hands and knees (Fig. 3). Computed tomography scans of the right kidney lesions showed almost no change during treatment (Fig. 4a, b), but the diameter of the left lung metastases sharply increased to 4.9 (Fig. 2d). Moreover, the absolute count of peripheral lymphocytes decreased from 2.75×10^9/L to 0.74×10^9/L after radiotherapy.

Radiological evaluation alone is not enough to distinguish pseudoprogression from HPD, so a biopsy of the lung metastasis was performed. It showed no infiltration of lymphocytes (Fig. 5 and Additional file 1: Fig. S1); thus, pseudoprogression was excluded. Subsequently, the patient received prednisone therapy. However, her general condition worsened and she received supportive care. She died of respiratory failure on the 70th day after administration of the third dose of nivolumab.

Discussion and conclusions

It is hypothesized that the therapeutic effect of radiotherapy combined with ICIs should be better. However, in this case, radiotherapy combined with an ICI led to a significant increase in the size of the left lung metastasis, suggesting that radiotherapy induced HPD.

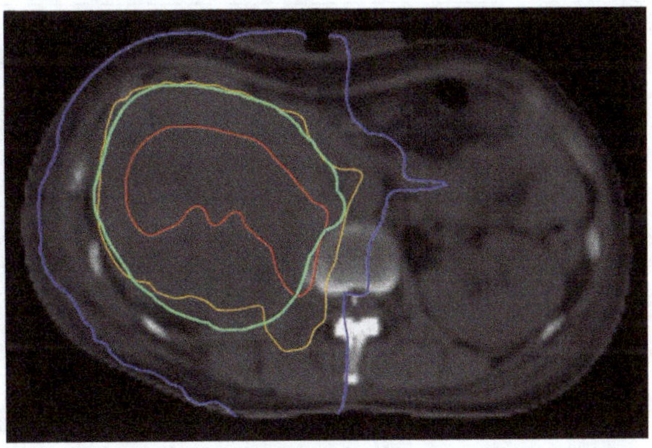

Fig. 1 The treatment plan isodose distribution for right kidney lesion. Red indicates the planning target volume of hypofraction, and green indicates the planning target volume of conventional fraction

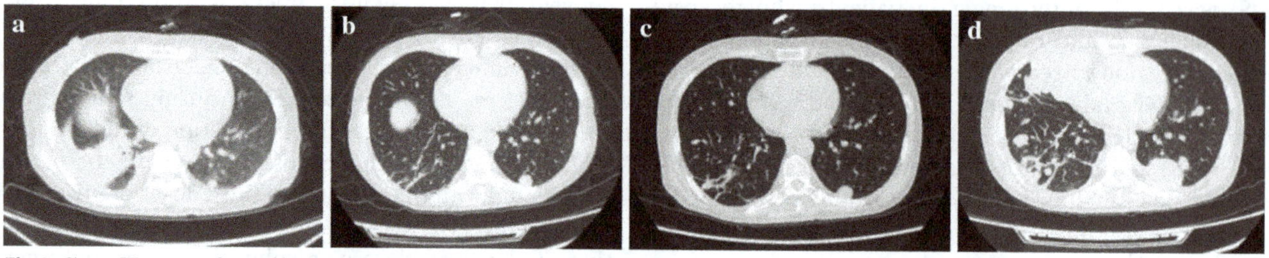

Fig.2 Chest CT scan performed before administration of the first dose of nivolumab (**a**), during radiotherapy (**b**), after radiotherapy (**c**), after administration of the third dose of nivolumab (**d**)

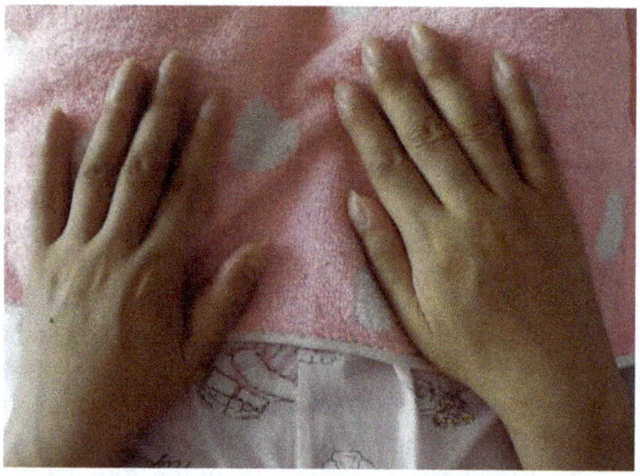

Fig.3 The patient's knuckles were deformed after administration of the third dose of nivolumab

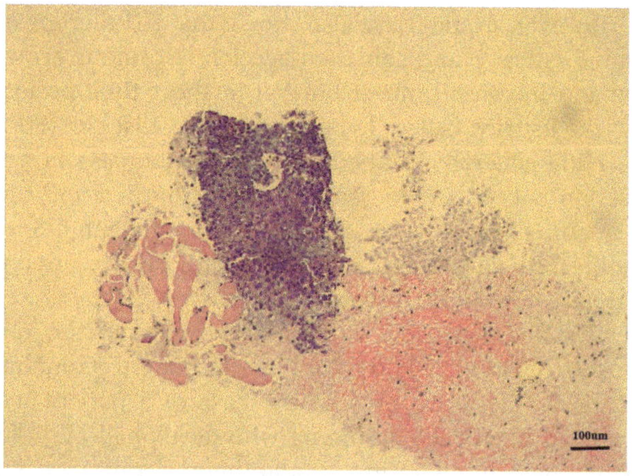

Fig.5 Haematoxylin and eosin staining of the lung metastasis biopsy sample showed no infiltration of lymphocytes

To date, there are few reports regarding HPD. In the literature, the incidence of HPD ranged from 1 to 7% for renal cell carcinoma and from 1 to 30% for other tumours [11]. Few studies have analysed the relationship between HPD and radiotherapy combined with ICIs, and their conclusions are controversial. Champiat et al. reported that ICI-related HPD occurred in twelve patients with malignant solid tumours. The authors found that HPD was not related to the type of previous treatment, including radiotherapy [9]. Ferrara et al. analysed the relevant factors in 56 advanced NSCLC patients with HPD and reached a similar conclusion [12]. However, in patients

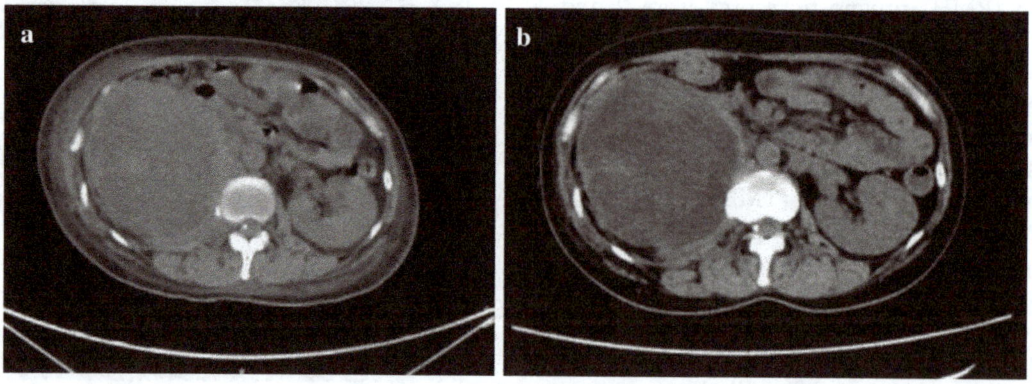

Fig.4 Abdominal CT scan performed before administration of the first dose of nivolumab (**a**), after administration of the third dose of nivolumab (**b**)

with recurrent and/or metastatic head and neck squamous cell carcinoma, the incidence of HPD was up to 29%. The authors of that study argued that radiotherapy might play a role since almost all cases of HPD occurred in patients who had at least one locoregional recurrence in an irradiated field [13]; however, they did not study the underlying mechanism. Nevertheless, their study reported the most information regarding the relationship between radiotherapy and HPD. To our knowledge, there are, in total, ten studies that involve radiotherapy and HPD (Table 1).

Because radiotherapy is considered a double-edged sword in anti-tumour immunity, some investigators have suggested that HPD results from radiotherapy, which impairs the function of immune cells and changes the tumour microenvironment. Du et al. reported the case of a patient with NSCLC who developed HPD following SBRT combined with an ICI [18]. By analysing the biopsies of the irradiated target lesion after radiotherapy and prior to ICI treatment, they found that the absence of tumour-infiltrating lymphocytes (TILs) and cancer-intrinsic PD-1 expression may be the main causes of HPD. Further studies have revealed that blockade of cancer-intrinsic PD-1 can enhance cancer survival in vitro and in vivo. The authors proposed that radiotherapy prior to ICI treatment can increase type I interferon production by either tumour cells or immune cells, which may in turn increase cancer-intrinsic PD-1 expression; however, they did not analyse the biopsies before radiotherapy, so there is insufficient evidence to support this theory. Ogata et al. reported the case of a patient with advanced gastric cancer who received nivolumab seven days after the completion of radiotherapy, whereupon he experienced HPD within the irradiation field [17]. They suggested that radiotherapy alters the immune environment and facilitates the occurrence of HPD, but did not investigate this further.

Although the expression of cancer-intrinsic PD-1 was not detected in our patient, the lymphocyte counts sharply decreased after radiotherapy, and the absence of TILs may have been the cause of HPD. This is consistent with the report of Alexander et al [14]. Cho et al. also reported that lymphopenia was indicative of poor prognosis in NSCLC patients who received ICIs, and this was significantly associated with radiotherapy [21].

Regulatory T cells (Tregs), which function to suppress tumour-specific immunity, have been confirmed as radioresistant lymphocyte subpopulations in many studies [22–26]. Kamada et al. found that PD-1 blockade can markedly increase the number of Tregs in HPD patients and result in inhibition of anti-tumour immunity [27]. Romano et al. investigated 15 patients with stage IV cutaneous melanoma who responded to CTLA-4-specific monoclonal antibody, and found that anti-CTLA-4 therapy may enhance immune responses by target Tregs in vivo [28]. To our knowledge, there are no reports of patients who developed HPD following radiotherapy combined with anti-CTLA-4 therapy. Therefore, this combination may reduce the occurrence of HPD and improve the curative effect. Unfortunately, in our patient, biopsy of the lung metastasis showed no lymphocytes, and we did not detect the Treg fraction in the peripheral blood. Moreover, we were concerned about the side effects of anti-CTLA-4 therapy, and regardless, the patient would not have been able to receive anti-CTLA-4 therapy because this drug was not available in China.

The choice of radiotherapy dose is the other key aspect of the combination therapy, and SBRT may be the best option [29]. Compared with conventional fractionated radiotherapy, preclinical studies confirmed that SBRT can promote the host anti-tumour immune

Table 1 Ten studies of HPD involved radiotherapy

Year	Author	Tumor types	The number of cases of HPD	Radiotherapy strategy	Type of ICB	Relationship between radiotherapy and HPD
2016	Champiat [9]	Solid tumors	12	Not described	Anti-PD-1 Anti-PD-L1	Unrelated
2016	Alexander [14]	Renal cancer	1	20 Gy in 5 fractions	Anti-PD-1	Unrelated
2017	Kato [15]	Endometrial stromal sarcoma	1	SBRT	Anti-PD-1	Not described
		Breast cancer	1	Not described	Anti-PD-1	Not described
2017	Saâda-Bouzid [13]	Head and neck cancers	10	Not described	Anti-PD-1 Anti-PD-L1	Related
2017	Yoshida T [16]	Lung cancer	1	60 Gy	Anti-PD-1	Related
2018	Ogata [17]	Gastric cancer	1	50.4 Gy in 28 fractions	Anti-PD-1	Related
2018	Du [18]	Lung cancer	1	8 Gy in 1 fraction	Anti-PD-1	Related
2018	Ferrara [12]	Lung cancer	56	Not described	Anti-PD-1 Anti-PD-L1	Not described
2019	Yilmaz [19]	Melanoma	1	Not described	Anti-PD-1	Related
2019	Bosch-Barrera [20]	Lung cancer	1	8 Gy in 1 fraction	Anti-PD-L1	Not described

response through several potential mechanisms, including normalisation of microvessels to alleviate tumour hypoxia, improvement in efficient delivery of drugs, abundant neoantigen exposure, and recruitment of anti-tumour immune cells to alter the immunosuppressive tumour microenvironment [29–32]. Several clinical studies have reported that the combination of SBRT with immunotherapy has shown favourable curative effect [6, 33, 34]. Two recent clinical trials also found that ICIs combined with SBRT show good prospects for the treatment of renal cell carcinoma [35, 36]; therefore, our patient was treated with SBRT at a dose of 24 Gy for 3 fractions. However, there were also two cases reported in which the patients developed HPD following SBRT combined with ICIs. One NSCLC patient was mentioned above in this paper [18]. Another patient with endometrial stromal sarcoma experienced HPD after treatment with nivolumab combined with SBRT [15]; however, the strategy of combined treatment administered in this case was not described in detail. The patient was found to have MDM2 amplifications and that was considered the primary cause of HPD. Nevertheless, our patient did not have any gene mutation associated with HPD, including MDM2/MDM4 and EGFR.

While two cases are not enough to conclude that SBRT was associated with HPD, studies have also suggested that SBRT can suppress the immune system. For example, research has found that SBRT can increase the relative number of Tregs [23]. However, Cho et al. reported that compared with SBRT, multiple courses of radiotherapy and high total dose significantly increased the risk of lymphopenia in patients receiving immunotherapy for NSCLC, who showed poorer PFS and OS than those who did not receive immunotherapy [21]. In an attempt to activate the immune system and directly kill the local tumour, we administered SBRT followed by the conventional fractioned radiotherapy. This type of radiotherapy strategy may be counterproductive. Moreover, Tang et al. reported that a larger target volume was associated with severe lymphopenia [37]. These factors may have caused lymphopenia and HPD in our patient.

The patient had received sorafenib and pazopanib as first- and second-line treatments, respectively. However, Zhao et al. found that sorafenib may cause the loss of T-cell immune response by inducing apoptosis and targeting LCK [38]. Sunitinib, another renal cancer-targeted drug, has been found to prevent T-cell-mediated immune response [39]. Despite the aforementioned issues, ICIs combined with targeted drugs have already been approved for the treatment of advanced renal cell carcinoma, and there are no reports indicating a higher rate of HPD than that in other solid tumours to date. Therefore, targeted drugs may not be a risk factor for HPD.

The TMB of our patient was very high. Although the prognostic role of TMB in cancer patients receiving ICIs is controversial, some studies have found that high TMB predicts better efficacy of ICIs [40, 41]. However, Kim et al. reported that HPD is not associated with TMB and PD-L1 expression [42]. In addition, our patient developed severe immune-related adverse events. Several studies have found that immune-related adverse events are associated with a better outcome after treatment with ICIs [43–45]. However, Kanjanapan et al. reported that HPD was not associated with immune-related adverse events [46]. Therefore, the positive correlative factors of the effect of ICIs may be irrelevant to HPD.

In conclusion, this report describes the development of HPD in a case of advanced renal cell cancer following the administration of radiotherapy combined with an ICI. We argue that radiotherapy may show bidirectional regulation effects on anti-tumour immune response, and if the immunosuppressive function of these treatments is dominant, combination with ICIs could result in treatment failure or even HPD. In contrast, the positive correlative factors of the effect of ICI, including TMB and PD-L1 expression and immune-related adverse events, may be irrelevant to HPD. Further research is needed to elucidate the mechanisms of these associations.

Abbreviations

CTLA-4: Cytotoxic T lymphocyte antigen; HPD: Hyperprogressive disease; ICI: Immune checkpoint inhibitor; NSCLC: Non-small cell lung cancer; OS: Overall survival; PD-1: Programmed death 1; PD-L1: Programmed death-ligand 1; PFS: Progression-free survival; SBRT: Stereotactic body radiation therapy; TIL: Tumour-infiltrating lymphocyte; TMB: Tumour mutation burden.

Supplementary Information

Additional file 1: Fig. S1. Haematoxylin and eosin staining of the lung metastasis biopsy sample showed no infiltration of lymphocytes.

Acknowledgements

Not applicable.

Authors' contributions

CL provided patient care, interpreted the data, and drafted the manuscript. JP contributed to the expansion of the literature review. ZS revised the initial draft and reviewed the manuscript. All authors read and approved the final manuscript.

Author details

[1] Department of Oncology, Zhuozhou Hospital, No.129, Fanyang Road, Zhuozhou City, Hebei Province, China. [2] College of Nursing, Hebei University of Chinese Medicine, Shijiazhuang, Hebei Province, China.

References

1. Frey B, Rubner Y, Wunderlich R, et al. Induction of abscopal anti-tumor immunity and immunogenic tumor cell death by ionizing irradiation-implications for cancer therapies. Curr Med Chem. 2012;19(12):1751.
2. Demaria S, Ng B, Devitt ML, et al. Ionizing radiation inhibition of distant untreated tumors (abscopal effect) is immune mediated. Int J Radiat Oncol Biol Phys. 2004;58(3):862–70. https://doi.org/10.1016/j.ijrobp.2003.09.012.
3. Shaverdian N, Lisberg AE, Bornazyan B, et al. Previous radiotherapy and the clinical activity and toxicity of pembrolizumab in the treatment of non-small-cell lung cancer: a secondary analysis of the KEYNOTE-001 phase 1 trial. Lancet Oncol. 2017;18(7):895–903. https://doi.org/10.1016/S1470-2045(17)30380-7.
4. Antonia SJ, Villegas A, Daniel D, et al. Overall survival with durvalumab after chemoradiotherapy in stage III NSCLC. N Engl J Med. 2018;379(24):2342–50. https://doi.org/10.1056/NEJMoa1809697.
5. Tang J, Yu JX, Vanessa M, et al. The clinical trial landscape for PD1/ PDL1 immune checkpoint inhibitors. Nat Rev Drug Discov. 2018;17:854–5.
6. Golden EB, Demaria S, Schiff PB, et al. An abscopal response to radiation and ipilimumab in a patient with metastatic non-small cell lung cancer. Cancer Immunol Res. 2013;1(6):365–72.
7. Koller KM, Mackley HB, Liu J, et al. Improved survival and complete response rates in patients with advanced melanoma treated with concurrent ipilimumab and radiotherapy versus ipilimumab alone. Cancer Biol Ther. 2016;18(1):36–42. https://doi.org/10.1080/15384047.2016.1264543.
8. Postow MA, Callahan MK, Barker CA, et al. Immunologic correlates of the abscopal effect in a patient with melanoma. N Engl J Med. 2012;366(10):925–31. https://doi.org/10.1056/NEJMoa1112824.
9. Champiat S, Dercle L, Ammari S, et al. Hyperprogressive disease is a new pattern of progression in cancer patients treated by anti-PD-1/PD-L1. Clin Cancer Res. 2017;23(8):1920–8. https://doi.org/10.1158/1078-0432.CCR-16-1741.
10. Wang X, Wang F, Zhong M, et al. The biomarkers of hyperprogressive disease in PD-1/PD-L1 blockage therapy. Mol Cancer. 2020;19(1):81. https://doi.org/10.1186/s12943-020-01200-x.
11. Kim JY, Lee KH, Kang J, et al. Hyperprogressive disease during anti-PD-1 (PDCD1)/PD-L1 (CD274) therapy: a systematic review and meta-analysis. Cancers. 2019;11(11):1699. https://doi.org/10.3390/cancers11111699.
12. Ferrara R, Mezquita L, Texier M, et al. Hyperprogressive disease in patients with advanced non-small cell lung cancer treated with PD-1/PD-L1 inhibitors or with single-agent chemotherapy. JAMA Oncol. 2018;4(11):1543. https://doi.org/10.1001/jamaoncol.2018.36762018-11-01.
13. Saâda-Bouzid E, Defaucheux C, Karabajakian A, et al. Palomar Coloma. Hyperprogression during anti-PD-1/PD-L1 therapy in patients with recurrent and/or metastatic head and neck squamous cell carcinoma. Ann Oncol. 2017;28(7):1605–11.
14. Alexander GS, Palmer JD, Tuluc M, et al. Immune biomarkers of treatment failure for a patient on a phase I clinical trial of pembrolizumab plus radiotherapy. J Hematol Oncol. 2016;9(1):96–7.
15. Kato S, Goodman A, Walavalkar V, et al. Hyperprogressors after immunotherapy: analysis of genomic alterations associated with accelerated growth rate. Clin Cancer Res. 2017;23(15):4242–50.
16. Yoshida T, Furuta H, Hida T. Risk of tumor flare after nivolumab treatment in patients with irradiated field recurrence. Med Oncol. 2017. https://doi.org/10.1007/s12032-017-0895-4.
17. Ogata T, Satake H, Ogata M, et al. Hyperprogressive disease in the irradiation field after a single dose of nivolumab for gastric cancer: a case report. Case Rep Oncol. 2018;11(1):143–50.
18. Du S, McCall N, Park K, et al. Blockade of tumor-expressed PD-1 promotes lung cancer growth. Oncoimmunology. 2018;7(4):e1408747. https://doi.org/10.1080/2162402X.2017.1408747.
19. Yilmaz M, Akovali B. Hyperprogression after nivolumab for melanoma: a case report. J Oncol Pharm Pract. 2020;26(1):244–51. https://doi.org/10.1177/1078155219845436
20. Bosch-Barrera J, Oliva E, Sais E, et al. Hyperprogression after first dose of immunotherapy in a patient with radioresistant metastasis from nonsmall cell lung cancer. Anticancer Drugs. 2019;30(10):1067–70.
21. Cho Y, Park S, Byun HK, et al. Impact of treatment-related lymphopenia on immunotherapy for advanced non-small cell lung cancer. Int J Radiat Oncol Biol Phys. 2019;105(5):1065–73.
22. Persa E, Balogh A, Safrany G, et al. The effect of ionizing radiation on regulatory T cells in health and disease. Cancer Lett. 2015;368(2):252–61. https://doi.org/10.1016/j.canlet.2015.03.003.
23. Schaue D, Ratikan JA, Iwamoto KS, et al. Maximizing tumor immunity with fractionated radiation. Int J Radiat Oncol Biol Phys. 2012;83(4):1306–10.
24. Qu Y, Jin S, Zhang A, et al. Gamma-ray resistance of regulatory CD4+CD25+ Foxp3+ T cells in mice. Radiat Res. 2010;173(2):148–57.
25. Muroyama Y, Nirschl TR, Kochel CM, et al. Stereotactic radiotherapy increases functionally suppressive regulatory T cells in the tumor micro-environment. Cancer Immunol Res. 2017;5(11):992–1004.
26. Wirsdorfer F, Cappuccini F, Niazman M, et al. Thorax irradiation triggers a local and systemic accumulation of immunosuppressive CD4+ FoxP3+ regulatory T cells. Radiat Oncol. 2014;9(1):98. https://doi.org/10.1186/1748-717X-9-98.
27. Kamada T, Togashi Y, Tay C, et al. PD-1+ regulatory T cells amplified by PD-1 blockade promote hyperprogression of cancer. Proc Natl Acad Sci USA. 2019;116(20):9999–10008.
28. Romano E, Kusio-Kobialka M, Foukas PG, et al. Ipilimumab-dependent cell-mediated cytotoxicity of regulatory T cells ex vivo by nonclassical monocytes in melanoma patients. Proc Natl Acad Sci USA. 2015;112(19):6140–5. https://doi.org/10.1073/pnas.1417320112.
29. Bernstein MB, Krishnan S, Hodge JW, et al. Immunotherapy and stereotactic ablative radiotherapy (ISABR): a curative approach? Nat Rev Clin Oncol. 2016;13(8):516–24.
30. Sun XW, Gan L, Na A, et al. Combination with stereotactic body radiotherapy offers a promising strategy to overcome resistance to immunotherapy in advanced renal cell cancer. J Oncol. 2019;2019:1–12. https://doi.org/10.1155/2019/1483406.
31. Lugade AA, Moran JP, Gerber SA, et al. Local radiation therapy of B16 melanoma tumors increases the generation of tumor antigen-specific effector cells that traffic to the tumor. J Immunol. 2005;174(12):7516–23.
32. Lee Y, Auh SL, Wang Y, et al. Therapeutic effects of ablative radiation on local tumor require CD8+ T cells: changing strategies for cancer treatment. Blood. 2009;114(3):589–95.
33. Hiniker SM, Chen DS, Reddy S, et al. A systemic complete response of metastatic melanoma to local radiation and immunotherapy. Transl Oncol. 2012;5(6):404–7.
34. LaPlant Q, Deselm C, Lockney NA, et al. Potential abscopal response to dual checkpoint blockade in RCC after reirradiation using dose-painting SBRT. Pract Radiat Oncol. 2016;7(6):396–9. https://doi.org/10.1016/j.prro.2017.04.009.
35. Masini C, Iotti C, De Giorgi U, et al. Nivolumab in combination with stereotactic body radiotherapy in pretreated patients with metastatic renal cell carcinoma: first results of the phase II NIVES study. 2020 Genitourinary Cancers Symposium. Abstract 613. Presented February 15, 2020.
36. Hammers HJ, Vonmerveldt D, Ahn C, et al. Combination of dual immune checkpoint inhibition with stereotactic radiation in metastatic renal cell carcinoma. 2020 Genitourinary Cancers Symposium. Abstract 614. Presented February 15, 2020.
37. Tang C, Liao Z, Gomez D, et al. Lymphopenia association with gross tumor volume and lung V5 and its effects on non-small cell lung cancer patient outcomes. Int J Radiat Oncol Biol Phys. 2014;89(5):1084–91.
38. Zhao W, Gu YH, Song R, et al. Sorafenib inhibits activation of human peripheral blood T cells by targeting LCK phosphorylation. Leukemia. 2008;22(6):1226–33.
39. Gu Y, Zhao W, Meng F, et al. Sunitinib impairs the proliferation and function of human peripheral T cell and prevents T-cell-mediated immune response in mice. Clin Immunol. 2010;135(1):55–62. https://doi.org/10.1016/j.clim.2009.11.013.
40. Cao D, Xu H, Xu X, et al. High tumor mutation burden predicts better efficacy of immunotherapy: a pooled analysis of 103078 cancer patients. Oncoimmunology. 2019;8(9):e1629258. https://doi.org/10.1080/2162402X.2019.1629258pmid:31428527.
41. Samstein RM, Lee CH, Shoushtari AN, et al. Tumor mutational load predicts survival after immunotherapy across multiple cancer types. Nat Genet. 2019;51(2):202–6. https://doi.org/10.1038/s41588-018-0312-8.

42. Kim CG, Kim KH, Pyo KH, et al. Hyperprogressive disease during PD-1/PD-L1 blockade in patients with non-small-cell lung cancer. Ann Oncol. 2019;30(7):1104–13.
43. Maher VE, Fernandes LL, Weinstock C, et al. Analysis of the association between adverse events and outcome in patients receiving a programmed death protein 1 or programmed death ligand 1 antibody. J Clin Oncol. 2019;37(30):2730–7. https://doi.org/10.1200/JCO.19.
44. Berner F, Bomze D, Diem S, et al. Association of checkpoint inhibitor-induced toxic effects with shared cancer and tissue antigens in non-small cell lung cancer. Jama Oncol. 2019;5(7):1043. https://doi.org/10.1001/jamaoncol.2019.0402.
45. Teraoka S, Fujimoto S, Morimoto T, et al. Early immune-related adverse events and association with outcome in advanced non-small cell lung cancer patients treated with nivolumab: a prospective cohort study. J Thorac Oncol. 2017;12(12):1798–805.
46. Kanjanapan Y, Day D, Wang L, et al. Hyperprogressive disease in early-phase immunotherapy trials: clinical predictors and association with immune-related toxicities. Cancer. 2019;125(8):1341–9. https://doi.org/10.1002/cncr.31999.

11

Calcitriol-mediated hypercalcemia as an immune-related adverse event in a patient receiving nivolumab and ipilimumab for metastatic renal cell carcinoma, case report

Kai Johnson, Majd Issa, Anish Parikh, Paul Monk, Ming Yin, Amir Mortazavi and Yuanquan Yang*

Abstract

Background: Severe hypercalcemia is often associated with uncontrolled malignancy through several mechanisms. However, calcitriol-mediated hypercalcemia is a rare etiology for advanced solid tumors.

Case presentation: We report a case of calcitriol-mediated hypercalcemia secondary to immune checkpoint inhibition in a responder with metastatic clear cell renal cell carcinoma (ccRCC). In this case, a 68 year old male with metastatic ccRCC to the liver within 4 months of right radical nephrectomy went on to develop hypercalcemia (12.8 mg/dL) shortly following 2 cycles of nivolumab and ipilimumab. Additional testing showed an elevated calcitriol level (142 pg/mL), low parathyroid hormone (PTH) and parathyroid hormone-related protein (PTHrP) levels, and a normal 25-hydroxyvitamin D level. FDG-PET imaging showed hypermetabolic mediastinal, hilar, and intra-abdominal lymphadenopathy, however the subsequent lymph node biopsy only showed reactive lymphoid cells without malignancy or granuloma. The hypercalcemia was resistant to initial therapy with calcitonin, hydration, and zoledronic acid but quickly responded to high-dose prednisone (1 mg/kg), followed by normalization of calcitriol levels. The patient was rechallenged with nivolumab and ipilimumab which provided a partial response after 4 cycles. He was maintained on low dose prednisone (10 mg daily) leading to a sustained resolution of his hypercalcemia.

Conclusion: This case suggests calcitriol-mediated hypercalcemia as a novel immune-related adverse event.

Keywords: Autoimmunity, Case report, Immunotherapy, Kidney neoplasms, Urologic neoplasms

Background

In the setting of malignancy, multiple mechanisms have been found to cause hypercalcemia. The most common of these are local osteolysis due to bony invasion from solid and hematologic malignancies (e.g., breast cancer), humoral hypercalcemia of malignancy due to paraneoplastic hormones (e.g., PTHrP), ectopic hyperparathyroidism, and calcitriol-secreting tumors (e.g., lymphoma) [1, 2]. Calcitriol-mediated hypercalcemia accounts for approximately 1% of cases of hypercalcemia in the setting of malignancy [3]. Under normal physiologic circumstances, vitamin D is stored in the liver as 25-hydroxyvitamin D. When hypocalcemic, it is released due to the presence of PTH before ultimately undergoing conversion to calcitriol by renal 1-α-hydroxylase. Calcitriol then signals for both increased calcium absorption via the intestines, as well as increased osteolytic activity in the bone. The cumulative effect leads to improved serum calcium levels. Certain malignancies are able to produce extra-renal 1-alpha-hydroxylase, leading to increased

*Correspondence: yuanquan.yang@osumc.edu
Medical Oncology, Ohio State University James Cancer Hospital, Suite 1335 Lincoln Tower, 1800 Cannon Drive, Columbus, OH 43210, USA

production of calcitriol. This is true most commonly with lymphoid malignancies, especially in the setting of progressive disease, whereas with solid tumors this is a rare occurrence [4]. In such rare cases involving solid tumors, alternative mechanisms for explaining calcitriol-mediated hypercalcemia must be explored, particularly when therapies themselves may play a role, such as in the case described below.

Case presentation

The case involves a 68 year old male with metastatic clear cell renal cell carcinoma (ccRCC). His medical history was significant for well-controlled hypertension, stage 3 chronic kidney disease, and psoriatic arthritis which was controlled with hydroxychloroquine maintenance. He was referred to our clinic after presenting to a local provider with acute gross hematuria. He underwent a CT urogram that revealed a 7.3 cm mass in the right kidney with renal vein invasion and small, non-specific pulmonary nodules in the bilateral lung bases. He underwent a right radical nephrectomy within a month of his initial diagnosis. Pathology revealed a 6 cm (pT3a pNx) WHO grade 4 renal cell carcinoma, clear cell type. The tumor extended to the resection margin of the renal vein. Adjuvant radiation was not recommended at that time and he was placed on surveillance. Restaging scans four months after surgery showed stable sub-centimeter pulmonary nodules and multiple new hypodense hepatic lesions, the largest being 5.7 × 4.4 cm involving the central right hepatic lobe. No bone metastases were identified on imaging. A liver biopsy confirmed the diagnosis of metastatic ccRCC. He was then initiated on nivolumab 3 mg/kg and ipilimumab 1 mg/kg shortly afterwards. He tolerated the first cycle well but did develop a grade 1 rash involving his chest within a week of the infusion. This resolved with use of topical steroids. Two days following his cycle 2 infusion, he began to develop arthralgias that were attributed to a flare of his known psoriatic arthritis. On day 7 of cycle 2, he noticed progressive fatigue and nausea. On day 14 of cycle 2, he had an episode of emesis and was brought back to our clinic given his progression of symptoms. Routine labs at the time revealed new hypercalcemia to 12.8 mg/dL (previously 9.6 mg/dL two weeks prior) and that he had developed an acute kidney injury (creatinine 3.62 mg/dL, up from baseline of 1.6 to 1.9 mg/dL). He was admitted to our inpatient service for further testing, part of which is summarized in Table 1.

His inpatient workup was significant for an elevated 1, 25-dihydroxyvitamin D3 (calcitriol) level of 142 pg/mL (reference 20–79 pg/mL) in the presence of low-normal 25-hydroxyvitamin D (25{OH} D) at 36.7 ng/mL (reference 30–100 ng/mL), suggesting alpha hydroxylation. Other hypercalcemia testing revealed an elevated phosphorus level of 5.4 mg/dL (reference 2.2–4.6 mg/dL), a suppressed parathyroid hormone (PTH) of less than 6.3 pg/mL (reference 14.0–72.0 pg/mL), a low parathyroid hormone-related peptide (PTHrP) of 0.7 pmol/L (reference ≤ 4.2 pmol/L), an elevated adrenocorticotropic hormone (ACTH) level of 273.0 pg/mL (reference 9.0–50.0 pg/mL), an elevated cortisol level of 37.03 mcg/dL (reference 3.09–22.40 mcg/dL), a normal alkaline phosphatase level of 110 U/L (reference 32–126 U/L), and a normal angiotensin-converting enzyme level of 62 ng/dL (reference 9–67 ng/dL). FDG-PET imaging showed multiple hypermetabolic mediastinal, hilar and intra-abdominal lymph nodes (max SUV of 15), as illustrated in Fig. 1. The liver lesions themselves *were* not FDG-avid but were stable in size, as were his prior lung nodules. He underwent a bronchoscopy with biopsy of four separate lymph nodes, none of which demonstrated malignancy nor granulomatous disease. He was initially treated with intravenous normal saline, calcitonin 4 units/kg every 12 h and 4 mg zoledronic acid. Despite seven days of aggressive treatment, his hypercalcemia persisted, as shown in Fig. 2. He was then started on 1 mg/kg of oral prednisone both for this calcitriol-mediated

Table 1 Summary of lab tests performed and their respective values along with reference ranges

Lab test	Lab value
1, 25-dihydroxyvitamin D3 (calcitriol)	142 pg/ml (reference 20–79 pg/ml)
25-hydroxyvitamin D (25{OH}D)	36.7 ng/mL (reference 30–100 ng/mL)
Phosphorous	5.4 mg/dL (reference 2.2–4.6 mg/dL)
Parathyroid hormone (PTH)	< 6.3 pg/mL (reference 14.0–72.0 pg/mL)
Parathyroid hormone-related peptide (PTHrP)	0.7 pmol/L (reference ≤ 4.2 pmol/L)
Adrenocorticotropic hormone (ACTH)	273.0 pg/mL (reference 9.0–50.0 pg/mL)
Cortisol	37.03 mcg/dL (reference 3.09–22.40 mcg/dL)
Angiotensin-converting enzyme level	62 ng/dL (reference 9–67 ng/dL)
Alkaline phosphatase	110 U/L (reference 32–126 U/L)

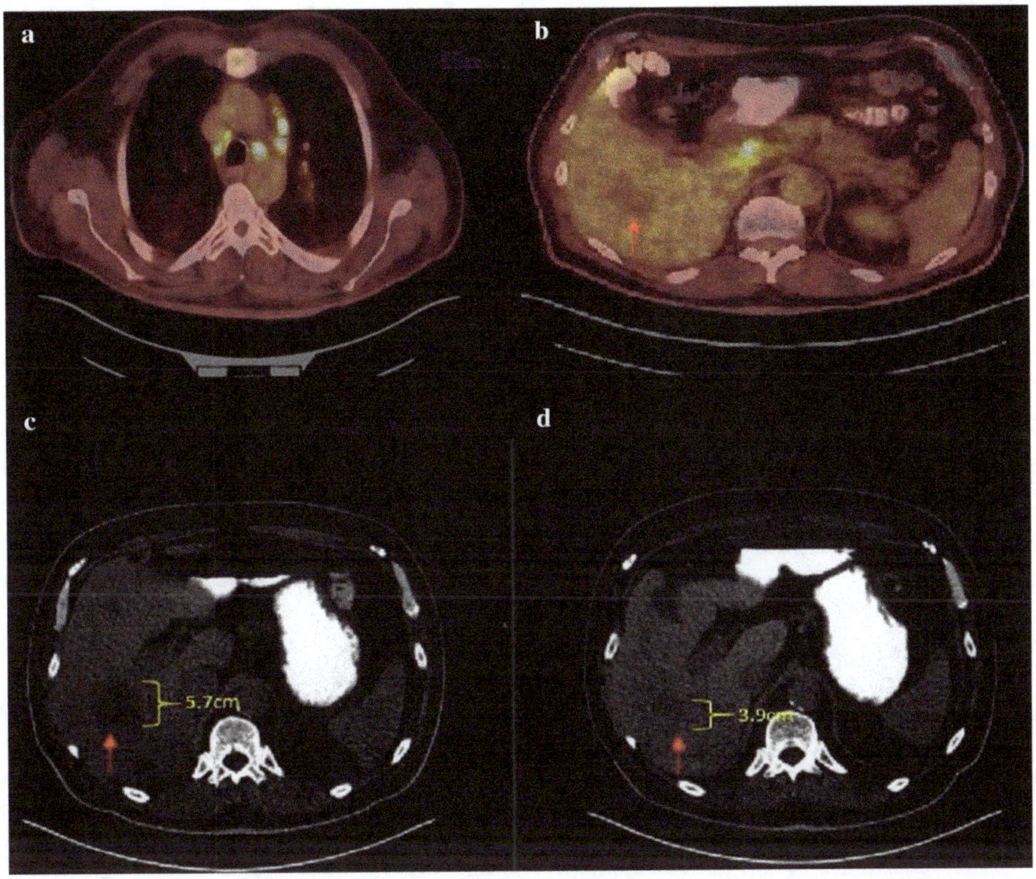

Fig. 1 **a** FDG-PET/CT demonstrating hypermetabolic mediastinal lymph nodes. **b** FDG-PET/CT showing a hypermetabolic portacaval lymph node, though the known liver metastasis was not FDG-avid (red arrow). Below these PET images, two CT scans of the abdomen & pelvis are shown: one before treatment was initiated (**c**) and one 6 months after treatment was completed (**d**). The dominant right liver lesion decreased from 5.7 × 4.4 cm to 3.9 × 3.6 cm in size (red arrow)

hypercalcemia as well as for his ongoing psoriatic arthritis flare. Within two days of starting systemic steroids, the patient's calcitriol level normalized (56.6 pg/mL), as did his calcium level (8.9 mg/dL). He reported notable relief of arthritic symptoms immediately. He was then discharged home and slowly weaned down to prednisone 10 mg daily, which was continued for control of his arthritis.

As an outpatient, he was re-challenged with nivolumab and ipilimumab 1 month later. Restaging CT scans after cycle 4 revealed an overall partial response, with the largest liver lesion shrinking by 32% in the long-axis (3.6 × 3.9 cm from 4.4 × 5.7 cm), as seen in Fig. 1. Prior to receiving cycle 6 nivolumab maintenance, routine lab work showed the development of immunotherapy-related hypothyroidism for which thyroid hormone replacement therapy was started. He remains on nivolumab maintenance therapy with ongoing partial response of his disease, no recurrent hypercalcemia, and no further immunotherapy-related adverse events (irAE) to date.

Discussion and conclusions

We report the first-known case of calcitriol-mediated hypercalcemia associated with immunotherapy. We come to this etiologic conclusion given the laboratory findings of a suppressed PTH, low PTHrP, and an elevated calcitriol level. In addition, multiple PET-avid mediastinal lymph nodes were biopsied and failed to demonstrate the presence of malignancy or granulomatous disease, though this does not definitively rule out either condition. Our suspicion that this may be an irAE is based on multiple factors, including onset soon after immunotherapy initiation, the concurrent worsening of his chronic autoimmune disorder (psoriatic arthritis), the rapid normalization of calcitriol levels with the introduction of high-dose glucocorticoid therapy, and partial responses noted on restaging scans. Given these findings, it seems likely that this episode of calcitriol-mediated hypercalcemia was in relation to immune checkpoint blockade.

Despite this likely association, the mechanism of dysregulated calcitriol production in the setting of

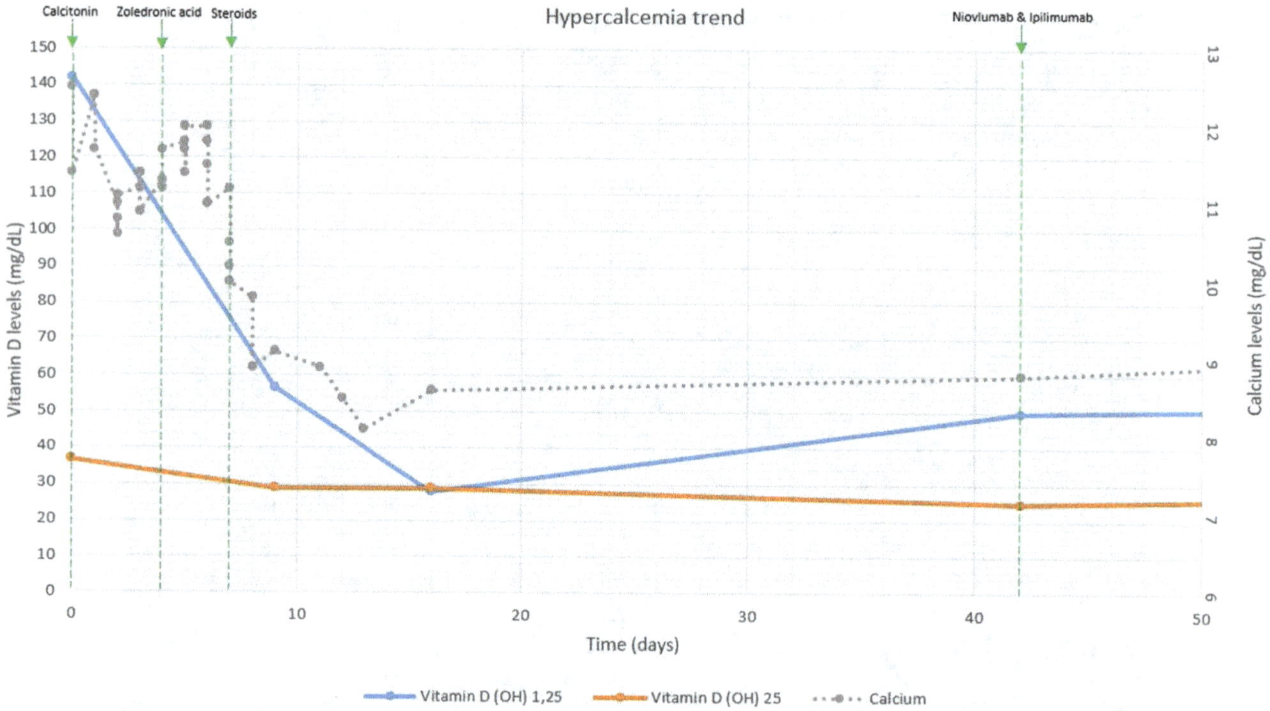

Fig. 2 This graph demonstrates the changes in levels of calcium (shown in gray), 1, 25(OH) D (shown in blue), and 25(OH) D (shown in orange) throughout the patient's hospitalization as various treatments were provided as labeled above. The X axis represents time measured in days. The left Y axis illustrates vitamin D levels in mg/dL. The right Y axis demonstrates the calcium levels in mg/dL. The green dashed lines indicate the start dates for the various treatments described above including steroids (prednisone), zoledronic acid, calcitonin, and immunotherapy (nivolumab and ipilimumab re-challenge)

immunotherapy is unclear. It is well-known that certain inflammatory conditions with granuloma formation, such as sarcoidosis, can present with calcitriol-induced hypercalcemia [5]. This process is mediated through the abnormal activation of macrophages, which play an important role in calcium homeostasis. They are an extra-renal source of calcitriol production through stimulation of their own unique 25(OH) D-hydroxylase enzyme, which is insensitive to PTH and is less susceptible to negative inhibition through its substrate as compared to its renal counterpart [6–8]. A subset of macrophages from cancer patients also express PD-1 [9]. The blockade of PD-1/PD-L1 with monoclonal antibodies can activate macrophages, increase phagocytosis activity and reduce tumor growth. It is possible that the calcitriol-mediated hypercalcemia of our patient was due to macrophage activation by nivolumab, an anti-PD-1 antibody. Furthermore, it is well-established that PD-1/PD-L1 blockade activates T cells. Activated T cells express an increased level of 25(OH) D-hydroxylase [10]. The local conversion of 25(OH) vitamin D to 1, 25$(OH)_2$ vitamin D is important for T cell function [11]. Corticosteroids help block hydroxylase enzymes responsible for this vitamin D conversion as well as inhibit osteoclast resorption through suppression of tumor cytokine production [12].

In conclusion, we report a rare case of calcitriol-mediated hypercalcemia as a novel immunotherapy-related adverse event in the absence of granulomas. Steroids played a central role in the management of this case. Additional study is needed to further characterize calcitriol production in response to immunotherapy within various immune cell types in vitro and the role of vitamin D supplementation in cancer immunotherapy.

Abbreviations

ccRCC: Clear cell renal cell carcinoma; PTH: Parathyroid hormone; PTHrP: Parathyroid hormone-related peptide; ACTH: Adrenocorticotropic hormone; SUV: Standardized uptake values; irAE: Immunotherapy-related adverse events.

Acknowledgements

We thank the patient for giving us permission to publish this report.

Authors' contributions

KJ, MI, and YY collected data, analyzed data, and prepared the manuscript; AP, PM, MY, and AM reviewed and edited the manuscript. All authors have read and approved the manuscript. All authors read and approved the final manuscript.

References

1. Clines GA, Guise TA. Hypercalcaemia of malignancy and basic research on mechanisms responsible for osteolytic and osteoblastic metastasis to bone. Endocr Relat Cancer. 2005;12:549–83.
2. Stewart AF. Hypercalcemia associated with cancer. N Engl J Med. 2005;352:373–9. https://doi.org/10.1056/NEJMcp042806.
3. Goldner W. Cancer-related hypercalcemia. J Oncol Pract. 2016;12(5):426–32. https://doi.org/10.1200/JOP.2016.011155.
4. Shallis RM, Rome RS, Reagan JL. Mechanisms of hypercalcemia in non-hodgkin lymphoma and associated outcomes: a retrospective review. Clin Lymphoma Myeloma Leuk. 2018;18(2):e123–9. https://doi.org/10.1016/j.clml.2017.12.006.
5. Adams JS, Sharma OP, Gacad MA, Singer FR. Metabolism of 25-hydroxyvitamin D3 by cultured pulmonary alveolar macrophages in sarcoidosis. J Clin Invest. 1983;72:1856–60.
6. Tobler A, Gasson J, Reichel H, Norman AW, Koeffler HP. Granulocyte-macrophage colony-stimulating factor: Sensitive and receptor-mediated regulation by 1,25-dihydroxyvitamin D3 in normal human peripheral blood lymphocytes. J Clin Invest. 1987;79:1700–5.
7. Monkawa T, Yoshida T, Hayashi M, Saruta T. Identification of 25-hydroxyvitamin D3 1alpha-hydroxylase gene expression in macrophages. Kidney Int. 2000;58(2):559–68. https://doi.org/10.1046/j.1523-1755.2000.00202.x.
8. Murayama A, Takeyama K, Kitanaka S, Kodera Y, Kawaguchi Y, Hosoya T, Kato S. Positive and negative regulations of the renal 25-hydroxyvitamin D3 1α-hydroxylase gene by parathyroid hormone, calcitonin, and 1α,25(OH)2D3 in intact animals. Endocrinology. 1999;140:2224–31.
9. Gordon SR, Maute RL, Dulken BW, Hutter G, George BM, McCracken MN, Gupta R, Tsai JM, Sinha R, Corey D, Ring AM, Connolly AJ, Weissman IL. PD-1 expression by tumour-associated macrophages inhibits phagocytosis and tumour immunity. Nature. 2017;545(7655):495–9. https://doi.org/10.1038/nature22396.
10. Bikle DD, Patzek S, Wang Y. Physiologic and pathophysiologic roles of extra renal CYP27b1: case report and review. Bone Rep. 2018;8:255–67. https://doi.org/10.1016/j.bonr.2018.02.004.
11. Kongsbak M, von Essen MR, Levring TB, et al. Vitamin D-binding protein controls T cell responses to vitamin D. BMC Immunol. 2014;15:35. https://doi.org/10.1186/s12865-014-0035-2.
12. Asonitis N, Angelousi A, Zafeiris C, Lambrou GI, Dontas I, Kassi E. Diagnosis, pathophysiology and management of hypercalcemia in malignancy: a review of the literature. Horm Metab Res. 2019;51(12):770–8. https://doi.org/10.1055/a-1049-0647 (**Epub 2019 Dec 11 PMID: 31826272**).

12

The diagnostic utility of diffusion weighted MRI imaging and ADC ratio to distinguish benign from malignant renal masses: Sorting the kittens from the tigers

Suresh de Silva[1,2*], Kathleen Rebecca Lockhart[3], Peter Aslan[3], Peter Nash[3], Anthony Hutton[1,3], David Malouf[3], Dominic Lee[3], Paul Cozzi[4], Fiona MacLean[5] and James Thompson[1,3]

Abstract

Background: MRI is playing an increasing role in risk stratification and non-invasive diagnosis of the undifferentiated small renal mass. This study was designed to assess the reliability of MRI in diagnostic evaluation of renal masses, specifically characterising lesions with diffusion weighted imaging (DWI) and apparent diffusion coefficient (ADC) values.

Methods: This is a retrospective analysis of patients undergoing MRI as part of their clinical workup for a renal mass suspicious for renal cell carcinoma (RCC) on CT or ultrasound followed by biopsy and/or surgical excision. All cases were conducted on 3 Tesla MRI, with conventional breath-held sequences, DWI and dynamic contrast enhanced phases. Tumour regions of interest were evaluated on ADC maps and compared with T2 weighted and post-contrast images.

Results: Of the 66 renal tumours included, 33 (50.0%) were Clear Cell RCC, 11 (16.7%) were Oncocytoma, nine (13.6%) were Angiomyolipoma (AML), nine (13.6%) were Papillary RCC and four (6.1%) were Chromophobe RCC. Oncocytoma had the largest ADC values, significantly larger than AMLs and all RCC subtypes ($p < 0.001$). The average ADC value was also significantly larger in Clear Cell RCCs compared to AMLs, and other RCC subtypes ($p < 0.001$).

Conclusions: MRI with DWI/ADC imaging may aid the differentiation of oncocytomas from RCCs and stratify RCC subtypes, Further studies are required to validate these findings.

Trial registration: Not applicable/retrospective study.

Keywords: Renal neoplasms, Radiology, Urology, Magnetic resonance imaging

Background

The incidental renal mass is a common diagnostic and management dilemma, since the widespread adoption of Computed Tomography (CT) and Ultrasound (US) in recent decades. Surgical resection is often considered the gold standard treatment as the majority are renal cell carcinomas (RCC). However, up to 33% of excised or biopsied renal masses have benign or indolent histopathology [1, 2]. If the nature of those masses could be reliably established by imaging then these patients could be spared the nephron loss, risks and costs of surgical intervention.

Conventional imaging cannot reliably differentiate benign or low-grade malignancies from high-grade malignancies. For example, benign oncocytomas, minimal fat angiomyolipomas (AMLs) and RCCs can have

*Correspondence: suresh.desilva@unsw.edu.au
[1] Faculty of Medicine, University of NSW, Kensington, NSW, Australia
Full list of author information is available at the end of the article

very similar CT and US characteristics [3]. Percutaneous biopsy aids pathological diagnosis, but risks include life-threatening bleeding, injury to surrounding organs, tumour seeding, sampling error underestimating overall grade and a significant non-diagnostic rate of 10–23% (often due to insufficient material) [1, 2]. Additionally, some masses are not amenable to biopsy (due to factors such as medial peri-hilar tumour location, predominately cystic composition, small size, single kidney, obesity or high bleeding risk).

MRI has developed an increasing role in non-invasive urologic tumour assessment (notably in prostate cancer), including the use of diffusion weighted imaging (DWI) with apparent diffusion coefficient values (ADC) [2–5]. DWI captures inherent differences between tissues in restricting water motion (Brownian motion) and ADC is a quantitative measure derived from DWI [6]. ADC is influenced by multiple factors including cellularity (validated in numerous studies, accounting for restricted diffusion in malignancy), cell membrane integrity, nuclear to cytoplasmic ratio and viscosity [7–9]. As renal tumour types vary with these structural properties, their ADC characteristics may allow for differentiation. There remains a paucity of published data in this area.

The aims of our study were to determine whether MRI ADC characteristics can be used to differentiate renal tumour types.

Methods

This is a retrospective analysis of patients derived from a prospectively reported database of consecutive patients who underwent mpMRI for a de novo renal mass suspicious for RCC on CT or ultrasound as part of their clinical workup, followed by either percutaneous biopsy and/or surgical excision for histopathological diagnosis. All included cases were conducted on 3 Tesla (T) MRI, with improved signal-to-noise ratio/ spatial resolution compared to older 1.5 T MRI scanners. The scope of this study was only the select group for whom MRI was clinically indicated. The majority of local renal mass cases would not have had MRI or been excluded for a variety of reasons including but not limited to: pathognomonic findings on conventional imaging, offered to but declined by the patient due to personal preference for upfront biopsy/excision, symptoms requiring definitive treatment precluding need for further imaging, advanced stage of/ metastatic cancer, a large tumour, contraindicated for MRI (e.g. non compatible medical implant or foreign body, significant chronic renal impairment, claustrophobia), the patient refusing to undergo subsequent biopsy/ excision therefore the histopathological diagnosis, or a lesion ideally suited to partial nephrectomy in which MRI would be unlikely to change management.

Local health district ethical approval was obtained; individual patient consents were not sought as clinical practice was not changed in any way and all data was collected retrospectively and deidentified.

Between June 2014 and June 2019, all patients who had MRI imaging for renal masses at the same imaging facility were evaluated In total 75 renal masses with MRI imaging were included. Six were excluded due to non-standard imaging parameters or poor quality images that were not interpretable. Three masses were excluded due to (1) the presence of organising haematoma or (2) equivocal or unclassified diagnosis on histopathology. Five renal masses were diagnostic of Angiomyolipomas (AML), due to the presence of macroscopic fat without necrosis or calcification. These were included without tissue diagnosis to provide data for this benign tumour type; biopsy would have been unethical given their pathognomonic imaging findings and risk of bleeding with prominent vascularity. This left a final study cohort of 66 renal masses.

All patients underwent MRI on a 3T Siemens Skyra, using a 30 channel body array place over the pelvis and using the posterior coil elements of the in-table spine array. Scans included the following conventional non-contrast breath held sequences: Axial in and out of phase T1, Axial and Coronal 2D T2- weighted Haste, and Axial and Coronal 3D fat suppressed T1-weighted volume interpolated breathhold examination (VIBE) sequence. Dynamic contrast enhanced VIBE sequences obtained following the administration of gadolinium were included. The contrast agent (dose correlating to patient weight) was administered as an IV bolus using a power injector (Bracco) followed by a 30 ml saline flush, with both the contrast and saline injected at 2mls per second. Contrast enhanced sequences were obtained at cortico-medullary, nephrographic and excretory phases.

All scans included a DWI sequence performed in the axial plane before administration of contrast. DWI scans were a three- scan trace, monopolar with three diffusion directions. Diffusion b values were 50, 400 and 800, the DWI sequence used was 2D echoplanar, spin echo free breathing with a scan time of ~ 4:30 min. Fat Suppression was used, with a TR of 6100 ms and TE at min (~ 61 ms) ADC maps were obtained. Distortion correction was used with a noise level of 10. Slice thickness was 5 mm and 36 slices were obtained with a 38 cm FOV, EPI factor of 102 and a bandwidth of 1860 Hz/Px.

Imaging data was analysed by one sub-specialist radiologist with 15 years' experience in evaluating body MRI imaging (SD). The ADC map of each renal mass was reviewed for the qualitative ADC value most representative of the tumour and a region of interest (ROI) then measured, expressed in units of mm^2/second. The

ADC maps were evaluated in conjunction with the T2 weighted and post contrast images to ensure placement of ROIs over solid tumour (not cystic/necrotic portions). A ROI of up to 50 mm^2 was measured. In masses where qualitatively there were two ADC values which were approximately equally represented in the mass, two ROI were measured, one in each region measuring up to $50mm^2$. The combined value of these two regions averaged to obtain the ADC value.

Histopathology specimens (either biopsies, or excised specimens from partial or radical nephrectomy) were fixed in formalin, and processed in the usual manner. Microscopic examination was initially via hematoxylin and exosin stained slides, with immunoperoxidase and special stains utilized as required. The histology was diagnosed by six specialist uropathologists, and all cases were centrally reviewed by one highly experienced professor of uropathology specialising in renal histopathology (FM). All participating pathologists were blinded to the imaging results.

SPSS version 23 was used for analysis. To compare ADC values across the five lesion types investigated, analysis of variance (ANOVA) was used, accompanied by pairwise comparison of means undertaken using Tamhane's T2 method, because ADC had been captured as a continuous variable measured on a ratio/interval scale while lesion type had been captured as a categorical variable with more than two (five) categories. Tamhane's T2 method was chosen as the variance was likely to be significantly different between at least two tumour types compared. The 5% level of significance defined statistical significance.

The data analyses generated are available within the presented study but specific datasets are kept confidential due to their nature of including clinical and radiological details. Further information regarding dataset analysis may be available from the corresponding author upon request.

All methods were carried out in accordance with relevant guidelines and regulations, including those of the local health district and ethics committee.

Results

Of the 66 patients with renal MRI examined for ADC characteristics, 33 (50.0%) were Clear Cell RCC, 11 (16.7%) were Oncocytoma, nine (13.6%) were Angiomyolipoma, nine (13.6%) were Papillary Type 1 RCC and four (6.1%) were Chromophobe RCC (Fig. 1). The renal masses had an average maximal dimension of 41 mm and a range of 9-126 mm.

Oncocytoma had the largest ADC values, followed in descending order by Clear Cell RCC, Chromopohobe RCC, Papillary RCC and Angiomyolipoma. This is summarised in Fig. 2. In terms of histopathological gold standard diagnosis, 39.6% of masses were diagnosed with partial nephrectomy, 45.3% with radical nephrectomy and 15.1% with core biopsy. One patient had a non-diagnostic biopsy (this case was excluded from the analysis as described in Methods) and this patient had definitive successful focal ablation with cryotherapy.

ANOVA results indicated that the average ADC value difference was statistically significant for at least two tumour types ($p < 0.001$) with the assumptions of homogeneity of variance not being violated at the 1% level of significance ($p > 0.01$) (Table 1). Average ADC value was 2.1609 ± 0.2104 for Oncocytoma, 1.5033 ± 0.1328 for Clear Cell RCC, 1.1075 ± 0.1034 for Chromophobe RCC, 0.7611 ± 0.0942 for Papillary RCC and 0.6989 ± 0.0757 for AML (Table 1). At the 5% level of significance, the normality of distribution assumption was not violated ($p > 0.05$) (Fig. 2). Post-hoc analysis indicated that Oncocytoma average ADC value was significantly larger than that of AMLs (d=1.46202, $p < 0.001$), Papillary (d=1.39980, $p < 0.001$), Chromophobe (d=1.05341, $p < 0.001$) and Clear Cell (d=0.65758, $p < 0.001$) RCCs (Table 1). Average ADC value obtained was also significantly larger for Clear Cell RCC than for AML (d=0.80444, $p < 0.001$), Papillary RCC (d=0.74222, $p < 0.001$) and Chromophobe RCC (d=0.39583, $p < 0.001$) (Table 1). Therefore, Oncocytoma can be differentiated from other tumours types investigated based on ADC values. Similarly, Clear Cell RCC can be differentiated from Angiomyolipoma, Papillary RCC and Chromophobe RCC. Although the box plots show some overlap, this is not the ultimate decision criteria as it is based on a sample, therefore significant p-values can still be obtained when there is overlap in box-plots. The ultimate decision criteria requires inferential testing/hypothesis testing where we have used the parametric ANOVA test and pairwise comparison. This enables the accurate assessment of the exact difference in groups with the results as noted above.

Discussion

Our results indicated that the average ADC of Oncocytomas was significantly higher than in all types of RCCs and AMLs, therefore able to be reliably identified and differentiated from other tumours. An ADC value of less than 1.9505 indicates the lesion is more likely to be an RCC or AML than an Oncocytoma. The addition of MRI in diagnostic workup could overcome some limitations of biopsy which is often unable to differentiate between oncocytoma and chromophobe RCC, and potentially avoid unnecessary surgery.

Other studies have found that Oncocytomas have significantly higher ADC values than clear cell RCCs but

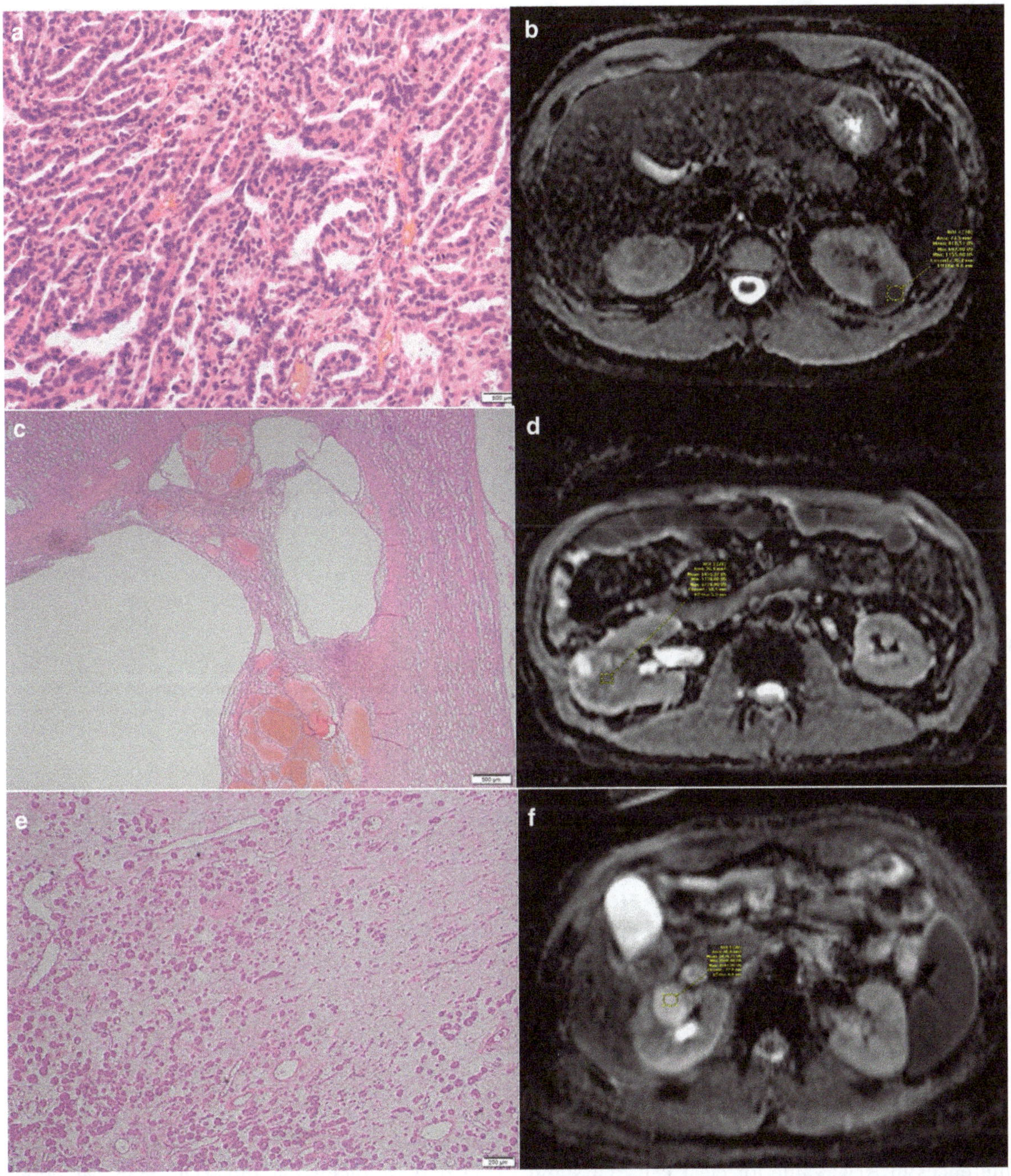

Fig. 1 **a** Microscopy slide shows the cellular nature of papillary RCC which contributes to these tumours showing diffusion restriction and the low ADC number. **b** ADC map demonstrates a papillary RCC in the left kidney with low/ dark signal and an ADC number of only 0.81. **c** Microscopy slide shows the cystic change that can be seen in clear cell RCCs which contributes to them having a higher ADC number than non-clear cell RCCs. **d** ADC map shows low to intermediate signal in the clear cell RCC in the R Kidney, with the signal lower than that of Oncocytomas but higher than non-clear cell RCCs. **e** The microscopy slide demonstrates oedema, a feature of Oncocytomas, the key characteristic which produces the free diffusion and high ADC number. **f** ADC map demonstrates high signal intensity in an Oncocytoma in the right kidney with an ADC number of 2.43

often within a similar range, making clarification between the two difficult even with MRI ADC mapping (although meta-analysis has supported the fact that ADC can differentiate between oncocytomas and malignant tumours in general) [10–13]. Our study, with the use of a 3T rather than 1.5 T MRI has demonstrated that oncocytomas and ccRCCs can be reliably discerned.

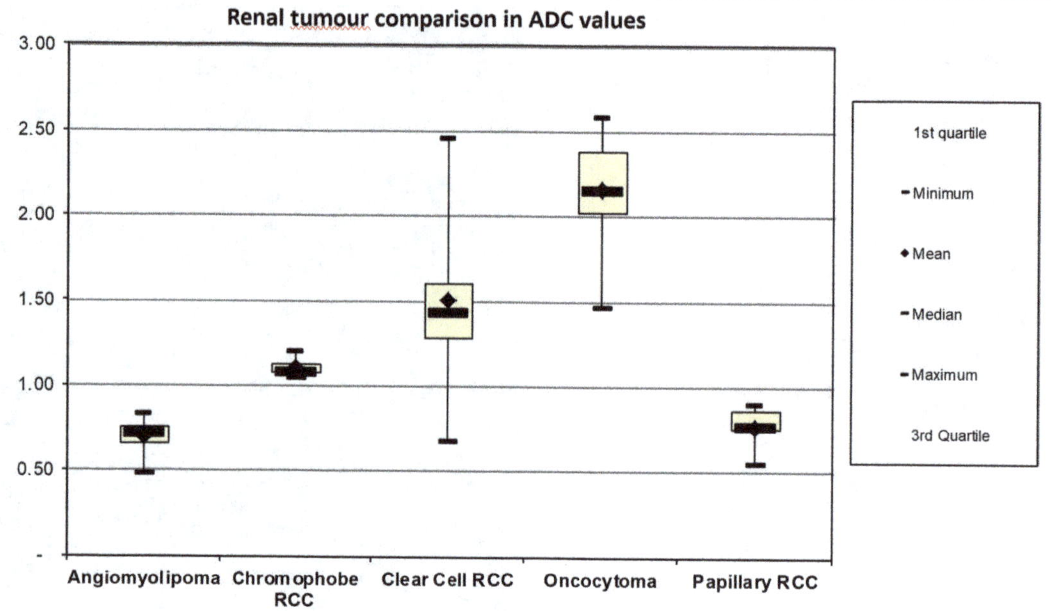

Fig. 2 Comparison of ADC values between renal tumours

Table 1 Renal mass comparison of ADC value

	Clear Cell RCC	Angiomyolipoma	Papillary RCC	Chromophobe RCC	Oncocytoma
Mean	1.50	0.69	0.76	1.11	2.16
Standard error	0.07	0.04	0.04	0.03	0.09
Median	1.44	0.71	0.77	1.09	2.16
Mode	1	1	N/A	N/A	2
Standard deviation	0.37	0.10	0.12	0.06	0.31
Sample variance	0.14	0.01	0.02	0.00	0.10
Kurtosis	1.04	2.44	(0.31)	2.32	1.24
Skewness	0.74	(1.14)	(0.75)	1.41	(0.86)
Range	2	0	0	0	1
Minimum	1	0	1	1	1
Maximum	2	1	1	1	3
Sum	50	6	7	4	24
Count	33	8	9	4	11

This study also demonstrates statistically significant differences in ADC value for clear cell RCCs and non-clear cell RCC subtypes. The average ADC value is significantly higher in clear cell RCC than papillary and chromophobe RCCs as well as AMLs. With an ADC measurement of less than 1.3705, the lesion is more likely to be a non-clear cell RCC of low malignant potential (chromophobe or type 1 papillary) than clear cell. This is consistent with the findings of other studies demonstrating the ADC difference between clear cell and non-clear cell RCC is statistically significant [10–12, 14].

Whereas most other groups have sampled/measured the darkest region on the ADC map we sampled the region most representative of the ADC in the mass. This may have improved diagnostic accuracy in this study. The technique we used to calculate the ADC value should be easily reproducible, and would lend itself to being part of a standardised protocol (although there is a general lack of protocol standardisation in renal MRI between imaging facilities currently). Renal MRI protocols are very much vendor specific and are influenced by several factors which include the strength of the magnet and the b values that are chosen to acquire the ADC calculations.

These differences will contribute to variations in the ADC value of different tumour types between different studies. This can be mitigated by further studies using the same parameters with a consistent vendor as in this study.

MRI is likely to play an increasing role in renal tumour diagnosis as urologists are commonly faced with the management dilemma of an incidental renal mass where invasive investigation or surgical excision may carry high risk when compared to the option of active surveillance with imaging. For example, when biopsy is either non-diagnostic, not feasible due to anatomic factors (e.g. antero-medial or peri-hilar tumour location) or relatively contra-indicated due to patient factors (single kidney, anticoagulation with a high risk of thrombosis if temporarily withheld) [1, 15–17]. Surgical excision via partial or radical nephrectomy carries significant risk of major complications, quality of life effects and cost/ resource burdens on health systems [18, 19].

For these cases, performing an mpMRI with DWI/ADC may indicate likely tumour type and subtype/s. If the DWI/ADC strongly suggests a benign or indolent tumour such as an Oncocytoma or the urologist and patient may reach a shared decision for initial surveillance of the renal mass ifthe risks of invasive procedures outweigh the risks of surveillance. Conversely, in cases where the differential diagnosis includes aggressive malignancy (e.g. Clear Cell RCC), the risks of biopsy or excision are justified.

Our study has several limitations. As a retrospective study, it has the potential to introduce bias in measurement or selection. However, it represents a continuous cohort with clearly rationalised exclusions. Furthermore, all imaging and histopathology were reported prospectively and these assessors blinded. Although we demonstrated a statistically significant difference in ADC for non-clear cell RCCs, only 13 of these subtypes were included in this cohort (due to their relatively low prevalence), and further studies are required with larger population cohorts to validate these findings. Additionally, analysis of ADC measurements were all performed by a single experienced radiologist with an interest in kidney MRI, so further studies should assess for inter reader variability. The imaging completed in this study was with 3T MRI, which is not yet globally available (potentially affecting reproducibility) although it is higher quality imaging than 1.5 T MRI. Finally, a percentage of patients had biopsy diagnosis rather than excision, which has the potential of being less reliable in histopathological diagnosis.

In the evaluation of Renal MRIs, there is an urgent need to develop and validate a consensus -Ki-RADS MRI scanning and reporting system (including analyses such as ADC value) in order to guide radiologists and urologists in diagnostic probability.

Conclusions

Our results suggest that renal MRI DWI/ADC imaging may aid the differentiation of oncocytomas and AMLs from RCCs and assist in stratifying RCC subtypes, especially in challenging cases where biopsy or surgery may be high risk or infeasible.

Abbreviations

MRI: Magnetic resonance imaging; DWI: Diffusion weighted imaging; ADC: Apparent diffusion coefficient; RCC: Renal cell carcinoma; CT: Computed tomography; T: Tesla; ROI: Regions of interest; ANOVA: Analysis of variance; AML: Angiomyolipoma; US: Ultrasound; mpMRI: Multiparametric magnetic resonance imaging; VIBE: Volume interpolated breathhold examination; 2D: Two-dimensional; TR: Repetition time; TE: Echo time; FOV: Field-of-view; EPI: Echo planar; Hz/Px: Hertz per pixel; CKD: Chronic kidney disease.

Acknowledgements

The authors would like to acknowledge the contribution of Mary O'Dwyer, senior MRI radiographer, I-MED radiology network.

Authors' contributions

SdS lead the project development, data collection and analysis, manuscript writing and editing. KL assisted in manuscript writing, data analysis, editing and submission. PA, PN, AH, DM, DL, PC were involved in data collection. FM contributed data collection and assisted with manuscript writing. JT provided guidance for project development, data analysis and manuscript editing. All authors have read and approved the manuscript.

Author details

[1]Faculty of Medicine, University of NSW, Kensington, NSW, Australia. [2]Department of Radiology, I-MED Radiology Network, Sydney, Australia. [3]Department of Urology, St George Hospital, Kogarah, NSW, Australia. [4]Hurstville Private Hospital, Hurstville, NSW, Australia. [5]Department of Anatomical Pathology, Sonic Healthcare, Ryde, NSW, Australia.

References

1. Mytsyk Y, Dutka I, Yuriy B, Maksymovych I, Caprnda M, Gazdikova K, et al. Differential diagnosis of the small renal masses: role of the apparent diffusion coefficient of the diffusion-weighted MRI. Int Urol Nephrol. 2018;50(2):197–204.
2. Pierorazio PM, Patel HD, Johnson MH, Sozio SM, Sharma R, Iyoha E, et al. Distinguishing malignant and benign renal masses with composite models and nomograms: a systematic review and meta-analysis of clinically localised renal masses suspicious for malignancy. Cancer. 2016;122(21):3267–76.
3. Akin IB, Altay C, Güler E, Çamlidağ I, Harman M, Danaci M, et al. Discrimination of oncocytoma and chromophobe renal cell carcinoma using MRI. Diagn Interv Radiol. 2019;25:5–13.
4. Shen L, Zhou L, Liu X, Yang X. Comparison of biexponential and monoex ponential DWI in evaluation of Fuhrman grading of clear cell carcinoma. Diagn Interv Radiol. 2017;23:100–5.
5. Ljungberg B, Bensalah K, Bex A, Canfield S, Dabestani S, Hofmann F, et al. Guidelines on renal cell carcinoma. Eur Urol. 2015;67(5):913–24.
6. Baliyan V, Das CJ, Sharma R, Gupta AK. Diffusion weighted imaging: techniques and applications. World J Radiol. 2016;8(9):785–98.
7. Gauvain KM, McKinstry RC, Mukherjee P, Perry A, Neil JJ, et al. Evaluating brain tumour cellularity with diffusion-tensor imaging. AJR Am J Roentgerol. 2001;177:449–54.
8. Guo AC, Cummings TJ, Dash RC, Provenzale MJ. Lymphomas and high grade astrocytomas, comparison of water diffusibility and histological

characteristics. Radiology. 2002;224:177–83.
9. Koh DM, Collins DJ. Diffusion-weighted MRI in the body: applications and challenges in Oncology. AJR Am J Roenterol. 2007;188:1622–35.
10. Taouli B, Thakur R, Mannelli L, Babb JS, Kim S, Hecht EM, et al. Renal lesions: characterisation with diffusion-weighted imaging versus contrast enhanced MR imaging. Radiology. 2009;251(2):398–407.
11. Hotker AM, Mazaheni Y, Wibmer A, Zheng J, Moskowitz CS, Tickoo SK, et al. Use of DWI in the differentiation of renal cortical tumours. AJR Am J Roentgenol. 2016;206:100–5.
12. Wang H, Cheng L, Zhang X, Wang D, Guo A, Gao Y, et al. Renal cell carcinoma: diffusion-weighted MRI imaging for subtype differentiation at 3.0 T. Radiology. 2010;257(1):135–43.
13. Lassel EA, Rao R, Schwenke C, Schenberg SO, Michaely HJ. Diffusion-weighted imaging of focal renal lesions: a meta-analysis. Eur Radiol. 2014;24:241–9.
14. Goyal R, Gersbach E, Yang XJ, Rohan SM. Differential diagnosis of renal tumours with clear cytoplasm: clinical relevance of renal tumor subclassification in the era of targeted therapies and personalized medicine. Arch Pathol Lab Med. 2013;137:467–80.
15. Canvasser NE, Kay FU, Xi Y, Pinho DF, Costa D, de Leon AD, et al. Diagnostic accuracy of multiparametric magnetic resonance imaging to identify clear cell renal cell carcinoma in cT1a renal masses. J Urol. 2017;198(4):780–6.
16. Sanchez A, Feldman AS, Hakimi AA. Current management of small renal masses, including patient selection, renal tumor biopsy, active surveillance, and thermal ablation. J Clin Oncol. 2018;36(36):3591–600.
17. Campi R, Sessa F, Corti F, et al. Triggers for delayed intervention in patients with small renal masses undergoing active surveillance: a systematic review. Minerva Urologica e Nefrologica/Ital J Urol Nephrol. 2020;72(4):389–407. https://doi.org/10.23736/s0393-2249.20.03870-9.
18. Yang Y. Partial versus radical nephrectomy in patients with renal cell carcinoma: a systematic review and meta-analysis. Urol J. 2020;17(2):109–17.
19. Minervini A, Mari A, Borghesi M, Antonelli A, Bertolo R, Bianchi G, Brunocilla E, Ficarra V, Fiori C, Longo N, Mirone V, Morgia G, Porpiglia F, Rocco B, Serni S, Simeone C, Tellini R, Volpe A, Carini M, Schiavina R. The occurrence of intraoperative complications during partial nephrectomy and their impact on postoperative outcome: results from the RECORd1 project. Minerva Urol Nefrol. 2019;71(1):47–54. https://doi.org/10.23736/S0393-2249.18.03202-2.

13

Radical prostatectomy outcomes in renal transplant recipients: A retrospective case series of Thai patients

Kun Sirisopana[1], Pocharapong Jenjitranant[1], Premsant Sangkum[1], Kittinut Kijvikai[1], Suthep Pacharatakul[2], Charoen Leenanupunth[1], Wachira Kochakarn[1] and Wisoot Kongchareonsombat[1*]

Abstract

Background: The incidence of prostate cancer in renal transplant recipients (RTR) is similar to the general population. Radical prostatectomy (RP) is the standard of care in the management of clinically localized cancer, but is considered complicated due to the presence of adhesions, and the location of transplanted ureter/kidney. To date, a few case series or studies on RP in RTR have been published, especially in Asian patients. This study aimed to evaluate the efficacy and safety and report the experience with RP on RTR.

Methods: We retrospectively reviewed data of 1270 patients who underwent RP from January 2008 to March 2020, of which 5 patients were RTR. All available baseline characteristics, perioperative and postoperative data (operative time, estimated blood loss (EBL), complications, length of hospital stay, complication), pathological stage, Gleason score, surgical margin status, and pre/postoperative creatinine were reviewed.

Results: Of the 5 RTR who underwent RPs (1 open radical prostatectomy (ORP), 1 laparoscopic radical prostatectomy (LRP), 2 robotic-assisted laparoscopic radical prostatectomies (RALRP), and 1 Retzius-sparing RALRP (RS-RALRP)) prostatectomy, the mean age ($\pm$SD) was 70 ($\pm$5.62) years. In LRP and RALRP cases, the standard ports were moved slightly medially to prevent graft injury. The mean operative time ranged from 190 to 365 min. The longest operative time and highest EBL (630 ml) was the ORP case due to severe adhesion in Retzius space. For LRP and RALRP cases, the operative times seemed comparable and had EBL of $\leq$300 ml. All RPs were successful without any major intraoperative complication. There was no significant change in graft function. The restorations of urinary continence were within 1 month in RS-RALRP, approximately 6 months in RALRP, and about 1 year in ORP and LRP. Three patients with positive surgical margins had prostate-specific antigen (PSA) persistence at the first follow-up and 1 had later PSA recurrence. Two patients with negative margins were free from biochemical recurrence at 47 and 3 months after their RP.

Conclusions: Our series suggested that all RP techniques are safe and feasible mode of treatment for localized prostate cancer in RTR.

Keywords: Prostate cancer, Radical prostatectomy, Laparoscopy, Robot-assisted laparoscopic surgery, Renal transplant recipients

*Correspondence: wisoot2002@hotmail.com
[1] Division of Urology, Department of Surgery, Faculty of Medicine, Ramathibodi Hospital, Mahidol University, 270 Thanon Rama VI, Thung Phaya Thai, Ratchathewi, Bangkok 10400, Thailand
Full list of author information is available at the end of the article

Background

Along with the improvement in renal transplantation techniques and post-transplantation care, the recipients live longer. Most renal transplant recipients (RTR) are aged older than 45 years [1], so prostate cancer screening and treatment are still important in these patients.

Prostate cancer is the fifth most common cancer in Thai men [2], and the number of cases continues to increase despite active screening. Unfortunately, the incidence of prostate cancer in RTR is similar to the general population [3]. Radical prostatectomy (RP) is the standard of care in the management of clinically localized cancer. Radical prostatectomy in RTR is considered complicated due to the presence of adhesions or the location of transplanted ureter/kidney. Radiotherapy, active surveillance, or watchful waiting are alternative options. However, radiotherapy is less recommended due to post-radiation complications. To date, there have been a few case series or studies on radical prostatectomy in renal transplant recipients (RTR) published [4–9], especially in Asian patients. This case series aimed to demonstrate our experience with RP for localized prostate cancer in RTR and evaluated the surgical and oncological outcomes.

Methods

Study Design and population

We retrospectively reviewed the data of 1270 patients who underwent RP from January 2008 to March 2020 at Ramathibodi Hospital, Bangkok, Thailand. There were 5 patients (0.39%) who underwent renal transplantations before RP. The RP approaches in those RTR patients were open radical prostatectomy (ORP) in 1 case, laparoscopic radical prostatectomy (LRP) in 1 case, Retzius-sparing robotic-assisted laparoscopic radical prostatectomy (RS-RALRP) in 1 case and robotic-assisted laparoscopic radical prostatectomy (RALRP) in 2 cases. The Committee for Research of the Faculty of Medicine, Ramathibodi Hospital, Mahidol University approved the study prior to commencing the study data review and collection (Approval certificate ID MURA2020/298). Individual informed consent was exempted by the committee due to the type of the research. The study adhered to STROBE guidelines. The principles of the Helsinki Declaration were followed during the study data collection, and the confidentiality of the patients' data was guaranteed.

Surgical techniques

We performed ORP in a retropubic fashion through a low midline incision (Fig. 1A) according to our regular ORP approach [10]. Briefly, the space of Retzius was developed using blunt and sharp dissection along the outside of the left umbilical ligament. At this step, special care was taken to avoid injury to the transplanted ureter and dissected only along the left umbilical ligament. Endopelvic fascia on both sides was bluntly opened, the puboprostatic ligament was dissected. The dorsal venous complex was sutured and ligated with Vicryl No.1. The bladder neck was incised with monopolar cautery, followed by pulling and traction of foley's catheter, dissection of seminal vesicle and vas deferens, and opening Denonvilliers' fascia. At the moment, the posterior surface of the prostate was freed. The lateral prostatic pedicles were dissected with monopolar cautery and ligated with non-nerve sparing, followed by incision of the urethra using Metzenbaum scissors. We performed vesicourethral anastomosis with interrupted sutures, using Vicryl No. 3/0, 6 sutures. Before the last suture, a new 20 Fr Foley's catheter insertion was performed through the urethra into bladder. The surgical areas were examined to ensure there is no active bleeding, followed by Silastic drain placement in the cul-de-sac.

The LRP was performed in an extraperitoneal fashion using 5 trocars with some modification from the standard port positions [10] to facilitate graft injury prevention (Fig. 1B, C). Firstly, we incised sub-umbilical and created extraperitoneal space with kidney shape balloon with a dissection balloon (PDB, Covidien, United States). Extra-pneumoperitoneum was developed by CO_2 insufflation to create an abdominal pressure of 15 mmHg, followed by the modified port placement as Fig. 1C, and trocar insertion under direct visualization. The patients were placed in thirty-degree standard Trendelenburg position with cushioning for the dependent zone. The Retzius space was carefully developed to avoid injury to the transplanted ureter. Endopelvic fascia on both sides was opened, followed by puboprostatic ligament dissection and bladder neck incision with monopolar cautery. We controlled the dorsal venous complex with Vicryl No.1 CT-1 needle. After that, the Foley's catheter was pulled to traction, followed by dissection of seminal vesicle and vas deferens and opening Denonvilliers' fascia to free the posterior surface of the prostate, respectively. We controlled the lateral prostatic by Hem-o-lock clip and dissected it with a vessel sealing device (LigaSure Impact Curved, Large jaw, Medtronic, United Kingdom) with non-nerve sparing, followed by urethra incision with cold scissors. We performed vesicourethral anastomosis with continuous watertight sutures with Vicryl 3/0. To ensure adequate insertion of 20 Fr Foley's catheter into the urinary bladder, we inserted the catheter before passing the anterior stitch. After completing the anastomosis, a closed suction drain was placed in the cul-de-sac. The specimen was retrieved through a sub-umbilical incision using a laparoscopic bag.

The RALRPs were performed using the Da Vinci Si Surgical System by transperitoneal technique with 5 trocars. In general, the procedures of RALRP in RTR were not different from RALRP in general patients but the trocars were placed slightly medially (Fig. 1E, F, G) from the standard port sites [10] (Fig. 1D) to deliver sufficient

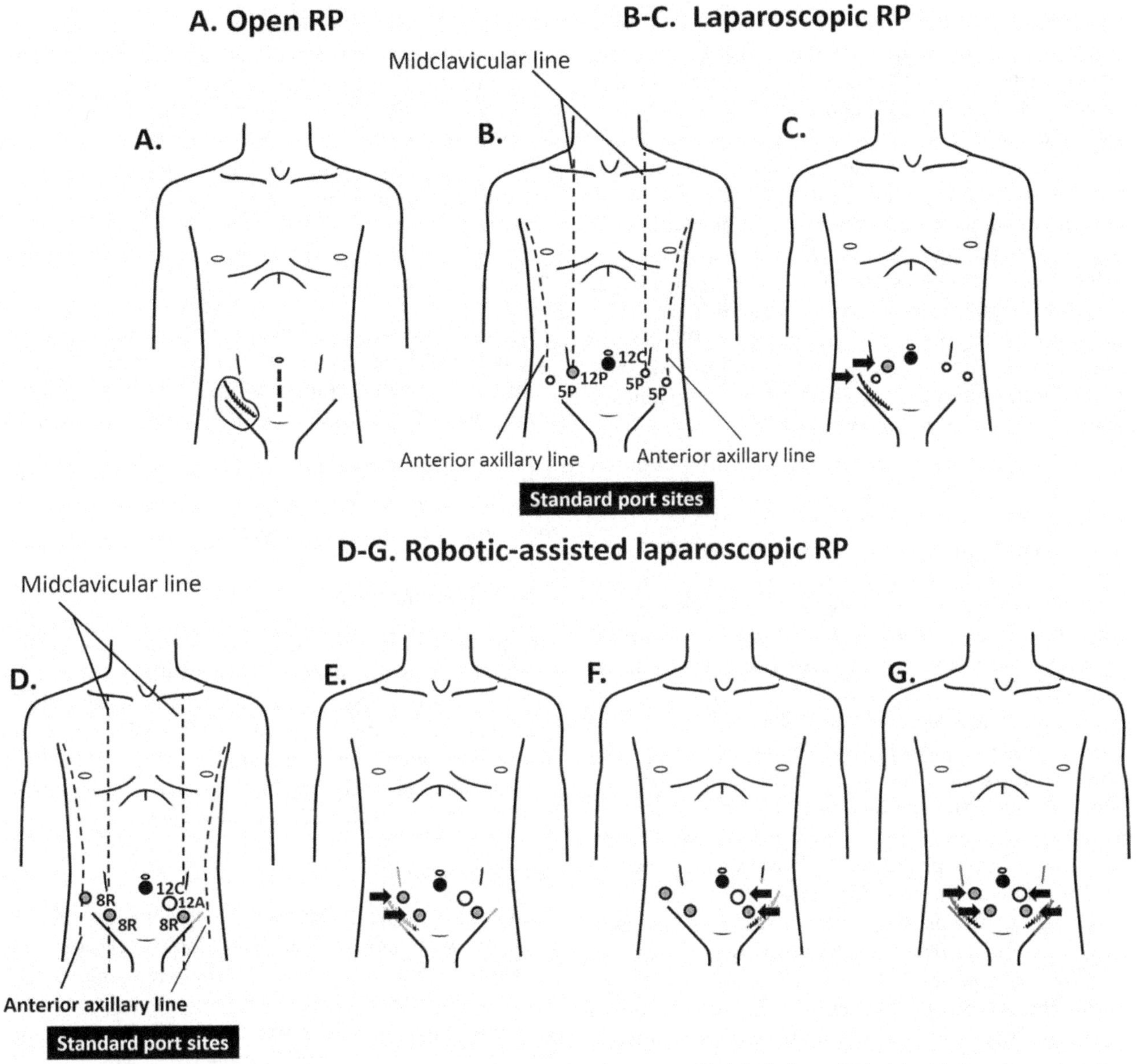

Fig. 1 Skin incision and port placement for the radical prostatectomy (RP). **A** Skin incision (dash line) of open RP in right-sided renal transplantation; **B** Laparoscopic port placement in general population; **C** Laparoscopic port placement in right-sided renal transplantation; **D** Robotic port placement in general population; **E–G** Robotic port placement in right-sided (**E**), left- sided (**F**), and both sides renal transplantation (**G**). Symbols: 12C,12 mm camera port; 12P, 12 mm laparoscopic port; 5P, 5 mm laparoscopic port; 8R, 8 mm robotic port, 12A, 12 mm assistant port, black arrow; direction of port modification/adjustment

access without graft injury. Veress needle is punctured at the sub-umbilical area to establish pneumoperitoneum. of 15 mmHg. A 12 mm sub-umbilical trocar was inserted into abdominal space to be used as a camera port to insert the resting trocar under direct visualization. On the right side, two robotic trocars were placed with at least 8 cm apart from each other (Arm 1, Arm 3). For the left side, a robotic trocar was placed (Arm 2), and the assistance 12 mm trocar was placed between the robotic port and the camera port. Robotic Arm 1, 2, and 3 were equipped with Monopolar scissors, Bipolar Maryland, and ProGrasp forceps, respectively. The patients were placed in thirty-degree standard Trendelenburg position with cushioning for dependent zone. A Retzius space was developed carefully to avoid injury to the transplanted ureter. Endopelvic fascia on each side was opened, followed by the puboprostatic ligament dissection. We controlled the dorsal venous complex using barbed suture No.1 (V-Loc PBT wound closure device, Medtronic, United Kingdom). The bladder neck incision was performed with monopolar and bipolar cautery then Foley's catheter was gently pulled to traction, followed by dissection of seminal vesicle and vas deferens, and opening Denonvilliers' fascia to free the posterior surface of prostate. The lateral prostatic pedicles were controlled with Hem-o-lock clip and dissected with monopolar and bipolar cautery. One case was performed with interfascial nerve-sparing and another case was non-nerve sparing. The urethra was then incised by cold scissors. A vesicourethral anastomosis with continuous watertight sutures, using barbed suture 3/0 (V-Loc PBT wound closure device, Medtronic, United Kingdom) was performed. The procedures for Foley's catheter insertion and specimen retrieval were the same as LRP.

The RS-RALRP was performed using the Da Vinci Si Surgical System with 5 trocars. A paraumbilical incision was made. The first 12-mm camera trocar was placed with the use of an open Hasson technique. CO_2 was insufflated to obtain pneumoperitoneum up to the level of 15 mmHg, and 2 other robotic trocars were placed in the left and right iliac fossae under direct visualization. The trocar in the right iliac fossa was inserted cautiously to avoid injury to graft. A 12-mm assistant port was placed in the left iliac fossa. The patient was placed in thirty-degree standard Trendelenburg position with cushioning for dependent zone. At the anterior surface of the Douglas space, parietal peritoneum was incised. Seminal vesicles and vas deferens were dissected. Denonvilliers' fascia was opened by the posterolateral surface of the prostate in an antegrade direction, reaching the prostatic apex. The bladder neck was incised. The anterior surface of the prostate was bluntly dissected from the dorsal venous complex without incision, followed by the incision of urethra with cold scissors. The vesicourethral anastomosis was performed with continuous watertight sutures, using barbed suture 3/0 (V-Loc PBT wound closure device, Medtronic, United Kingdom). Before passing the posterior stitch, the 20 Fr Foley's catheter was passed into the bladder and the anastomosis was completed. A closed suction drain was placed in the prevesical space. The specimen was retrieved with the use of laparoscopic bag through a paraumbilical incision. The peritoneum at the Douglas space was closed.

All RPs were done by 2 experienced senior instructor surgeons without pelvic lymphadenectomy. The surgeons and patients worked and made decisions together to select the procedure techniques.

Baseline characteristics and preoperative parameters

The patients' age, body weight (kgs), height (cms), body mass index (BMI), Gleason score (GS) of the biopsy specimen, initial prostate-specific antigen (PSA) level, clinical T stage (TNM classification), prostate cancer risk group (according to the National Comprehensive Cancer Network [NCCN] Clinical Practice Guidelines in Oncology: Prostate Cancer Version 2, 2020) [11], graft localization, type of donor and time from transplantation to RP were collected from the patients' medical records, including histo-pathological reports, and imaging study reports.

Surgical outcomes

Surgical outcomes included type of procedure, undergoing nerve-sparing, operative time, estimated blood loss (EBL), perioperative complications, including transfusion rate, adjacent organ injury of the bladder, rectum, ureter, bowel, or blood vessel, length of hospital stay (days, which were determined by subtracting the date of admission from the date of discharge) and post-operative complication (Clavien-Dindo classification).

Oncological outcomes

The prostate weight (g), GS of the specimen, pathological T stage, and the margin status were evaluated by an experienced uropathologist in accordance with the NCCN guidelines. A positive surgical margin (PSM) was simply defined as cancer cells extending to the inked surface of the specimen [12]. The follow-up period and post-operative course were collected from medical records.

Statistical analysis

Sample size calculation was not applied. All RTR patients, who underwent RP, were included in the study. Descriptive statistics, i.e. frequency with proportion or percentage, mean with SD, and range, were used to present the study data. There were no comparisons between RP approaches due to small sample size. Statistical analysis was performed using StataSE, version 20 (IBM, New York, NY, USA).

Results

Baseline characteristics

Five patients were included in this study. The baseline characteristics and preoperative parameters are demonstrated in Table 1. The mean patients' age at the time of RP ($\pm$SD) was 70 ($\pm$5.62) years (ranged from 64–79 years). Risk group stratification in these patients was low (1/5), favorable intermediate (1/5), unfavorable intermediate (1/5), high risk (1/5) and very high risk (1/5). The kidney allografts were implanted in the right iliac fossa in the first 3 cases (Case 1, 2, and 3), in the left iliac fossa in the 4th case (Case 4), and the last case (Case 5) had renal grafts on both sides of iliac fossa. The first 2 cases and Case 4 received kidney from deceased

Table 1 Baseline characteristics

	Case 1	Case 2	Case 3	Case 4	Case 5
Age (years)	67	64	74	66	79
BMI (kg/m^2)	26.99	22.86	29.92	23.88	28.21
Biopsy Gleason score	4+5	3+3	3+4	4+4	3+3
Preoperative PSA (ng/ml)	25.66	10.84	11.53	130	9.63
Clinical T stage	T3b	T1c	T1c	T3a	T1c
NCCN Prostate cancer risk group	Very high	Favorable intermediate	Unfavorable intermediate	High	Low
Graft localization	Right	Right	Right	Left	Both sides
Donor	DDKT	DDKT	LRKT	DDKT	DDKT and LRKT
Time from transplantation to RP (years)	13	9	21	8	13

BMI, body mass index; DDKT, deceased-donor kidney transplantation; LRKT, living-related kidney transplantation; NCCN, National Comprehensive Cancer Network; PSA, prostate-specific antigen; RP, radical prostatectomy

donors, Case 3 from living related donor and Case 5 from deceased donor for the left side and living related donors for the right side. There was no adjustment in the immunosuppressive regimen during the surgery, but a watchful follow-up by nephrologist was performed for the purpose of early detection of complication. Table 1 presents the patients' baseline characteristics.

Surgical outcomes

The RP approaches were performed with non-nerve sparing, except for Case 5 that performed RP with unilateral nerve-sparing. The surgical data and outcomes were demonstrated in Table 2. The mean operative time (±SD) was 237 (±64.47) minutes (ranged from 190 to 365 min). The longest operative time was Case 1 who underwent ORP (365 min) with the EBL of 630 mls due to severe adhesion in Retzius space. For LRP (210 min) and RALRP (210, 190, and 210 min), the operative times seemed comparable.

There was no perioperative complication in all 5 patients. The postoperative course of the patients was uneventful, excepted for Case1 and Case 2 that required blood transfusion, due to anemia and postoperative fever in post-operative day 1 which subsided in the next day.

In Case 1 and 2, the urethral catheter was removed on post-operative day 13 and 14, respectively after cystogram while the others were removed on post-operative day 7. The differences in urethral catheter retention duration depended on the surgeon's confidence, but was not from complication. In the first and second case of RP in RTR patients (Case 1 and Case 2), the surgeon decided to retain the catheter for approximately two weeks post-operation to ensure the anastomosis healing from the open and laparoscopic complexity. In the latter cases (Cases 3, 4, and 5), the surgeon decided to retain the catheter for 1 week after RP because they were confident that one week was sufficient to secure the anastomosis after RP using the Da Vinci Si Surgical System. The restorations of urinary continence after surgery were within 1 month in RS-RALRP (Case 3), approximately 6 months in RALRP (Case 4 and 5), and about 1 year in ORP (Case 1) and LRP (Case 2).

Wound related complication was not encountered in all patients. Means length of hospital stay (±SD) was 7.8 (±2.79) days (ranged from 5 to 13 days). The longest hospital stay (13 days) was Case 1 who was the first case in our experience.

Oncological outcomes

The oncological outcomes were also demonstrated in Table 2. Pathological analysis revealed GS 3+3 (1/5), 3+4 (1/5), 4+3 (1/5) and 4+5 (2/5). The pathological tumor stage (pT) was T2a (2/5), T2c (1/5) and T3b (2/5). Three patients had positive surgical margin, consisting of Case 1 who underwent ORP, had pathological GS of 4+5 and pT3b, Case 3 who underwent RS-RALRP, had the GS of 4+3 and pT2c, and Case 4 who underwent RALRP, had the GS of 4+5 and pT3b.

The follow-up period of the 5 patients ranged from 6 to 129 months. Case 1 (GS 4+5, pT3b and margin positive disease) had PSA persistence without distant metastasis and was treated with androgen deprivation therapy (ADT) until the patient died in 2016 from progressive allograft dysfunction with uremia (total follow-up period 129 months). Case 2 (GS 3+3, pT2a and negative margin) had remained recurrence free with total follow-up period of 47 months, until 2014, when the patient presented at hospital with the sigmoid colon cancer with gut obstruction and died from septic shock. Case 3 (GS 4+3, pT2c and margin positive disease) experienced a biochemical recurrence at 13 months post-operation. The patient was treated with ADT

Table 2 Intraoperative, post-operative and oncological outcomes

	Case 1	Case 2	Case 3	Case 4	Case 5
Operative date	23-Nov-05	11-June-10	08-Apr-15	06-Dec-18	05-Mar-20
Type of RP	ORP	LRP	RS-RALRP	RALRP	RALRP
Nerve sparing	No	No	No	No	Unilateral
Operative time (min)	365	210	210	190	210
EBL (mLs)	630	300	250	150	100
Prostate specimen weight (g)	34.8	40	24	23.5	30
Perioperative complication	None	None	None	None	None
Complication by Clavien-Dindo classification	2	2	1	1	1
Complication	Blood transfusion and postoperative fever	Blood transfusion and postoperative fever			
LOS (days)	13	6	8	5	7
Pathological Gleason score	4+5	3+3	4+3	4+5	3+4
Pathological T stage	T3b	T2a	T2c	T3b	T2a
Marginal status	Positive	Negative	Positive	Positive	Negative
Follow-up period (months)	129	47	63	31	6
Creatinine (mg/dl)					
Preoperative	1.3	1	1.41	0.66	1.11
1 day postoperative	1.2	0.8	1.38	0.57	0.87
3 days postoperative	1.12	Not measured	0.88	0.58	0.79
7 days postoperative	1.25	Discharged	1.06	Discharged	0.78
The last available Cr	1.6 Year 2016	1.28 Year 2014	1.74 Year 2020	0.65 Year 2020	1.05 May-20
Survival/oncological status	PSA persistence, on ADT until death in 2016 due to progressive allograft dysfunction with uremia	Recurrence free until death in 2014 due to sigmoid colon carcinoma with gut obstruction and septic shock	PSA recurrence at 13 months. Then on ADT, PSA < 0.003 at the follow up on 9 June 2020	PSA persistence, on ADT. PSA of 0.85 at the follow-up on 25 May 2020	Recurrence free at the follow-up on May 2020
Return of urinary continence after surgery	1 year	1 year	1 month	6 months	6 months

ADT, androgen deprivation therapy; Cr, creatinine; EBL, estimated blood loss; LRP, laparoscopic radical prostatectomy; LOS, length of hospital stay; ORP, open radical prostatectomy; PSA, prostate-specific antigen; RALRP, robotic-assisted laparoscopic radical prostatectomy; RP, radical prostatectomy; RS-RALRP, Retzius-sparing robotic-assisted laparoscopic radical prostatectomy

without adjuvant radiation therapy due to worrisome complication of radiation and remained on ADT, with undetectable PSA (follow-up period 63 months). Case 4 (GS 4+5, pT3b and margin positive disease) encountered PSA persistence without distant metastasis and was treated with ADT alone and remain on ADT, with PSA level of 0.85 (follow-up period 31 months). Case 5 (GS 3+4, pT2a and negative margin) had remained recurrence free with the total follow-up of 6 months. Additionally, graft function as represented by the serum creatinine level was stable before, during and after surgery in all patients as shown in Table 2.

Discussion

Although improving in transplantation techniques and post-transplantation care, cancer remains a major adverse feature. The prevalence of prostate cancer in RTR is similar to the general population [3]. However, some studies showed the prevalence of genitourinary cancer is the second most common cancer in RTR [13], especially prostate cancer as the fifth most common cancer [14] with the prevalence range from 0.72 to 3.1% [7, 9]. In Thailand, the incidence of prostate cancer has been increasing and impactful as the fifth most common cancer in Thai men [2].

The prognosis and natural history of prostate cancer in RTR are not associated with worse outcomes than non-RTR. The standard treatments should be proposed to this population with satisfying surgical and oncological out comes [15, 16]. There are several treatments for prostate cancer, including active surveillance, RP, radiotherapy, hormonal therapy, and watchful waiting. Each option is viable and should be a shared decision with patients.

In our experience, we do not believe that RP should be avoided in selected patients even with the history of abdominal surgery. Some previous literature revealed that prior abdominal surgery does not impact surgical outcomes and complications [17]. Even, there are potentially risks of injury due to smaller working space, adhesion, and transplanted renal and ureter, the surgery itself is possible. Moreover, a systematic review also showed that RP is the preferred treatment of localized prostate cancer [15].

Despite all these difficulties, multiple approaches of radical prostatectomy, including retropubic [18, 19], perineal [20], laparoscopic [21–23] and robotic-assisted [6, 24, 25] have been used in the treatment of prostate cancer in RTR, with comparable outcomes. Classically, radical retropubic prostatectomy was performed and obtained good results, although a study reported a graft injury event during retraction [26]. In our study, we performed retropubic ORP with partial bladder mobilization only along contralateral side of the umbilical ligament to avoid injury to the transplanted ureter. The perineal approach is also a viable procedure with some edge, including less manipulation of transplanted kidney and ureter [20]. However, we did not use this approach in our series. In Shah et al. [27] reported the first case of LRP in localized prostate cancer in RTR. In our experience, we used the extraperitoneal approach with medial port insertion from the standard port placement to avoid injury to transplanted graft and ureter.

Recently, the robotic-assisted procedure has become more routinely used. In Jhaveri et al. [28] presented the first RALRP in RTR with technical adjustment to mitigate graft injury. In our series, the surgical modification includes slight medial movement of trocars placement with an assistant port on contralateral side to renal graft, initiating the Retzius space dissection from the contralateral side with limited ipsilateral dissection, and constant awareness of vesicoureteral anastomosis to avoid injury to transplant graft. However, Wagener et al. [29] suggested that routine placement of trocar was also feasible. In Mistretta et al. [9] reported the use of RS-RALRP in RTR with modification of 12 mm assistant port to provide more medial and cranial respect to the standard set to avoid injury to graft. We performed RS-RALRP with medial placement of 5 trocars similar to RALRP and also preferred this approach more than others due to the anatomical safety. Additionally, if severe tension is encountered when performing vesicourethral anastomosis, we suggest using continuous watertight sutures by including some pelvic floor muscle into the stitch to prevent cutting through surrounding organ/tissues.

To cope with the difficulties for vesicourethral anastomosis, we performed the anastomosis by continuous watertight suturing technique with V-Loc™ in RALRP and RS-RALRP. The anastomosis was quite simple in RALRP and RS-RALRP, because the Da Vinci Surgical System provided more visualization and accessibility to the suturing area to meticulously handle the anastomosis. In LRP, the same anastomosis technique as RALRP and RS-RALRP was performed, but it took a longer duration due to less clear visualization of the operative field and more difficulty to handle the suturing. In ORP, we used the parachute technique with Vicryl 3/0, 6 stitches for the anastomosis. The results from the present study showed that the patient who underwent RS-RALRP or RALRP was more likely to regain urinary continence earlier than those who underwent ORP or LRP.

In our series, all RPs in RTR were performed without lymphadenectomy to keep the procedure to be generally simple and less time consuming. In addition, the lymphadenectomy can cause collateral damage to the vascular and ureterovesical anastomosis of the transplanted kidney. The lymphadenectomy also does not provide better overall survival outcomes [30]. Although this procedure may be required in some cases, we suggest evaluating each patient individually based on the future need for a second transplant.

In terms of marginal status, there were 3 out of 5 patients having PSM. Two PSM patients (Case 1 and Case 4) were high and very high-risk group patients, while another patient (Case 3) was in the unfavorable intermediate-risk group. The patient Case 3 was our first RTR patient performing RS-RALRP and our early experience in RS-RALRP approach. The two negative surgical margin patients were favorable intermediate and low-risk group patients. The presence of PSM seemed to be likely related to the extent and severity of the disease.

Radiotherapy, including intensity-modulated radiation therapy or low dose rate prostate brachytherapy, is also feasible and acceptable minimally invasive treatment for selected RTR [31, 32]. However, some complications were encountered such as incontinence, urethral stricture, and obstruction of distal ureter, resulting in decreased graft function [33, 34]. There are several limitations of our study. We did not perform comparison among the

RP approaches due to small number of patients. To our knowledge, our series demonstrated the first largest series in Thailand about RP in RTR that includes all different techniques. Multicenter studies were suggested in the future to confirm the safety of RP in RTR.

Conclusions

The results from this series suggested that radical prostatectomy was a feasible and safe operation for the treatment of localized prostate cancer in renal transplant recipients. Moreover, minimally invasive techniques, especially robotic-assisted laparoscopic radical prostatectomy, provided advantage because they allowed greater visualization and handling of instruments in a restricted working space.

Abbreviations

BMI: Body mass index; GS: Gleason score; LRP: Laparoscopic radical prostatectomy; NCCN: National Comprehensive Cancer Network; ORP: Open radical prostatectomy; PSA: Prostate-specific antigen; RALRP: Robotic-assisted laparoscopic radical prostatectomy; RP: Radical prostatectomy; RS-RALRP: Retzius-sparing robotic-assisted laparoscopic radical prostatectomy; RTR: Renal transplant recipients.

Acknowledgements

The authors would like to thank Ms. Wijittra Matang, Ms. Yada Phengsalae and Ms. Kornkanok Somboonpun for continued support and encouragement, Ms. Threechada Boonchan for drawing figures, and Mr. Stephen Pinder for English proofreading.

Authors' contributions

KS: Methodology, formal analysis, data curation, writing the initial draft, and performing the radical prostatectomy. PJ: Data curation, review and editing the manuscript, and performing the radical prostatectomy. PS: Performing the radical prostatectomy, data validation, review and editing the manuscript. KK: Performing the radical prostatectomy, review and editing the manuscript. SP: Performing the radical prostatectomy, review and editing the manuscript. CL: Performing the radical prostatectomy, review and editing the manuscript. WcK: Review and editing the manuscript. WsK: Conceptualization, methodology, performing the radical prostatectomy, supervision, data interpretation, writing the initial manuscript, and finalize manuscript. All authors have read and approved the manuscript.

Author details

[1]Division of Urology, Department of Surgery, Faculty of Medicine, Ramathibodi Hospital, Mahidol University, 270 Thanon Rama VI, Thung Phaya Thai, Ratchathewi, Bangkok 10400, Thailand. [2]Division of Urology, Department of Surgery, Police Hospital, Bangkok, Thailand.

References

1. Wolfe R. The state of kidney transplantation in the United States. Semin Dial. 2005;18(6):453–5.
2. Sangrajrang S, Laowahutanont P, Sangariyavanich E, Pecthrith W. Hospital based cancer registry. Bangkok, Thailand: Information Technology Division, National Cancer Institute; 2018. https://www.nci.go.th/th/File_download/Nci%20Cancer%20Registry/Hospital-Based%20NCI2%202016%20Web.pdf. Accessed 10 July 2020.
3. Mohammed Shahait M, Jackman SV. Urologic complication of renal transplantation. 12th ed. Amsterdam: Elsevier; 2020.
4. Marra G, Dalmasso E, Agnello M, Munegato S, Bosio A, Sedigh O, Biancone L, Gontero P. Prostate cancer treatment in renal transplant recipients: a systematic review. BJU Int. 2018;121(3):327–44.
5. Léonard G, Pradère B, Monléon L, Boutin JM, Branchereau J, Karam G, Rigaud J, Bruyère F. Oncological and postoperative outcomes of robot-assisted laparoscopic radical prostatectomy in renal transplant recipients: a multicenter and comparative study. Transplant Proc. 2020;52(3):850–6.
6. Iwamoto K, Iizuka J, Hashimoto Y, Kondo T, Takagi T, Hata K, Unagami K, Okumi M, Ishida H, Tanabe K. Radical prostatectomy for localized prostate cancer in renal transplant recipients: 13 cases studied at a single center. Transplant Proc. 2018;50(8):2539–44.
7. Iizuka J, Hashimoto Y, Kondo T, Takagi T, Inui M, Nozaki T, Omoto K, Shimizu T, Ishida H, Tanabe K. Robot-assisted radical prostatectomy for localized prostate cancer in Asian renal transplant recipients. Transplant Proc. 2016;48(3):905–9.
8. Smith DL, Jellison FC, Heldt JP, Tenggardjaja C, Bowman RJ, Jin DH, Chamberlin J, Lui PD, Baldwin DD. Robot-assisted radical prostatectomy in patients with previous renal transplantation. J Endourol. 2011;25(10):1643–7.
9. Mistretta FA, Galfano A, Di Trapani E, Di Trapani D, Russo A, Secco S, Ferro M, Musi G, Bocciardi AM, de Cobelli O. Robot assisted radical prostatectomy in kidney transplant recipients: surgical, oncological and functional outcomes of two different robotic approaches. Int Braz J Urol. 2019;45(2):262–72.
10. Sangkum P, Sirisopana K, Jenjitranant P, Kijvikai K, Pacharatakul S, Leenanupunth C, Kochakarn W, Kongchareonsombat W. Neoadjuvant androgen deprivation therapy effects on perioperative outcomes prior to radical prostatectomy: eleven years of experiences at ramathibodi hospital. Res Rep Urol. 2021;13:303–12.
11. NCCN Clinical Practice Guidelines in Oncology Prostate Cancer Version 2. 2020. https://www.nccn.org/professionals/physician_gls/pdf/prostate_blocks.pdf. Accessed 10 July 2020.
12. Silberstein JL, Eastham JA. Significance and management of positive surgical margins at the time of radical prostatectomy. Indian J Urol. 2014;30(4):423–8.
13. Sforza D, Parente A, Pellicciaro M, Morabito M, Iaria G, Anselmo A, Lindfors ER, Corrado F, Cacciatore C, Del Fabbro D, et al. Prostate cancer recurrence in kidney transplant recipient 15 years after radical prostatectomy: a case report. Transplant Proc. 2019;51(9):2995–7.
14. Pendón Ruiz de Mier V, Navarro Cabello MD, Martínez Vaquera S, Lopez Andreu M, Aguera Morales ML, Rodriguez Benot A, Aljama Garcia P. Incidence and long-term prognosis of cancer after kidney transplantation. Transplant Proc. 2015;47(9):2618–21.
15. Hevia V, Boissier R, Rodríguez-Faba Ó, Fraser-Taylor C, Hassan-Zakri R, Lledo E, Regele H, Buddde K, Figueiredo A, Olsburgh J, et al. Management of localised prostate cancer in kidney transplant patients: a systematic review from the EAU guidelines on renal transplantation panel. Eur Urol Focus. 2018;4(2):153–62.
16. Pettenati C, Jannot AS, Hurel S, Verkarre V, Kreis H, Housset M, Legendre C, Méjean A, Timsit MO. Prostate cancer characteristics and outcome in renal transplant recipients: results from a contemporary single center study. Clin Transplant. 2016;30(8):964–71.
17. Kishimoto N, Takao T, Yamamichi G, Okusa T, Taniguchi A, Tsutahara K, Tanigawa G, Yamaguchi S. Impact of prior abdominal surgery on the outcomes after robotic—assisted laparoscopic radical prostatectomy: single center experience. Int Braz J Urol. 2016;42(5):918–24.
18. Antonopoulos IM, Nahas WC, Piovesan AC, Falci R Jr, Kanashiro H, Alvarez GA, Srougi M. Radical retropubic prostatectomy for localized prostate cancer in renal transplant patients. Urology. 2008;72(6):1362–5.
19. Kleinclauss FM, Neuzillet Y, Tillou X, Terrier N, Guichard G, Petit J, Lechevallier E. Morbidity of retropubic radical prostatectomy for prostate cancer in renal transplant recipients: multicenter study from Renal Transplantation Committee of French Urological Association. Urology. 2008;72(6):1366–70.
20. Yiou R, Salomon L, Colombel M, Patard JJ, Chopin D, Abbou CC. Perineal approach to radical prostatectomy in kidney transplant recipients with localized prostate cancer. Urology. 1999;53(4):822–4.

21. Maestro MA, Gómez AT, Alonso YGS, Ledo JC, de la Peña BJ, Martínez-Piñeiro L. Laparoscopic transperitoneal radical prostatectomy in renal transplant recipients: a review of the literature. BJU Int. 2010;105(6):844–8.
22. Robert G, Elkentaoui H, Pasticier G, Couzi L, Merville P, Ravaud A, Ballanger P, Ferrière JM, Wallerand H. Laparoscopic radical prostatectomy in renal transplant recipients. Urology. 2009;74(3):683–7.
23. Thomas AA, Nguyen MM, Gill IS. Laparoscopic transperitoneal radical prostatectomy in renal transplant recipients: a review of three cases. Urology. 2008;71(2):205–8.
24. Jenjitranant P, Sangkum P, Sirisreetreerux P, Viseshsindh W, Patcharatrakul S, Kongcharoensombat W. Retzius space preservation technique for robotic-assisted laparoscopic radical prostatectomy in a kidney transplant patient: first case in Thailand and our first experience. Transplant Proc. 2016;48(9):3130–3.
25. Moreno Sierra J, Ciappara Paniagua M, Galante Romo MI, Senovilla Pérez JL, Redondo González E, Galindo Herrero MI, Novo Gómez N, Blázquez Izquierdo J. Robot assisted radical prostatectomy in kidney transplant recipients. Our clinical experience and a systematic review. Urol Int. 2016;97(4):440–4.
26. Doerfler A, Vaessen C, Gosseine PN, Barrou B, Richard F. Laparoscopic radical prostatectomy in kidney transplant patient: our first experience-a case report. Transplant Proc. 2009;41(2):713–5.
27. Shah KK, Ko DS, Mercer J, Dahl DM. Laparoscopic radical prostatectomy in a renal allograft recipient. Urology. 2006;68(3):672.e675-677.
28. Jhaveri JK, Tan GY, Scherr DS, Tewari AK. Robot-assisted laparoscopic radical prostatectomy in the renal allograft transplant recipient. J Endourol. 2008;22(11):2475–9.
29. Wagener N, Nyarangi-Dix JN, Teber D, Zeier M, Hohenfellner M. Applicability of robot-assisted laparoscopic radical prostatectomy in renal allograft recipients. Transplant Proc. 2012;44(5):1287–92.
30. Fujimoto N, Shiota M, Tomisaki I, Minato A, Yahara K. Reconsideration on clinical benefit of pelvic lymph node dissection during radical prostatectomy for clinically localized prostate cancer. Urol Int. 2019;103(2):125–36.
31. Iizuka J, Hashimoto Y, Hashimoto Y, Kondo T, Takagi T, Nozaki T, Shimizu T, Akimoto T, Ishida H, Karasawa K, et al. Efficacy and feasibility of intensity-modulated radiation therapy for prostate cancer in renal transplant recipients. Transplant Proc. 2016;48(3):914–7.
32. Iizuka J, Hashimoto Y, Hashimoto Y, Kondo T, Takagi T, Nozaki T, Shimizu T, Akimoto T, Ishida H, Karasawa K, et al. Efficacy and feasibility of low-dose rate brachytherapy for prostate cancer in renal transplant recipients. Transplant Proc. 2016;48(3):910–3.
33. Gojdic M, Zilinska Z, Krajcovicova I, Lukacko P, Grezdo J, Obsitnik B, Breza J Sr, Trebaticky B. Radiotherapy of prostate cancer in renal transplant recipients: single-center experience. Neoplasma. 2019;66(1):155–9.
34. Mouzin M, Bachaud JM, Kamar N, Gamé X, Vaessen C, Rischmann P, Rostaing L, Malavaud B. Three-dimensional conformal radiotherapy for localized prostate cancer in kidney transplant recipients. Transplantation. 2004;78(10):1496–500.

Expression pattern and regulatory effect of lysine-specific demethylase 2A gene in clear cell renal cell carcinoma

Jiannan Wang[1], Tan Li[2], Xiang Li[1], Yixia Zhang[1] and Xuemei Wang[1*]

Abstract

Background: Our study aimed to explore the expression and the biological role of lysine-specific demethylase 2A (KDM2A) in clear cell renal cell carcinoma (ccRCC).

Methods: In vitro, KDM2A expression was measured by qRT-PCR and western blot. A total of 50 patients with ccRCC were included, and KDM2A expression in ccRCC tissues was assessed by qRT-PCR and immunohistochemistry. The effects of KDM2A expression on cell biological behavior were examined by cell counting kit-8 assay, transwell assay and flow cytometry, respectively. The prognostic value of KDM2A in ccRCC was evaluated by Kaplan–Meier method.

Results: The KDM2A expression was significantly upregulated in ccRCC cell line ($P<0.05$). Compared with para cancer tissues, ccRCC samples showed a higher KMD2A mRNA level and a larger proportion of high KDM2A expression (all $P<0.05$). High KDM2A mRNA expression was more likely to occur in ccRCC tissues with tumor size > 7 cm ($P=0.005$) and T3-T4 stage ($P=0.047$). Knockdown of KDM2A significantly suppressed the proliferation and invasion, and promoted the apoptosis of ccRCC cells (all $P<0.05$). Moreover, Kaplan–Meier survival analysis revealed that higher level of KDM2A expression in ccRCC patients was associated with lower survival rate ($P=0.004$).

Conclusions: Our findings demonstrated a vital role of KDM2A in the pathogenesis of ccRCC, which provides a new perspective to understand the underlying molecular mechanisms in ccRCC.

Keywords: Lysine-specific demethylase 2A, Renal cell carcinoma, Expression, Cell biological behavior, Survival rate

Background

Kidney cancer is a common malignancy of urinary system, whereas renal cell carcinoma (RCC) is the most common kidney neoplasm and contains a cluster of heterogeneous tumors which originate from the renal tubular epithelial cells [1, 2]. At present, the accepted treatment of RCC is mainly surgical resection. Clear cell renal cell carcinoma (ccRCC) is the most frequent subtype of RCC, which nearly accounts for about 75% of RCC [3]. It derives from the proximal tubular epithelium and is characterized by the worst clinical process and prognosis among the classes of RCC. However, the genetic and epigenetic background of changes that occur during the initiation and development of ccRCC remains poorly understood [4]. Therefore, to illuminate the molecular mechanisms underlying ccRCC tumorigenesis and progression so as to identify novel biological makers and targets for effective treatments for ccRCC is of great significance.

Covalent histone modifications play a critical part in the regulation of chromatin dynamics and functions [5]. Histone methylation is an important form of epigenetic modification and occurs on both lysine and arginine

*Correspondence: wxmlmt@163.com
[1] Department of Ultrasound, The First Hospital of China Medical University, No. 155 NanjingBei Street, Heping District, Shenyang 110001, Liaoning Province, People's Republic of China
Full list of author information is available at the end of the article

residues. Through the methylation of different histone sites, gene expressions can be regulated by influencing the activation and inhibition of transcription [6]. The constant level of covalent histone methylation is under the control of histone methyltransferases and demethylases [7]. The lysine-specific demethylase 2A gene (KDM2A), found on chromosome 11q13.2, is a member of the KDM histone lysine demethylase family, which exhibits specificity for removal of methyl groups of histone H3K36 by binding directly to CpG islands in gene promoters [7]. The dysfunction of KDM2A has been reported in various cancers, and its loss-of-function mouse mutants are embryonically lethal [7]. However, KDM2A has a complex and tissue-specific role in tumorigenesis and tumor progression. An increasing number of studies have described that KDM2A exerts an oncogenic role in a wide range of tumor types, including breast cancer, gastric cancer and lung cancer, and can enhance the growth and motility of cancer cells to promote tumor progression [8–12]. On the contrary, Frescas et al. found that KDM2A expression was often decreased in prostate cancer compared with normal prostate tissue [13]. However, its expression pattern and biological function in ccRCC have not yet been elucidated.

The current study aimed to investigate the expression pattern of KDM2A in vitro and in vivo, and determine the biological impact of KMD2A in ccRCC cell line. Then, the prognostic role of KDM2A in ccRCC was evaluated on the basis of survival data from TCGA. All together may provide novel insight into the development of therapeutic strategies for ccRCC.

Methods

Patients and samples

Fifty patients with ccRCC who underwent radical nephrectomy at the First Hospital of China Medical University from January 2018 to October 2018 were enrolled in the study. ccRCC tissues and corresponding para cancer tissues were obtained from renal operation and immediately stored at − 80 °C. The para cancer tissues were taken from a location 5 cm away from the tumor. For some patients with a large tumor with the remaining para cancer tissues being less than 5 cm, the renal tissues more than 3 cm away from the tumor were taken and pathologically proven to be cancer-free. No patients had received any preoperative adjuvant therapy, such as radiotherapy, chemotherapy, immunotherapy, targeted therapy, interventional embolization, and so on, or had a history of other malignant tumors. Demographic and clinical data of ccRCC patients are summarized in Table 1. This study was approved by the Ethics Committee of the First Hospital of China Medical University (Shenyang, China). Written informed consent was obtained from each subject.

Table 1 Baseline characteristics of ccRCC patients (n = 50)

Parameters	ccRCC
Gender, n (%)	
Male	29 (58%)
Female	21 (42%)
Age, years	58.78 ± 8.85
< 60, n (%)	28 (56%)
≥ 60, n (%)	22 (44%)
Location, n (%)	
Left	22 (44%)
Right	28 (56%)
BMI (kg/m^2)	24.79 ± 3.22
< 24, n (%)	20 (40%)
≥ 24, n (%)	30 (60%)
Tumor size(cm)	6.20 ± 2.38
≤ 7, n (%)	35 (70%)
> 7, n (%)	15 (30%)
Smoking, n (%)	
No	39 (78%)
Yes	11 (22%)
Thrombus of renal vein, n (%)	
No	46 (92%)
Yes	4 (8%)
TNM stage, n (%)	
T_1	27 (54%)
T_2	11 (22%)
T_3	10 (20%)
T_4	2 (4%)
T_1–T_2	38 (76%)
T_3–T_4	12 (24%)
ISUP grade, n (%)	
1	4 (8%)
2	31 (62%)
3	8 (16%)
4	7 (14%)
1–2	35 (70%)
3–4	15 (30%)
Symptoms, n (%)	
No	32 (64%)
Yes	18 (36%)
Hypertension, n (%)	
No	29 (58%)
Yes	21 (42%)

Cell culture and transfection

Human ccRCC cells (786-O) and Human kidney proximal tubular cells (HK-2) were purchased from the Cell

Bank of the Chinese Academy of Sciences (Shanghai, China). 786-O cells were cultured in RPMI 1640 medium (HyClone, Logan, UT, USA) containing 10% fetal bovine serum (FBS) (HyClone, Logan, UT, USA). HK-2 cells were cultured in DMEM/F12 medium (HyClone, Logan, UT, USA) containing 10% FBS. The cells were cultured at 37 °C in an incubator with 5% CO2. si-KMD2A and si-NC (GenePharma, Shanghai, China) were transfected into 786-O cells using Lipofectamine 2000 transfection reagent (Invitrogen, Grand Island, NY, USA) following the manufacturer's protocol.

Western blotting assay

The cells were lysed in cold RIPA Lysis Buffer (Beyotime, Shanghai, China), and the protein concentration was determined using a BCA Protein Assay Kit (Beyotime, Shanghai, China). After boiling in loading buffer at 95 °C for 5 min, 40 μg per lane of proteins were separated by 8% SDS-PAGE and then transferred to polyvinylidene difluoride membranes (Millipore, Billerica, MA, USA). The membranes were blocked using 5% (W/V) non-fat milk in Tris-buffered saline containing 0.1% (V/V) Tween-20 at room temperature for 1 h and then incubated overnight at 4 °C with the primary antibodies: rabbit anti-human KDM2A (1:1,000; Abcam, Cambridge, MA, USA) and rabbit anti-human β-actin (1:3,000; Proteintech, Rosemont, IL, USA). After several washings, the membranes were then incubated with HRP-conjugated affinipure goat anti-rabbit secondary antibody (1:5,000; Proteintech, Rosemont, IL, USA) for 45 min at 37 °C. The protein bands were visualized using a super ECL plus kit (US Everbright, Suzhou, China). The levels of protein expression were evaluated by ImageJ software (version 1.41; National Institutes of Health, Bethesda, MD, USA).

qRT-PCR

All the tissues were used to determine KDM2A mRNA level. Total mRNAs of ccRCC and paracancer tissues were extracted using TRIzol reagent (Invitrogen, Carlsbad, CA, USA.) following the manufacturer's protocols. Reverse-transcribed cDNA synthesis was performed with BioTeke Super RT kit (BioTeke, Beijing, China). Real-time PCR was conducted using 2 × Power Taq PCR MasterMix (BioTeke, Beijing, China) and SYBR Green (BioTeke, Beijing, China) according to the manufacturer's instructions. β-actin acted as an internal control. The primers were synthesized as follows: KDM2A Forward 5′-GGCAGTAGGAATCAAGGACC-3′, Reverse 5′-ACCCGACAGCAGTGAGTAGA-3′; β-actin: Forward 5′-CACTGTGCCCATCTACGAGG-3′, Reverse 5′-TAA TGTCACGCACGATTTCC-3′. PCR conditions were as follows: initial denaturation at 94 °C for 5 min, followed by 40 cycles of 94 °C for 15 s, 60 °C for 20 s, and 72 °C for 30 s. Each reaction was set up 3 times and the expression level of KDM2A was quantified using the $2^{-\Delta\Delta Ct}$ method.

Immunohistochemistry (IHC)

All the tissues were fixed in 4% paraformaldehyde, embedded in paraffin, and sectioned at 4 μm. Then, the slides were treated with xylene to remove the paraffin, followed by hydration with ethanol and the addition of EDTA for antigen retrieval. Endogenous peroxidase blocker solution was added to incubate for 10 min, and the sections were rinsed with phosphate buffer saline (PBS) 3 times. To avoid nonspecific binding, normal goat serum was added to block tissue collagen for 10 min. Sections were incubated with KDM2A monoclonal antibody (1:250; Abcam, Cambridge, MA, USA) for 1 h at room temperature. After washing 3 times with PBS, the sections were incubated with biotinylated secondary goat anti-rabbit antibody, and then with streptavidin–biotin peroxidase for 10 min each. Finally, the diaminobenzidine solution was used to stain the sections, which were then counterstained with hematoxylin.

The KDM2A IHC score was determined by both the intensity and percentage of cellular staining. The staining intensity was divided into scores of 0 (negative), 1 (mild), 2 (moderate), 3 (strong), and the percentage was classified as 1 (0–25%), 2 (26–50%), 3 (51–75%), and 4 (>75%). The intensity and percentage were multiplied to calculate the total IHC staining score, which was assigned as negative staining (−, 0), mild staining (+, 1–4), moderate staining (++, 5–8), severe staining (+++, 9–12). An IHC score ≥ 5 was defined as high expression, while a score of less than 5 was defined as low expression. Two independent observers were employed to assess and examine immunostaining.

Cell counting kit-8 (CCK-8) assay

Cells were seeded in 96-well plates at 3,000 cells per well and cultured for 24, 48 and 72 h. Then, 10 μl of CCK-8 (Dojindo Molecular Technologies, Kumamoto, Japan) was added and subsequently incubated for 1 h at 37 °C. The absorbance (optical density value) was measured at 450 nm.

Transwell assay

The cells were seeded at a density of 1×10^4 cells/well into the upper transwell chamber (Corning, NY, USA), which contained 200 μl serum-free medium, and 800 μl of the medium containing 20% FBS was added to the lower chamber. Following 48 h of incubation at 37 °C, the cells remaining on the upper membrane were removed with a sterile cotton swab. The chambers were fixed at room temperature with 4% paraformaldehyde for 20 min, and then stained with 0.1% crystal violet (Solarbio, Beijing, China) for 30 min. The numbers of stained cells were counted in five different fields using an inverted microscope at a magnification of × 200.

Cell apoptosis measured by flow cytometry

The cell apoptosis was assessed using an Annexin V-fluorescein isothiocyanate (FITC) /propidium iodide (PI) Apoptosis Detection Kit (Wanleibio, Shenyang, China). The cells were rinsed twice with sterile phosphate buffer saline and resuspended in 500 ul binding buffer. Subsequently, stained the cells with 5 μl Annexin V-FITC and 10 μl PI in the darkness for 15 min. Analysis was performed using a NovoCyte flow cytometer (ACEA Biosciences, San Diego, CA, USA).

Kaplan–Meier curve

Survival data from TCGA was obtained to clarify the prognostic value of KDM2A in ccRCC. They were submitted to OncoLnc (http://www.oncolnc.org/) and Kaplan–Meier curve was plotted for prognostic analysis.

Statistical analysis

Statistical analysis was performed using SPSS version 23 (IBM, Armonk, NY, USA). Quantitative data were expressed as the mean ± standard deviation (SD), and counting data were represented by the number and rate. The Kolmogorov–Smirnov test was performed to test whether the data were normally distributed. χ^2 test or Fisher's exact test was performed to compare the categorical variables. Differences between groups were calculated by independent sample t-test or one-way ANOVA. $P < 0.05$ was considered to indicate a statistically significant difference.

Results

Baseline characteristics of ccRCC patients

The patients' baseline characteristics are presented in Table 1. There were 29 (58%) male and 21 (42%) female cases with an average age of 58.78 years. TNM stage T1-T2 and T3-T4 accounted for 38 (76%) and 12 (24%) of all the patients, respectively. As for the International Society of Urological Pathology (ISUP) grade, 35 patients (70%) were classified as grade 1–2, while 15 patients (30%) were classified as grade 3–4. Moreover, most patients had no clinical symptoms.

KDM2A expression in ccRCC cell lines and tissues

As shown in Fig. 1, qRT-PCR and western blot were used to exam KDM2A expression in cell lines. The mRNA and protein expression of KDM2A were both significantly upregulated in 786-O cells in comparison with HK-2 cells ($P < 0.05$).

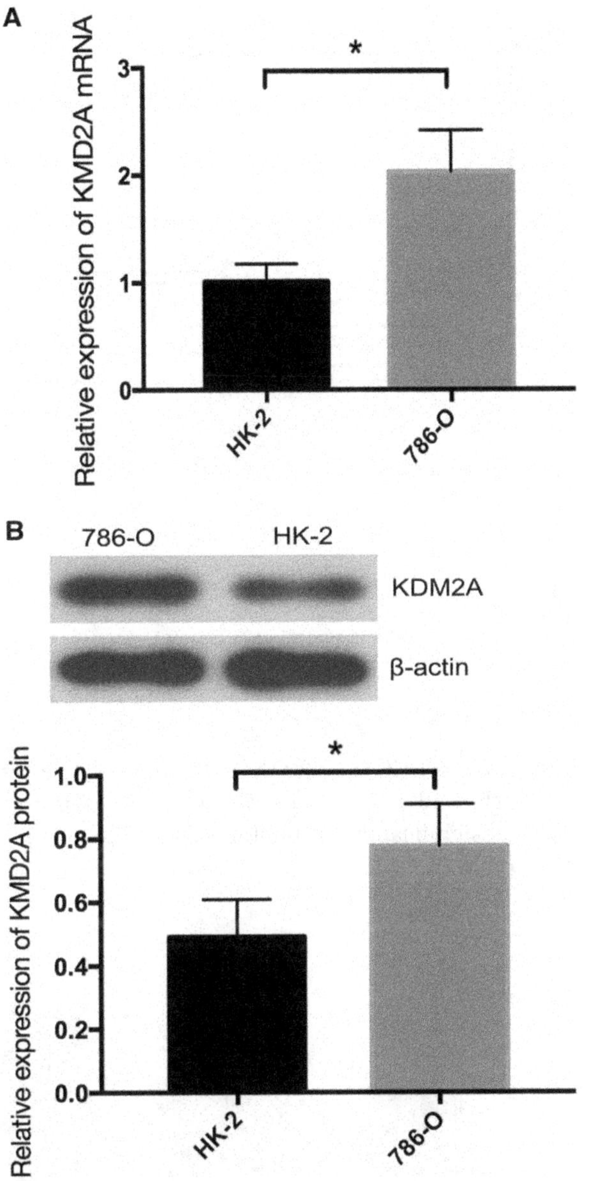

Fig. 1 KDM2A expression in cell lines. **a** qRT-PCR analysis and **b** western blot analysis indicated that KDM2A mRNA and protein expression levels were higher in 786-O cells compared with HK-2cells. *$P < 0.05$

KDM2A mRNA expression was around 2.59-fold higher in ccRCC samples than that in para cancer samples with a significant difference ($P < 0.05$; Fig. 2). According to the median ratio of KDM2A mRNA level (2.61) in tumor tissues, ccRCC patients were classified into the high and low KDM2A mRNA expression groups. IHC analysis revealed that KDM2A protein was predominantly located in the cell nucleus and ccRCC samples had significantly higher KDM2A expression levels than para cancer tissues (Fig. 3). In addition, based on IHC

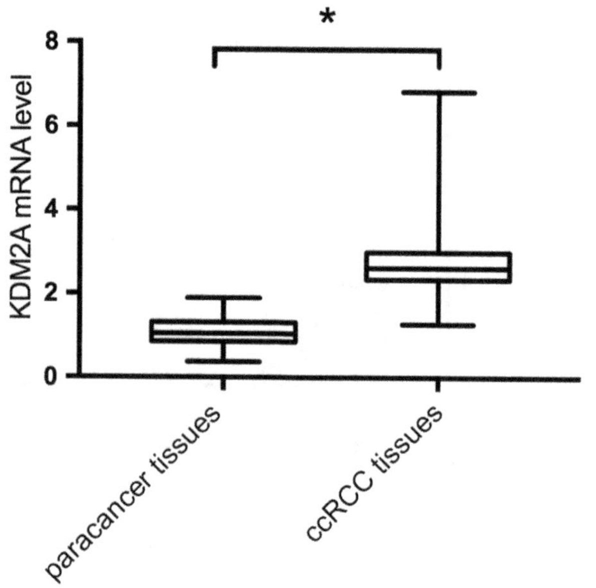

Fig. 2 KDM2A mRNA expression was detected by qRT-PCR and shown to be about 2.59-fold higher in ccRCC samples than in para cancer samples. $*P<0.05$

results, all the ccRCC samples were immunopositive, 90% of which showed a high expression of KDM2A protein, which was significantly higher than that in para cancer tissues (Table 2).

Furtherly, we analyzed the correlations of KDM2A mRNA and protein expression with clinical features in ccRCC and found that the high expression of KDM2A mRNA was more likely to occur in ccRCC tissues with tumor size > 7 cm ($P=0.005$) and T3-T4 stage ($P=0.047$) (Table 3). However, there was no significant association between KDM2A protein expression and clinical features in ccRCC (Table 4).

Knockdown of KDM2A suppresses the proliferation and invasion, and promotes the apoptosis of ccRCC cells

A loss-of function experiment was performed to determine the biological role of KDM2A in ccRCC. The efficiency of knockdown was confirmed by qRT-PCR and western blot analysis. The results showed that transfection with si-KDM2A notably decreased the mRNA and protein expression of KDM2A in 786-O cells compared to control and si-NC groups (Fig. 4a, b). CCK-8 and transwell assays revealed that si-KDM2A significantly inhibited the proliferative and invasive ability of 786-O cells when compared with control and si-NC groups, respectively ($P<0.05$) (Fig. 4c, d). The results of flow cytometry demonstrated that 786-O cells transfected with si-KDM2A had an apoptosis percentage of 32.10 ± 2.60%, which was significantly higher than control and si-NC group with cell apoptosis rate of 5.66 ± 2.46% and 6.83 ± 1.31%, respectively ($P<0.05$) (Fig. 4e).

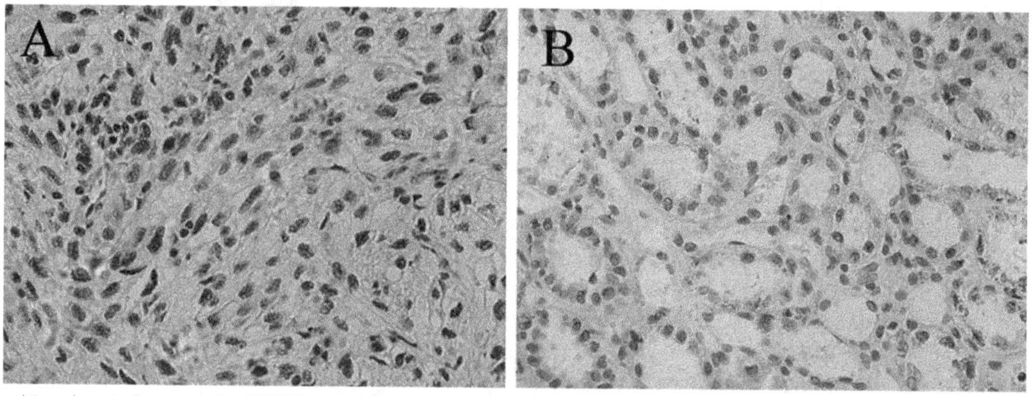

Fig. 3 Immunohistochemical staining for KDM2A protein expression in ccRCC and para cancer tissues (Magnification, × 400). **a** High expression of KDM2A in ccRCC tissues. **b** Low expression of KDM2A in para cancer tissues

Table 2 IHC analysis displayed the expression of KDM2A protein in ccRCC and para cancer tissues

Group	(−)	(+)	(++)	(+++)	*P*	Low, n (%)	High, n (%)	*P*
Para cancer tissues	8 (16%)	17 (34%)	14 (28%)	11 (22%)	Reference	25 (50%)	25 (50%)	Reference
ccRCC tissues	0 (0%)	5 (10%)	19 (38%)	26 (52%)	< 0.001	5 (10%)	45 (90%)	< 0.001

Table 3 Association between KDM2A mRNA expression and clinical features in ccRCC

Parameters	n	KDM2A mRNA expression in ccRCC		P
		Low, n (%)	High, n (%)	
Gender				
Male	29	12 (41.4%)	17 (58.6%)	0.152
Female	21	13 (61.9%)	8 (38.1%)	
Age, years				
< 60	28	13 (46.4%)	15 (53.6%)	0.569
≥ 60	22	12 (54.5%)	10(45.5%)	
Location				
Left	22	12 (54.5%)	10 (45.5%)	0.569
Right	28	13 (46.4%)	15 (53.6%)	
BMI (kg/m²)				
< 24	20	7 (35.0%)	13 (65.0%)	0.083
≥ 24	30	18(60.0%)	12 (40.0%)	
Tumor size (cm)				
≤ 7	35	22 (62.9%)	13(37.1%)	0.005
> 7	15	3 (20.0%)	12 (80.0%)	
Smoking				
No	39	20 (51.3%)	19 (48.7%)	0.733
Yes	11	5 (45.5%)	6 (54.5%)	
Thrombus of renal vein				
No	46	24 (52.2%)	22 (47.8%)	0.602
Yes	4	1 (25.0%)	3 (75.0%)	
TNM stage				
T_1–T_2	38	22 (57.9%)	16 (42.1%)	0.047
T_3–T_4	12	3 (25.0%)	9 (75.0%)	
ISUP grade				
1–2	35	19(54.3%)	16 (45.7%)	0.355
3–4	15	6 (40.0%)	9 (60.0%)	
Symptoms				
No	32	15 (46.9%)	17 (53.1%)	0.556
Yes	18	10 (55.6%)	8 (44.4%)	
Hypertension				
No	29	16 (55.2%)	13 (44.8%)	0.390
Yes	21	9 (42.9%)	12 (57.1%)	

Table 4 Association between KDM2A protein expression and clinical features in ccRCC

Parameters	n	KDM2A mRNA expression in ccRCC		P
		Low, n (%)	High, n (%)	
Gender				
Male	29	1 (3.4%)	28 (96.6%)	0.181
Female	21	4 (19.0%)	17 (81.0%)	
Age, years				
< 60	28	3 (10.7%)	25 (89.3%)	1.000
≥ 60	22	2 (9.1%)	20 (90.9%)	
Location				
Left	22	2 (9.1%)	20 (90.9%)	1.000
Right	28	3 (10.7%)	25 (89.3%)	
BMI (kg/m²)				
< 24	20	0 (0%)	20 (100%)	0.149
≥ 24	30	5 (16.7%)	25 (83.3%)	
Tumor size (cm)				
≤ 7	35	5 (14.3%)	30 (85.7%)	0.304
> 7	15	0 (0%)	15 (100%)	
Smoking				
No	39	5 (12.8%)	34 (87.2%)	0.495
Yes	11	0 (0%)	11 (100%)	
Thrombus of renal vein				
No	46	5 (10.9%)	41 (89.1%)	1.000
Yes	4	0 (0%)	4 (100%)	
TNM stage				
T_1–T_2	38	5 (13.2%)	33 (86.8%)	0.440
T_3–T_4	12	0 (0%)	12 (100%)	
ISUP grade				
1–2	35	4 (11.4%)	31 (88.6%)	1.000
3–4	15	1 (6.7%)	14 (93.3%)	
Symptoms				
No	32	4 (12.5%)	28 (87.5%)	0.768
Yes	18	1 (5.6%)	17 (94.4%)	
Hypertension				
No	29	4 (13.8%)	25 (86.2%)	0.567
Yes	21	1 (4.8%)	20 (95.2%)	

The prognostic value of KDM2A in ccRCC patients

Kaplan–Meier survival analysis suggested that higher expression of KDM2A in ccRCC patients was related to lower survival rate ($P = 0.004$, Fig. 5).

Discussion

In the current study, we are the first, to our knowledge, to make a comprehensive evaluation of KDM2A expression pattern and regulatory effect in ccRCC. We found that KDM2A level was upregulated in ccRCC cell line and tissues, and knockdown of KDM2A suppressed ccRCC cells to proliferate and invade and promoted their apoptosis. Moreover, high KDM2A mRNA expression in ccRCC was associated with large tumor size, advanced TNM stage and a poor survival prognosis. Our research may provide a theoretical basis for further pathological studies and the improvement of novel therapeutic approaches for ccRCC patients.

The occurrence and development of ccRCC is a complicated multi-step biological process, which may involve the instability of the genome, the gradual accumulation of gene mutations, epigenetic mechanism alterations, and

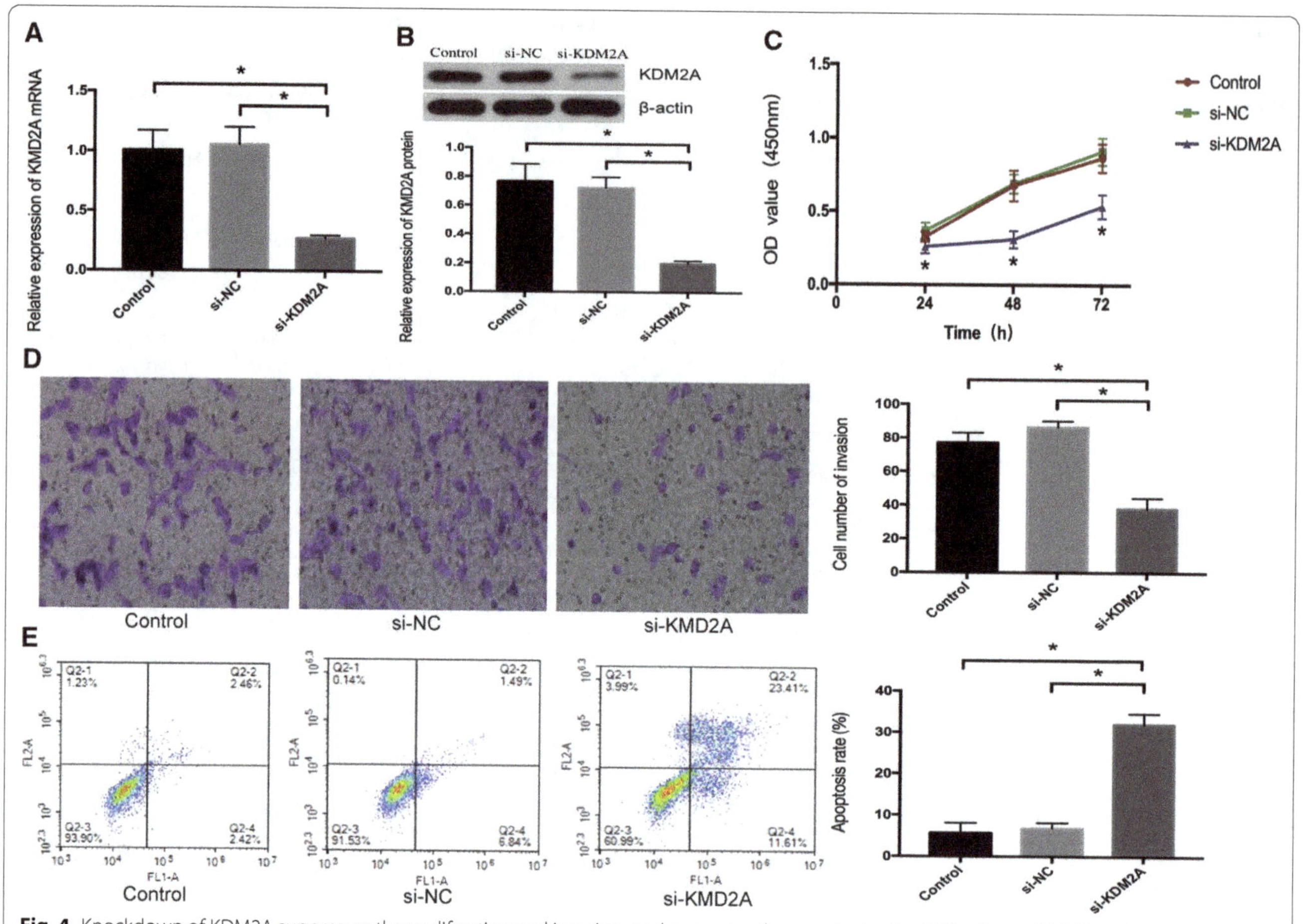

Fig. 4 Knockdown of KDM2A suppresses the proliferation and invasion, and promotes the apoptosis of ccRCC cells. **a** qRT-PCR analysis and **b** western blot analysis showed that KDM2A mRNA and protein expression levels in 786-O cells transfection with si-KDM2A were notably downregulated than control and si-NC groups. **c** The proliferative ability of 786-O cells transfected with si-KDM2A was determined by CCK-8 assay. **d** Representative image of transwell assay, quantitative measurement of the number of transmembrane cells indicates that knockdown of KDM2A reduces cellular invasion (Magnification, × 200). **e** The results of flow cytometry demonstrated that 786-O cells transfected with si-KDM2A had a higher apoptosis percentage (32.10 ± 2.60%) than control (5.66 ± 2.46%) and si-NC (6.83 ± 1.31%) group. *$P < 0.05$

abnormal gene expression [14, 15]. Histone lysine methylation was regarded as a central modification for the post-transcriptional regulation of chromosome structure and DNA replication, repair, and transcription procedure [16], and was relevant to the activation or silencing of gene expression [17]. KDM2A can specifically catalyze the demethylation of histone H3K36, which is a conserved epigenetic marker influencing gene transcription, alternative splicing, and DNA repair [18, 19]. During cell mitosis, KDM2A plays a role in maintaining genomic stability and centromeric integrity [13]. Meanwhile, the overexpression of KDM2A might antagonize the senescence of embryonic fibroblasts and promote somatic reprogramming [18]. The deletion of KDM2A could also inhibit the proliferation of stem cells from apical papilla [16]. In addition, Xu et al. found that KDM2A might be an important regulator of cell proliferation and cell cycle via impacting TGF-β signaling pathway [20].

Emerging studies have shown that the level of KDM2A expression is up-regulated in a variety of tumor cells and affects the biological behavior of tumor cells. In the present study, KDM2A expression in ccRCC was evaluated using multiple methods, which have never been reported before. Our results found that the mRNA and protein expression levels of KDM2A in ccRCC cells and tissues were significantly upregulated. Moreover, an elevated percentage of high KDM2A mRNA expression was markedly demonstrated in ccRCC tissues with tumor size > 7 cm and T3-T4 stage. Furthermore, we investigated the functional role of KDM2A in ccRCC cells, revealing that KDM2A silencing significantly suppressed the proliferation and invasion, and induced the apoptosis of 786-O cells. Based on the survival data from TCGA, it was demonstrated that ccRCC individuals with high KDM2A level would have a relatively worse survival prognosis. Our results indicated that KDM2A may play a

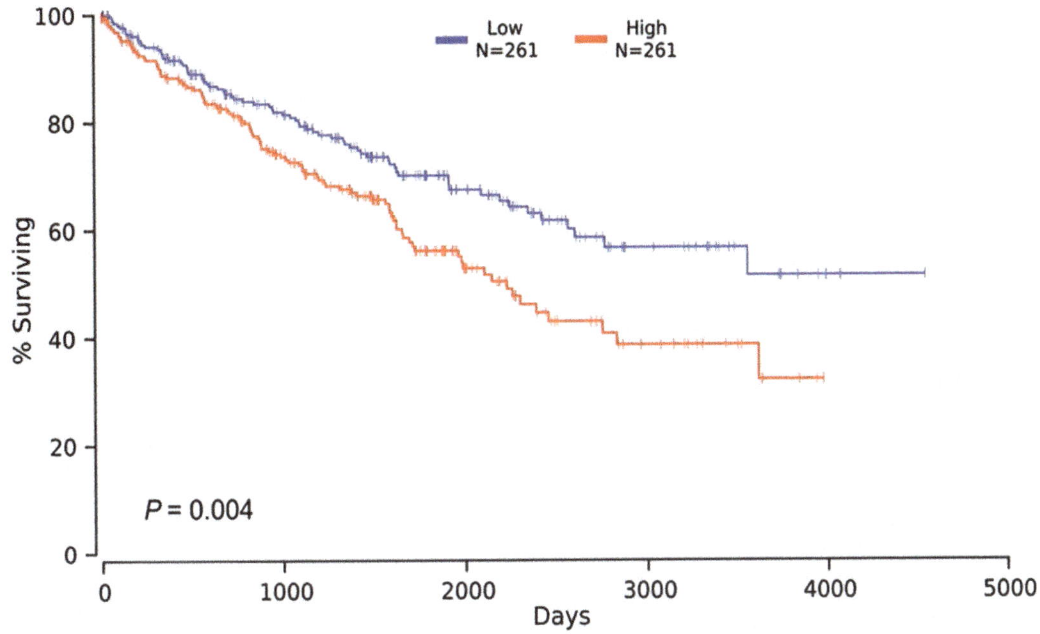

Fig. 5 Kaplan–Meier survival curve was performed to assess the prognostic value of KDM2A in ccRCC

key role in the initiation and progression of ccRCC, and could serve as a diagnostic and prognostic biomarker for this disease.

Similarly, gastric cancer tissues have been found to have an increased level of KDM2A expression and forced expression of KDM2A promoted cell growth and migration [8]. In breast cancer, KDM2A was found to be highly expressed and significantly correlated with shortened survival of breast cancer patients [11, 21]. In non-small cell lung cancer (NSCLC), Wagner et al. demonstrated that KDM2A was overexpressed and could promote the proliferation and metastasis of NSCLC cells by regulating the activity of ERK1/2 pathway, which was related to a poor prognosis of NSCLC patients [9]. An up-regulated expression of KDM2A was also shown to play a critical role in the onset and progression of cervical cancer and promote the proliferation and invasion of cervical cancer cells [22, 23]. However, Frescas et al. revealed a lower level of KDM2A expression in prostate carcinomas compared to normal prostate tissue [13]. These diverse observations may be attributed to the heterogeneity of disease and a variety of sample sizes.

Some limitations existed in our study. Firstly, there was a lack of comparison with normal kidneys. Secondly, due to the lack of prognostic information in our ccRCC patients, the prognostic results only relied on the data from TCGA. In addition, we did not verify our work in animals. Further studies that include a larger number of subjects with detailed clinical information are necessary to confirm our findings.

Conclusions

In summary, we observed the high expression of KDM2A in ccRCC cell line and tissues. High KDM2A mRNA expression was positively correlated with tumor size and TNM stage, and had an adverse effect on the overall survival of ccRCC patients. Additionally, the knockdown of KDM2A decreased cell proliferation and invasion, and increased the apoptosis in ccRCC. Our results unravel a new regulatory mechanism involved in ccRCC pathogenesis and progression, and KDM2A may be a potential marker for the diagnosis and prognosis of ccRCC patients.

Abbreviations

KDM2A: Lysine-specific demethylase 2A; ccRCC: Clear cell renal cell carcinoma; RCC: Renal cell carcinoma; FBS: Fetal bovine serum; IHC: Immunohistochemistry; PBS: Phosphate buffer saline; CCK-8: Cell counting kit-8; FITC: Fluorescein isothiocyanate; PI: Propidium iodide; SD: Standard deviation; ISUP: International Society of Urological Pathology; NSCLC: Non-small cell lung cancer.

Acknowledgements

Not applicable.

Authors' contributions

JW performed the experiments and wrote the manuscript. TL analyzed the data and revised the manuscript. XL participated in the experiments. YZ collected the tissue samples and clinical data. XW conceived and supervised the study. All authors read and approved the final manuscript.

Author details

[1]Department of Ultrasound, The First Hospital of China Medical University, No. 155 NanjingBei Street, Heping District, Shenyang 110001, Liaoning Province, People's Republic of China. [2]Department of Cardiovascular Ultrasound, The First Hospital of China Medical University, Shenyang 110001, People's Republic of China.

References

1. Siegel RL, Miller KD, Jemal A. Cancer statistics, 2020. CA Cancer J Clin. 2020;70(1):7–30.
2. Wang Y, Zhang Y, Wang P, Fu X, Lin W. Circular RNAs in renal cell carcinoma: implications for tumorigenesis, diagnosis, and therapy. Mol Cancer. 2020;19(1):149.
3. Feng C, Xiong Z, Jiang H, Ding Q, Fang Z, Hui W. Genetic alteration in notch pathway is associated with better prognosis in renal cell carcinoma. BioFactors. 2016;42(1):41–8.
4. Godlewski J, Kiezun J, Krazinski BE, Kozielec Z, Wierzbicki PM, Kmiec Z. The immunoexpression of YAP1 and LATS1 proteins in clear cell renal cell carcinoma: impact on patients' survival. Biomed Res Int. 2018;2018:2653623.
5. Tsukada Y, Fang J, Erdjument-Bromage H, Warren ME, Borchers CH, Tempst P, et al. Histone demethylation by a family of JmjC domain-containing proteins. Nature. 2006;439(7078):811–6.
6. Mikkelsen TS, Ku M, Jaffe DB, Issac B, Lieberman E, Giannoukos G, et al. Genome-wide maps of chromatin state in pluripotent and lineage-committed cells. Nature. 2007;448(7153):553–60.
7. Ladinovic D, Novotna J, Jaksova S, Raska I, Vacik T. A demethylation deficient isoform of the lysine demethylase KDM2A interacts with pericentromeric heterochromatin in an HP1a-dependent manner. Nucleus. 2017;8(5):563–72.
8. Huang Y, Liu Y, Yu L, Chen J, Hou J, Cui L, et al. Histone demethylase KDM2A promotes tumor cell growth and migration in gastric cancer. Tumour Biol. 2015;36(1):271–8.
9. Wagner KW, Alam H, Dhar SS, Giri U, Li N, Wei Y, et al. KDM2A promotes lung tumorigenesis by epigenetically enhancing ERK1/2 signaling. J Clin Invest. 2013;123(12):5231–46.
10. Wang F, Liang S, Liu X, Han L, Wang J, Du Q. LINC00460 modulates KDM2A to promote cell proliferation and migration by targeting miR-342-3p in gastric cancer. Onco Targets Ther. 2018;11:6383–94.
11. Chen JY, Luo CW, Lai YS, Wu CC, Hung WC. Lysine demethylase KDM2A inhibits TET2 to promote DNA methylation and silencing of tumor suppressor genes in breast cancer. Oncogenesis. 2017;6(8):e369.
12. Dhar SS, Alam H, Li N, Wagner KW, Chung J, Ahn YW, et al. Transcriptional repression of histone deacetylase 3 by the histone demethylase KDM2A is coupled to tumorigenicity of lung cancer cells. J Biol Chem. 2014;289(11):7483–96.
13. Frescas D, Guardavaccaro D, Kuchay SM, Kato H, Poleshko A, Basrur V, et al. KDM2A represses transcription of centromeric satellite repeats and maintains the heterochromatic state. Cell Cycle. 2008;7(22):3539–47.
14. Maher ER. Genomics and epigenomics of renal cell carcinoma. Semin Cancer Biol. 2013;23(1):10–7.
15. Rydzanicz M, Wrzesinski T, Bluyssen HA, Wesoly J. Genomics and epigenomics of clear cell renal cell carcinoma: recent developments and potential applications. Cancer Lett. 2013;341(2):111–26.
16. Gao R, Dong R, Du J, Ma P, Wang S, Fan Z. Depletion of histone demethylase KDM2A inhibited cell proliferation of stem cells from apical papilla by de-repression of p15INK4B and p27Kip1. Mol Cell Biochem. 2013;379(1–2):115–22.
17. Barski A, Cuddapah S, Cui K, Roh TY, Schones DE, Wang Z, et al. High-resolution profiling of histone methylations in the human genome. Cell. 2007;129(4):823–37.
18. Pfau R, Tzatsos A, Kampranis SC, Serebrennikova OB, Bear SE, Tsichlis PN. Members of a family of JmjC domain-containing oncoproteins immortalize embryonic fibroblasts via a JmjC domain-dependent process. Proc Natl Acad Sci USA. 2008;105(6):1907–12.
19. Rogawski DS, Grembecka J, Cierpicki T. H3K36 methyltransferases as cancer drug targets: rationale and perspectives for inhibitor development. Future Med Chem. 2016;8(13):1589–607.
20. Xu WH, Liang DY, Wang Q, Shen J, Liu QH, Peng YB. Knockdown of KDM2A inhibits proliferation associated with TGF-beta expression in HEK293T cell. Mol Cell Biochem. 2019;456(1–2):95–104.
21. Liu H, Liu L, Holowatyj A, Jiang Y, Yang ZQ. Integrated genomic and functional analyses of histone demethylases identify oncogenic KDM2A isoform in breast cancer. Mol Carcinog. 2016;55(5):977–90.
22. Ou R, Zhu L, Zhao L, Li W, Tao F, Lu Y, et al. HPV16 E7-induced upregulation of KDM2A promotes cervical cancer progression by regulating miR-132-radixin pathway. J Cell Physiol. 2019;234(3):2659–71.
23. Holland D, Hoppe-Seyler K, Schuller B, Lohrey C, Maroldt J, Durst M, et al. Activation of the enhancer of zeste homologue 2 gene by the human papillomavirus E7 oncoprotein. Cancer Res. 2008;68(23):9964–72.

15

Acute myocardial infarction and arterial embolism in a patient with newly diagnosed renal mass: Management dilemmas!

Benedikt Martin[1*], Andreas Greinacher[2], Robin Bülow[5], Fabian Hammer[3], Andreas Hoene[4], Martin Burchardt[1] and Uwe Zimmermann[1]

Abstract

Background: Cancer is often associated with a hypercoagulable state and new thrombosis is often the first clinical manifestation of cancer. Surgical treatment of the primary tumor is crucial since it provides the only curative approach in most cases, but management of patients is highly complex, especially in the presence of new antiplatelet drugs and/or anticoagulants. Paraneoplastic syndromes (PNS) represent a frequent complication of renal cell carcinomas (RCC) and include different hematological symptoms in patients, whilst occlusion of arterial blood vessels displays a rare form of PNS accompanying renal tumors.

Case presentation: We report the case of a 62-year old man who was initially hospitalized due to acute coronary syndrome. He subsequently underwent coronary angioplasty treatment including multiple stenting and treatment with ticagrelor and aspirin. Post-interventional, acute arterial thrombotic emboli of several limb arteries required thrombectomy. By computer tomography we identified a renal lesion suspicious for an RCC and suspected a PNS as underlying cause of the thrombotic complications. Triple anticoagulant therapy was maintained with therapeutic dose low molecular weight heparin (LMWH), aspirin, and clopidogrel, by which we replaced ticagrelor. Surgery was postponed for 4 weeks. We paused LMWH, aspirin and clopidogrel only at the day of surgery and perioperatively restored hemostasis by transfusion of two platelet concentrates. Laparoscopic nephrectomy was uneventful. Pathology confirmed a clear cell RCC. The patient fully recovered whilst slowly reducing anticoagulation dose.

Conclusions: A multidisciplinary team approach of experts in urology, cardiology and hemostasis was key in managing this patient since a personalized thrombosis consult was needed to minimize the risk of reinfarction due to in-stent thrombosis. We report a therapeutic protocol that may be helpful for the management of similar cases. Furthermore, the finding of thrombotic arterial occlusions in larger blood vessels represents a novel complication of PNS in RCC and adds to the varied possible manifestations of this clinical chameleon.

Keywords: Acute arterial thrombotic emboli, Paraneoplastic syndrome, Clear cell renal cell carcinoma

Background

Cancer induces a prothrombotic state. In about 25% of patients above the age of 50 years presenting with acute thrombosis, undiagnosed cancer is the underlying cause. Sometimes cancer is associated with massive hyper

*Correspondence: benedikt.martin@med.uni-greifswald.de
[1] Department of Urology, University Medicine Greifswald, Ferdinand-Sauerbruch-Str., 17475 Greifswald, Germany
Full list of author information is available at the end of the article

coagulopathy requiring removal of the tumor. Surgical treatment of cancer in a patient with recent thromboembolic complications is highly complex, as continuation of anticoagulation and antiplatelet therapy increases the bleeding risk, while cessation of these drugs increases the risk for re-thrombosis.

Renal cell carcinoma is the most common primary tumor of the kidney while it accounts for around 2–3% of all cancers worldwide [1]. Today it is most frequently diagnosed incidentally through radioimaging such as CT or MRI scans, whereas the classical symptom trias of haematuria, palpable tumor and flank pain leads to diagnosis in only 10% of patients [2]. Paraneoplastic syndromes are reported to occur in up to 68% of patients with RCC and can be subdivided into endocrinological and non-endocrinological forms, with hypertension, polycythaemia and hypercalcaemia being primary symptoms of manifestation [3]. Thus far, acute arterial occlusion has rarely been observed accompanying RCCs and has not been reported in larger peripheral blood vessels.

We report a patient who developed myocardial infarction and massive acute thrombotic emboli in main arteries due to a supposed paraneoplastic syndrome caused by an incidentally found clear cell RCC. We present the clinico-pathological outcome of an interdisciplinary approach.

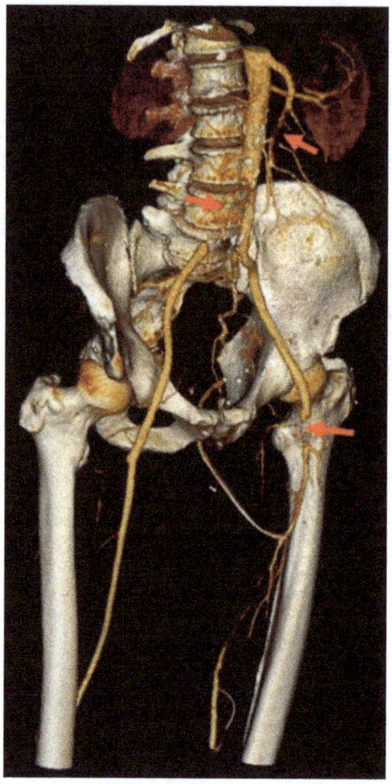

Fig. 1 3D-Reconstruction of CT images showing several arterial thrombotic embolies with incomplete vascular occlusion. Red darts indicate a branch of the upper mesenterial artery, the right common iliac artery and the left femoral artery from top to bottom

Case presentation

A 62-year old male with a history of metabolic syndrome including arterial hypertension, diabetes type 2, hyperlipidemia, obesity and sleep apnea syndrome was initially admitted to our hospital due to acute coronary syndrome. ST-elevated myocardial infarction was diagnosed followed by primary percutaneous coronary intervention (PCI) including angioplasty treatment and application of a singular drug-eluting stent in the right coronary artery. Post-interventional, dual anti-platelet therapy (DAPT) using ticagrelor and aspirin was initiated as well as thrombosis prophylaxis with LMWH. Initial blood testing was normal, particularly erythrocytosis, thrombocytosis and coagulopathy were excluded. As the patient remained instable, at day 3 a second PCI was performed and six drug-eluting stents placed in the left anterior descending artery. At day 10, the patient complained about severe pain in both legs. A thoracoabdominal CT scan showed several acute arterial thrombotic emboli, including incomplete occlusion of the right common iliac artery, the left femoral artery, several arteries of the lower leg and a main branch of the upper mesenteric artery (Fig. 1). Incidentally, the CT scan also showed a left renal tumor highly suspicious for a renal cell carcinoma, accompanied by a large renal cyst (Fig. 2). Platelet count was 149 Gpt/l and acute heparin-induced

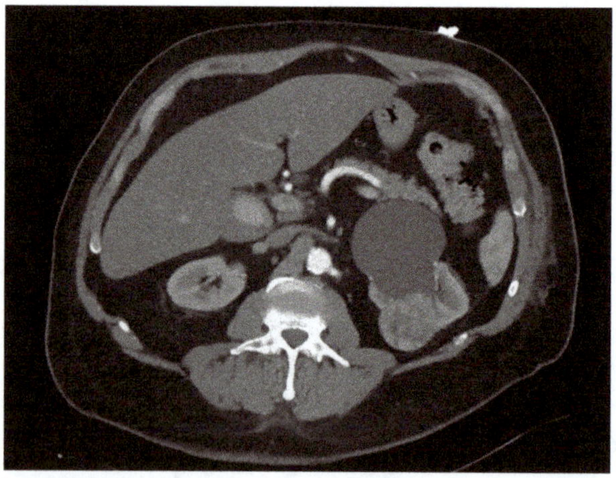

Fig. 2 Abdominal CT scan showing a renal tumor of the left side with adjacent renal cyst

thrombocytopenia (HIT) was considered very unlikely [4].

Therapeutic anticoagulation using unfractionated heparin was started in addition to the ongoing antiplatelet therapy. As this did not result in improvement of the leg perfusion arteriectomy was performed removing most of the occluding material. Histo-pathology confirmed fresh thrombotic emboli. Due to the radiologic suspect of an RCC, a PNS as cause of the massive coagulopathy was suspected.

In a multidisciplinary conference including cardiology, thrombosis consult, vascular surgery and urology, following issues were defined:

The risk for in-stent thrombosis of the seven drug-eluting coronary stents was considered very high in the absence of effective DAPT.

Minimally invasive, surgical total nephrectomy was considered as the intervention with the lowest bleeding risk, which however could not be performed on triple therapy with heparin, ticagrelor and aspirin.

The triple therapy had resulted in a decrease of the D-dimer and stabilization of the platelet count. It was therefore decided to keep the patient on triple anticoagulation therapy for four weeks to allow beginning of endothelialization of the coronary stens and of the altered limb arteries. Ticagrelor is a reversible P2Y12 inhibitor, which is present in the circulation in high concentration. Although the half-life of the drug is only 8 h, it takes about 72–96 h until the high drug levels are decreased to a level, which allows platelet transfusion without inhibition of the transfused platelets [5]. We therefore switched ticagrelor to clopidogrel. Clopidogrel is a direct P2Y12 inhibitor. When it binds to platelets, platelet ADP receptor is irreversibly inhibited for the life span of the platelet, but the active metabolite of clopidogrel has a short half-life of only 1–2 h.

DAPT and LMWH (enoxaparin 1 mg per KG body weight b.i.d) were maintained for 4 weeks and platelet counts, D-dimer and anti-factor Xa were monitored on a weekly basis to assure sufficient anticoagulation. Aspirin, clopidogrel and LMWH were stopped 24 h before surgery. According to the Greifswald bridging protocol, two platelet concentrates were transfused immediately before surgery [6]. Laparoscopic surgery was then performed without bleeding complications. Aspirin and LMWH in prophylactic dose (dalteparin 5000 aFXaU) were restarted six hours after surgery and clopidogrel 48 h after surgery. On the second postoperative day dalteparin was escalated to 5000 aFXa b.i.d. (half therapeutic dose) and therapeutic dose LMWH resumed at day 5. Pathology confirmed clear cell renal cell carcinoma pT3a L0 V0 R0 G2. After an uneventful postsurgical course, the patient was discharged at day eight after surgery. In the post-hospital setting, clopidogrel and aspirin were maintained for one year as indicated after myocardial infarction, while LMWH was stepwise reduced under control of repeated D-Dimer blood testing to prophylactic dose and could eventually be terminated after 6 weeks.

Discussion and conclusions

This patient exemplifies the dilemma of management of patients with newly diagnosed cancer complicated by acute thromboembolic complications, especially if the thrombotic state of the patient is induced by a paraneoplastic syndrome. In-stent thrombosis of the newly implanted coronary stents was considered to be of highest risk for myocardial infarction of this patient. As aggressive triple therapy with antiplatelet drugs and therapeutic dose anticoagulation stabilized the procoagulatory state, a wait and watch strategy for four weeks was considered acceptable. During this time control of anticoagulation was monitored by three parameters: D-dimer as an indicator for progression of fibrin formation, the platelet count as parameter for increased thrombin generation and consumptive coagulopathy, and aFXa levels for compliance and exclusion of consumption of heparin by acute phase proteins. As these parameters remained stable no dose escalation of LMWH was performed. Ticagrelor is recommended as first line P2Y12 inhibitor in patients with acute coronary syndrome. However, a major disadvantage of ticagrelor is its long presence in the circulation. After the last intake the drug persists for 72–96 h. As a small molecule it distributes not only in the intravascular space but also in the interstitial fluid from which it redistributes into the vasculature. Cessation of antiplatelet therapy for 72–96 h before surgery was inacceptable in this patient due to the high risk of in-stent or limb artery thrombosis four weeks after multiple arterial occlusions. Therefore, treatment was a switched from ticagrelor to clopidogrel (while aspirin and LMWH were maintained). Although clopidogrel inhibits platelets irreversible, its active metabolite has a short half-life. This allowed maintenance of antiplatelet therapy until 24 h before surgery, just skipping the morning dose at the day of surgery and subsequently restoring platelet function by platelet transfusion for the peri-interventional period. From on six hours after surgery antiplatelet and anticoagulatory treatment were restarted and escalated stepwise while the patient was carefully monitored for bleeding symptoms.

PNS in renal cell carcinoma are a common phenomenon with a wide variety of disease-associated symptoms [3, 7]. Among the many possible manifestations, vascular and haematological syndromes play a major role. Hypertension is a frequent symptom of PNS and is found in 7–35% of patients. It is assumed to have multiple causes such as combined polycythaemia, increased erythropoietin (EPO) expression or abnormal renin secretion of renal tumor mass [8]. A possible rare reason of acute emboli and stroke can be found in PNS-related polycythaemia which occurs in 8% of RCC patients due to elevated EPO blood levels produced by tumorous renal tissue [9]. Several other haematological abnormalities associated to PNS in RCC have been reported including thrombocytopenia or leukocytosis and are thought to be due to excessive tumor production of transmitters such as IL-6 or granulocyte colony stimulating factor [3].

Much more rarely, PNS-associated arterial ischemia and emboli have been reported in RCC. Few cases of acute digital ischaemia have been described showing classical symptoms of Raynaud's phenomenon. In these patients, tumor progression is more aggressive compared to the average patient cohort [10]. In another report, a fatal outcome of pulmonary tumor thrombotic microangiopathy based on a papillary RCC was identified, in which tumorous microemboli formed in the pulmonary arterioles and subsequently lead to right heart failure [11]. Venous thrombosis in central retinal veins or the upper caval vein are further manifestations of PNS, probably aggravated by elevated levels of antiphospholipid and anticardiolipin antibodies [12, 13].

Besides the incidentally identified RCC, other possible etiologies of limb artery emboli are thrombosis at the site of femoral artery puncture during PCI. An antiphospholipid syndrome which occurs as PNS or HIT had been excluded during the acute phase by negative antibody tests. The authors view the fact of total symptom resolution after nephrectomy is partial proof for the role of the tumor in disease progression as it is typical for PNS [14]. Nevertheless, PNS remains an exclusion diagnosis and the assumption of it being the underlying cause of the depicted symptoms must be seen as speculative. Additional and more specific biochemical investigations to support the diagnosis of PNS except those mentioned have not been performed in this study.

In conclusion, PNS in renal cell carcinoma can be perceived as a clinical chameleon showing a wide variety of symptoms. Unexplained arterial thrombosis seems to be another manifestation of PNS. Although elimination of the primary cause by surgical tumor removal is most important, a multidisciplinary treatment approach is often required to manage the multiple complications of PNS.

Abbreviations

DAPT: Dual anti-platelet therapy; EPO: Erythropoetin; HIT: Heparin-induced thromboyctopenia; LMWH: Low molecular weight heparine; PCI: Percutaneous coronary intervention; PNS: Paraneoplastic syndrome; RCC: Renal cell carcinoma.

Acknowledgements

Not applicable.

Authors' contributions

BM collected the case's details and was responsible for the initial drafts as well as recommended corrections. AG provided the specific thrombosis consult and literature concerning blood coagulation and was a major contributor in writing the manuscript. RB analyzed the raw radiological images and created the reconstructive footage. FH, AH and MB all contributed to the case by medical advice during the interdisciplinary conference in which further treatment was concluded as well as critical reading and corrections in all stages of the manuscript. UZ performed the surgical removal of the renal tumor, initiated the publication and was a major contributor for this case report through all steps of writing this manuscript. All authors read and approved the final manuscript.

Author details

[1]Department of Urology, University Medicine Greifswald, Ferdinand-Sauerbruch-Str., 17475 Greifswald, Germany. [2]Department of Transfusion Medicine, University Medicine Greifswald, Ferdinand- Sauerbruch-Str., 17475 Greifswald, Germany. [3]Department of Cardiology, KMG Clinic Guestrow, Friedrich-Trendelenburg-Allee 1, 18273 Guestrow, Germany. [4]Department of Vascular Surgery, University Medicine Greifswald, Ferdinand-Sauerbruch- Str., 17475 Greifswald, Germany. [5]Department of Radiology, University Medicine Greifswald, Ferdinand-Sauerbruch-Str., 17475 Greifswald, Germany.

References

1. Bray F, Ferlay J, Soerjomataram I, Siegel RL, Torre LA, Jemal A. Global cancer statistics 2018: GLOBOCAN estimates of incidence and mortality worldwide for 36 cancers in 185 countries. CA Cancer J Clin. 2018;68:394–424.
2. Lee CT, Katz J, Fearn PA, Russo P. Mode of presentation of renal cell carcinoma provides prognostic information. Urol Oncol Semin Orig Investig. 2002;7:135–40.
3. Hegemann M, Kroeger N, Stenzl A, Bedke J. Rare and changeable as a chameleon: paraneoplastic syndromes in renal cell carcinoma. World J Urol. 2018;36:849–54.
4. Greinacher A. Clinical practice. Heparin-induced thrombocytopenia. N Engl J Med. 2015;373(3):252–61. https://doi.org/10.1056/NEJMcp1411 910.
5. Godier A, Taylor G, Gaussem P. Inefficacy of platelet transfusion to reverse ticagrelor. N Engl J Med. 2015;8(2):196–7.
6. Baschin M, Selleng S, Hummel A, Diedrich S, Schroeder HW, Kohlmann T, Westphal A, Greinacher A, Thiele TJ. Preoperative platelet transfusions to reverse antiplatelet therapy for urgent non-cardiac surgery: an observational cohort study. Thromb Haemost. 2018;16(4):709–17.
7. Ding G, Feng C, Song N, Fang Z, Xia G, Jiang H, Hua L, Ding Q. Paraneoplastic symptoms: cachexia, polycythemia, and hypercalcemia are, respectively, related to vascular endothelial growth factor (VEGF) expression in renal clear cell carcinoma. Urol Oncol. 2013;31:1820–5.
8. Moein MR, Dehghani VO. Hypertension. A rare presentation of renal cell carcinoma. J Urol. 2000;164:2019.
9. Sacco E, Pinto F, Sasso F, Racioppi M, Gulino G, Volpe A, Bassi P. Paraneoplastic syndromes in patients with urological malignancies. Urol Int. 2009;83:1–11.
10. Kampoli K, Gardeli D, Mouktaroudi M, Fanouriakis A, Lazaris AM, Koumarianou A. Paraneoplastic digital ischemia in clear-cell renal-cell carcinoma: report of a case and review of the literature. Urologia. 2019;86:156–60.
11. Story M, Kwon SK, Robinson R, Fortis S. Acute cor pulmonale due to pulmonary tumour thrombotic microangiopathy from renal cell carcinoma. BMJ Case Rep. 2017;2017:bcr-2017.
12. Adrean SD, Schwab IR. Central retinal vein occlusion and renal cell carcinoma. Am J Ophthalmol. 2003;136:1185–6.
13. May M, Seehafer M, Helke C, Uberrück T, Gunia S, Hoschke BV. cava superior Syndrom mit beidseitiger Jugularis- und Subklaviavenenthrombose—Paraneoplastische Manifestation eines Nierenzellkarzinoms. Urologe A. 2003;42:1374–7.
14. Lee CM, Sim A, Kurugulasigamoney G, Ng LG. Heart failure as the first manifestation of renal cell carcinoma. Korean J Urol. 2015;56:82–5.

16

The role of angioembolization in the management of blunt renal injuries

Giovanni Liguori[1], Giacomo Rebez[1*], Alessandro Larcher[2], Michele Rizzo[1], Tommaso Cai[3] and Carlo Trombetta and Andrea Salonia[2]

Abstract

Background: Recently, renal angioembolization (RAE) has gained an important role in the non-operative management (NOM) of moderate to high-grade blunt renal injuries (BRI), but its use remains heterogeneous. The aim of this review is to examine the current literature on indications and outcomes of angioembolization in BRI.

Methods: We conducted a search of MEDLINE, EMBASE, SCOPUS and Web of Science Databases up to February 2021 in accordance with PRISMA guidelines for studies on BRI treated with RAE. The methodological quality of eligible studies and their risk of bias was assessed using the Newcastle–Ottawa scale

Results: A total of 16 articles that investigated angioembolization of blunt renal injury were included in the study. Overall, 412 patients were included: 8 presented with grade II renal trauma (2%), 97 with grade III renal trauma (23%); 225 with grade IV (55%); and 82 with grade V (20%). RAE was successful in 92% of grade III–IV (294/322) and 76% of grade V (63/82). Regarding haemodynamic status, success rate was achieved in 90% (312/346) of stable patients, but only in 63% (42/66) of unstable patients. The most common indication for RAE was active contrast extravasation in hemodynamic stable patients with grade III or IV BRI.

Conclusions: This is the first review assessing outcomes and indication of angioembolization in blunt renal injuries. The results suggest that outcomes are excellent in hemodynamic stable, moderate to high-grade renal trauma.

Keywords: Renal, Blunt, Angioembolization, Trauma, Kidney

Key points

Angioembolization is effective and safe in stable grade III–IV blunt renal trauma.
Grade I–II blunt renal injuries need RAE very occasionally.
A few hemodynamically unstable and or grade V patients might benefit from RAE but the data is not robust enough to support angioembolization as a standard of care in these subgroups.

Introduction

Renal angioembolization (RAE) is an effective, minimally invasive treatment that was first developed in the 1970s [1]. Renal injuries occur in approximately 10% of all abdominal trauma [2] and the kidney is the third most commonly injured solid organ. Every year, up to 245.000 renal injuries occur worldwide; blunt trauma is responsible for 80–90% of them [2, 3]. Over the last few decades,

*Correspondence: giacomorebez@gmail.com
Azienda Sanitaria Universitaria Giuliano-Isontina, Strada di Fiume 447, 34149 Trieste, Italy
Full list of author information is available at the end of the article

non-operative management (NOM), including observation, transfusion, bed rest and/or renal angiography with embolization (RAE), has become increasingly popular, especially for low-grade (I–II) and intermediate grade (III) blunt renal injuries (BRI). High-grade renal trauma has traditionally been managed via surgical exploration and published evidence is unclear about the role of NOM for higher grades (IV and V) [4–6]. Over the last few decades, the management of patients with multiple injuries has improved thanks to specialized trauma units and NOM has become the treatment of choice for most renal injuries [7]. Hemodynamic stability is one of the most important criteria to decide between operative and non-operative strategies in renal injuries [8]. As a whole, primary conservative management is associated with a lower rate of nephrectomies, without increasing the immediate or long-term morbidity. The improved staging of injury severity, thanks to advancing radiographic techniques, has enhanced the use of NOM [9]. Furthermore, selective treatment with interventional radiology procedures has eventually reduced the need for surgical interventions in patients with both blunt and penetrating renal injuries [9, 10]. Hemodynamic stability is one of the most important criteria to decide between operative and non-operative strategies in renal injuries [8] Angioembolization has an important role in the management of high-grade BRI [11, 12] but currently, its use remains heterogeneous. The aim of this review is to evaluate the efficacy of angioembolization in blunt renal trauma in current literature, with the aim of understanding the indications and outcomes of RAE in patients with moderate- to high grade renal trauma.

Methods

PRISMA guidelines [13] were followed, and a literature search was performed using PUBMED, EMBASE, SCOPUS, Web of Science. Articles either published or e-published on angioembolization for BRI between January 2009 and February 2021 were searched. The Mesh terms used for the search were: "renal" ("kidney"); "trauma" ("injury"); "embolization"; "angiography"; ("Renal Angio Embolization" or "RAE"). An additional manual search of EMBASE, as well as bibliographies of each included study, was done to identify studies not covered by the initial search.

Study eligibility

Studies were selected on the following criteria: (1) patients age > 18 years; (2) studies reporting outcomes of upfront RAE; (3) English language; (4) studies reporting indications, techniques and/or embolic materials. The exclusion criteria were as follows: (1) reviews or editor letters and single case report; (2) non-English language publications; (3) studies involving angioembolization of open injury, penetrating trauma, paediatric patients or iatrogenic injury; and (4) studies with insufficient or unconfirmed information.

Preferred Reporting Items for Systematic Review and Meta-Analysis (PRISMA) guidelines were followed to perform this review. The titles were screened to evaluate whether they met the inclusion criteria. These studies were divided into three different categories: included, probably relevant and excluded. Included and relevant studies were re-evaluated to check eligibility.

Data extraction and quality assessment

Data including the first author, publication year, number of patients, age, sex, indications, materials, and outcome of interest were extracted by two autonomous reviewers into standardized MS Office Excel. The risk of bias and the methodological quality of eligible studies were assessed using the Newcastle–Ottawa scale [14] which weighs nine items across the domains of selection, comparability and outcome for cohort studies. Each of these three items was assessed and graded (1 or 2 points). In this analysis, studies with NOS scores of 1–3, 4–6, and 7–9, were defined as of low, intermediate, and high quality, respectively. Poor quality studies were not excluded from the review. Two authors independently extracted the data and gave each study a quality assessment; any discordances were resolved through discussion to reach an agreement.

Results

Using these search criteria, an initial selection of 1057 articles was considered. After title screening and manual reduplication, we narrowed down to 943 eligible for abstract review. Full-text evaluation for the remaining 131 citations identified by abstract review or by a manual search of the references list was done (Fig. 1). A total of 16 articles that investigated angioembolization in blunt renal injury were included in the study.

Quality assessment of the included studies

Most studies (68.7%) were graded as intermediate or high quality and full details of the NOS quality appraisal score for each study are summarized in the Additional file 1: Table S1 Quality assessment using the modified Newcastle-Ottawa scale of included cohort studies. Selection and confounding were important sources of error, with only 2 (12.5%) studies attaining the maximum score for selection and no study reaching the maximum score for comparability; 31.2% of cohort designs scored 3/3 for outcome measurement. No prospective studies were available in the current literature.

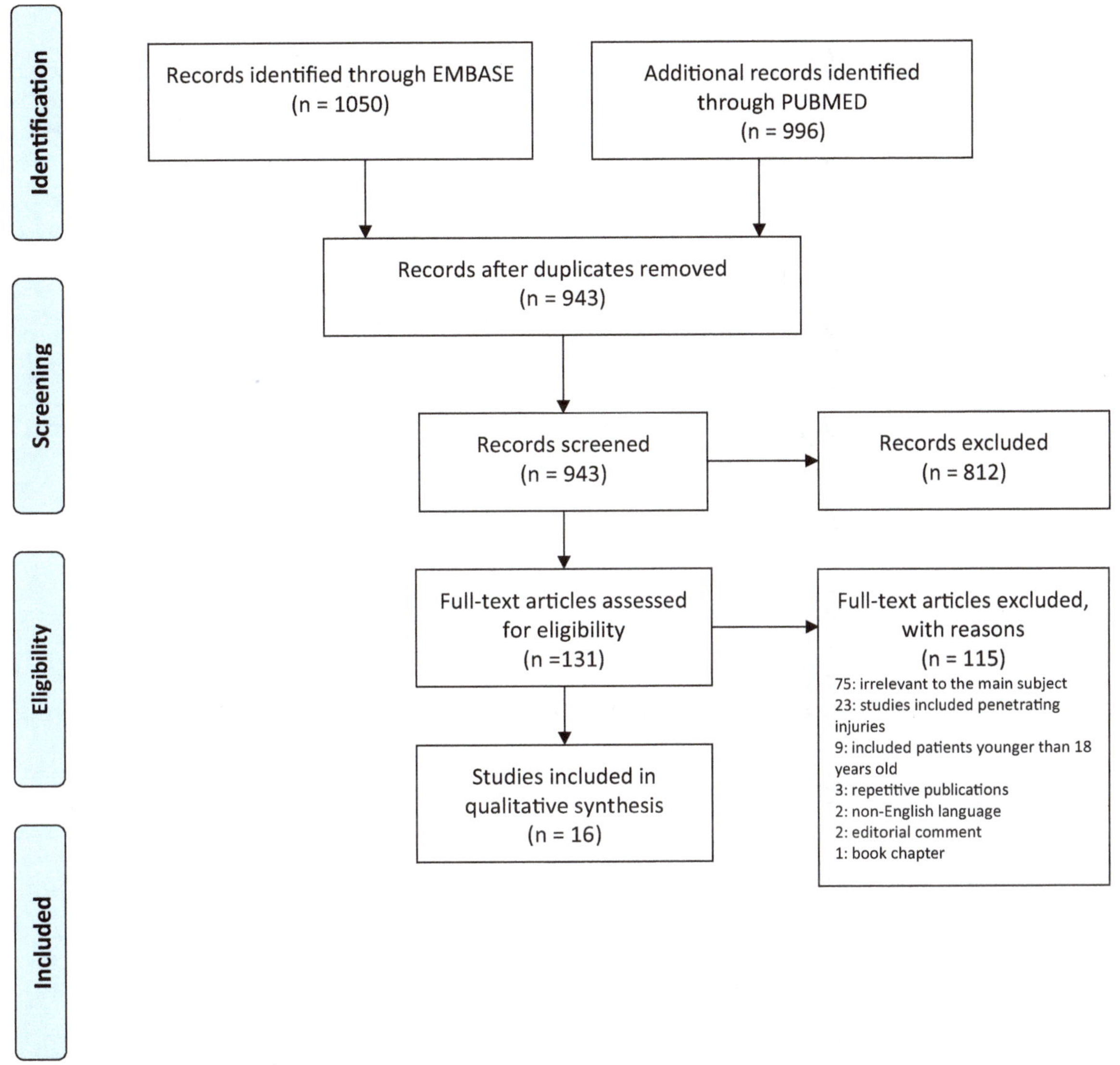

Fig. 1 PRISMA flow diagram

Success rate

The clinical success was defined as the absence of repeat RAE, salvage nephrectomy or death for each patient. All 412 patients identified in this review underwent unilateral RAE achieving clinical success in 354 of them (85%) range 75–100% (Tables 1, 2). Overall, 34 patients (8%) experienced surgical exploration for RAE failure: 31 patients underwent salvage nephrectomy (91%) and 3 patients underwent partial nephrectomy (9%). A second embolization, after the failure of the first attempt, was performed in 17 patients and was effective in all of them. The reason for RAE repetition was presence of pseudoaneurysm in 7 cases, recurrence of bleeding in 7 cases, persistent gross haematuria in 3 cases and arteriovenous fistula occurrence in one case, with an overall success rate of 100%. Moreover, 2 patients required subsequent angioplasty after [15] embolization to control arterial bleeding and 4 patients required a more proximal vessel embolization to stop angiographic extravasation [12, 16]. Overall, 404 patients with moderate to high grade renal injuries were included (Table 2): 97 presented with grade III renal trauma (23%); 225 with grade IV (55%); and 82 with grade V (20%). RAE was successful in 92% of cases (294/322) with grade III-IV renal trauma and 76% (63/82) of cases with grade V trauma (76%). Regarding haemodynamic status, success rate was achieved in 312/346 (90%)

Table 1 Summary of patient's characteristics and clinical outcomes

Year	References	Number of patients	AAST II	AAST III	AAST IV	AAST V	1st embolization success rate (%)	2nd embolization success rate	Salvage Nephrectomy	Perioperative mortality
2009	Brewer [24]	9	0	0	0	9	100	Not performed	RAE successful	12% (1)
2010	Fu [20]	14	0	2	11	1	85	100%	RAE successful	0%
2010	Menaker [36]	22	2	2	17	1	73	Not performed	27% (6)*	0%
2010	Stewart [6]	2	0	0	0	2	100	Not performed	RAE successful	0%
2011	Charbit [19]	10	0	1	4	5	90	Not performed	10% (1)	0%
2012	Van Der Vlies [39]	6	0	1	2	3	100	Not performed	16% (1)	0%
2013	Van de Wilden [12]	25	0	0	20	5	92	100%	RAE successful	0%
2014	Saour [18]	10	0	1	4	5	90	Not performed	10% (1)	0%
2014	Rao [30]	16	0	12	3	1	93	Not performed	7% (1)	6% (1)
2015	Vozianov [16]	20	2	11	7	0	90	100%	RAE successful	0%
2018	Yanagi [21]	17	0	0	17	0	100	Not performed	RAE successful	17% (3)
2019	Pretorius [37]	7	0	3	4	0	85	100%	RAE successful	0%
2020	Chen [38]	7	4	0	3	0	100	Not performed	RAE successful	12% (1)
2020	Desai [17]	15	0	1	12	2	86	Not performed	13% (2)	0%
2020	Xu [15]	62	0	28	20	14	95	Not performed	1.6% (1)	1.6% (1)
2021	Baboudjian [23]	170	0	35	101	34	77	100%	12% (22)	3.5% (6)

*Menaker performed 3 partial nephrectomies

Table 2 Outcomes of RAE sorted by hemodynamic status (a) and by AAST category (b)

Patients' characteristics	Number of patients	RAE Success	RAE Failure
(a) Hemodynamic status			
Overall	412 (100%)	354 (85%)	58 (15%)
Hemodynamic stable patients	346 (85%)	312 (90%)	34 (9%)
Hemodynamic unstable patients	66 (15%)	42 (63%)	24 (37%)
(b) AAST category			
Overall	412 (100%)	354 (85%)	58 (15%)
Grade V	82 (19%)	63 (76%)	19 (24%)
Grade III–IV	322 (77%)	294 (92%)	28 (8%)
Grade II	8 (2%)	8 (100%)	0

of stable patients, and only in 42/66 (63%) of unstable patients.

Overall, thirteen patients deceased (3%). Seven were hemodynamic unstable patients and died for causes related to the trauma: 4 deaths occurred within 24 h after RAE for uncontrolled bleeding, 1 patient died after surgery and 2 patients died for acute circulation failure despite a successful RAE. The other six patients died during hospitalization for other causes.

Complications were poorly reported. Urinoma was diagnosed as an early complication in 3 patients all successfully managed with ureteral stenting. Four retroperitoneal abscesses were reported and successfully drained. Moreover, two atrophic kidneys were reported as long-term complications by Desai [17]. No patient required dialytic treatment after discharge. Renal function outcome was reported in 3 studies. Xu [15] stated that Grade 3 and 4 lesions did not have a significant decrease in renal function while grade 5 treated with RAE had a significant decrease in glomerular filtration rate (78.8 ± 11.0 vs 72.5 ± 5.6 after RAE). Vozianov [16] reported 2 patients (10%) with a significant drop of renal function at 3 months follow up. Saour [18] reported no significant decrease of renal function after embolization. A brief analysis was performed excluding the lowest quality studies based on risk score ≤ 3. The sub analysis showed an overall success rate of 85% (281/334), success rate in unstable patient of 68% (39/57) while surgical treatment was required in 32 patients (10%).

Indications for RAE

The most common indication for RAE was contrast extravasation in stable patients with kidney trauma III to V grade. CT criteria, such as absence of major visceral injuries, perirenal hematoma rim distance, discontinuity of Gerota's fascia, or intravascular contrast extravasation were used to select patients for RAE [12, 19, 20]. Failure of conservative management due to unresponsive to fluid resuscitation hypotension or persistent gross haematuria represent further indication [16, 21–23].

Non operative management with angioembolization was described in hemodynamically unstable patients with high-grade renal injuries, [6, 15, 23, 24] without evidence of other intra-abdominal injuries requiring surgical exploration. Factors predictive of RAE failure were evaluated in one manuscript [23] which reported as significant predictors of RAE failure gross haematuria, hemodynamic instability, grade V trauma, and urinary extravasation.

Technique of RAE

Pre-procedure diagnostic work-up All patients were primarily screened with CT scan to identify the bleeding site. Angiography was performed prior to embolization to define the precise site of bleeding and the actual possibility to perform angioembolization.

Timing All patients underwent RAE within 24–48 h of hospital admission in an urgency/emergency setting.

Route Most RAE were performed through femoral approach, using 4–6 F sized arterial sheaths [25]. Radial or brachial approach was rare but necessary in case of iliac artery occlusion or unusual anatomic conditions [26].

Selective catheterization Selective embolization was performed on angiographic findings, after comparing CT and the arteriogram findings. Comparison between CT and arteriogram allowed the choice between selective embolization or embolization of the proximal branches of the renal artery [6, 19, 24].

Embolizing agents the selection mostly depends on interventional radiologists' preference and diameter of the bleeding vessel. The most popular material was coils (Table 3).

Table 3 Embolizing materials

Year	Author	Number of patients	Gelfoam	Pva	Microcoils	NBCA	Microcoils + Gelfoam	Success rate (%)
2009	Brewer [24]	9	44% (4)	0	66% (5)	0	0	100
2010	Stewart [6]	10	0	0	100% (10)	0	0	100
2011	Charbit [19]	10	40% (4)	0	60% (6)	0	0	90
2015	Vozianov [16]	20	30% (6)	70% (14)	0	0	0	90
2018	Yanagi [21]	17	47% (8)	0	11% (2)	5% (1)	35% (6)	100
2020	Desai [17]	15	0	0	86% (13)	0	0	85

Embolizing materials were selected according to radiologist's preference and diameter of embolized vessel

Discussion

We present the first systematic review conducted to assess the management and outcomes of RAE in blunt renal injuries. The current analysis suggests that urological outcomes are overall excellent in stable, moderate to high-grade renal trauma without concomitant major visceral injuries. Our findings are consistent with latest guidelines since hemodynamic stability is the main criterion for non-operative management of kidney trauma [27–31]. Angioembolization has a key role in the non-operative management, but no validated criteria to predict RAE efficacy are available in the current literature and its practice remains heterogeneous in blunt renal injuries [23, 32]. We analysed contemporary published articles of patients undergoing RAE for blunt renal trauma. Overall, among the 412 patients with kidney trauma treated with angioembolization, 354 patients (85%) achieved clinical success and avoided further treatments. These results reinforce the current management strategies for renal trauma. A large proportion of high-grade renal trauma could be safely managed with RAE. Moreover, RAE is considered as the first choice for hemodynamically stable patients, achieving an overall 90% success rate (including patients with grade V renal trauma). Conversely, the indications for embolization therapy in grade V are still debated since those injuries are uncommon and most studies lack an appropriate sample size to create statistical significance and deliver valid recommendations. In our review, the success rate for grade V is 73%, but the lack of categorization into renal pedicle injury versus shattered kidney may lead to a misinterpretation. Even if we could assume that RAE has a realistic chance of success in a shattered kidney with extravasations from secondary kidney artery branches, the success rate might be very low if the main renal artery is injured, and the embolization would not be selective. Unfortunately, the patient's selection was not based on a shared protocol, but on the clinical judgment of the trauma-surgeon and radiologist. Furthermore, these decisions could not be retrieved from the trauma registry or electronic medical record, resulting in a selection bias. Baboudijan et al. [23], the largest study to date, retrospectively analysed 170 patients with moderate- to high-grade renal trauma treated with upfront RAE. The authors found that RAE treatment was successful in 131 patients (77%). Subgroup analysis showed RAE efficacy of 64.7% for grade V trauma, 59.6% for patients with hemodynamic instability and 45% for patients with both grade V trauma and hemodynamic instability. Contrarywise, the decision to perform angioembolization or surgery is usually based on the presence of concomitant injuries, the hemodynamic status and the grade of the lesion. Overall, in our review, RAE was reported successful in 42 hemodynamically unstable patients with a 63% success rate. Unfortunately, the lack of a control group managed by surgery, prevented drawing strong conclusions around the role of RAE in hemodynamic unstable patients. Hemodynamic instability was defined by Brewer [24] as not responding to Advanced Trauma Life Support protocol, (i.e. presenting with or experiencing the development of hypotension, tachycardia or acidosis, and not responding to 2 l crystalloid and initial blood resuscitation). However, other authors did not define the hemodynamic instability, leading to a possible selection bias. According to Loggers' review [33], in the current literature there is no consensus on the definition of hemodynamic stability in blunt trauma. Moreover, all patients who died for causes related to kidney trauma were unstable at presentation; therefore, despite the encouraging success rate, this data is still not robust enough to support this treatment as a standard of care.

Overall, only 8 patients (2%) underwent RAE with a grade II renal injury. As a whole, grade I-II are the most frequent types of blunt trauma and usually benefit from a truly conservative approach without embolization. These patients should not be treated routinely with RAE, owing to the risk of inducing unnecessary renal infarctions and overtreatment [34]. In this review, we noted that second RAE or salvage nephrectomy after RAE failure were associated with a high success rate. Both procedures appear to be safe since only one patient (1/33) died after salvage nephrectomy, and none died after the second attempt of RAE. Moreover, three patients underwent RAE before laparotomy for other purposes. These results imply that a first attempt of angioembolization would not prevent the success of a secondary salvage nephrectomy or repeat RAE. The sub-analysis performed without the lowest quality studies showed very similar results to the overall analysis, reinforcing the overall results of this review.

Only one study [23] analysed predictive factors of angioembolization failure. Persistent gross haematuria, hemodynamic instability, and active urine extravasation were associated with RAE failure. Finally, numerous general indications among different embolizing agents have been described (Table 3) [35]; however, the failure rate could not be related to the type of materials.

There are several limitations in this review that should be acknowledged. First of all, a meta-analytic approach was not performed due to the heterogeneity of the studies and the lack of prospective ones. Moreover, retrieved data did not allow us to perform a comprehensive comparative evaluation of RAE vs. observation vs. surgery. Indeed, all studies except one [15] lacked a control group with similar clinical presentation of trauma but managed with either surgery or observation, preventing any solid conclusion on the relative role of RAE. Likewise, very few data on complication were available, and if available still were hardly comparable due to different measurements (i.e., eGFR vs serum creatinine) or different timing (pressure within 24 h of RAE vs at 1–3 months of follow up).

Conclusions

The use of angioembolization is very limited in low grade blunt renal trauma, where truly conservative management with active monitoring are optimal therapies in the vast majority of cases. Instead, an indication is in stable patients with grade III-IV blunt renal trauma which are likely to benefit from RAE with a very high success rate. Based on very recent studies, the use of embolization is expanding to unstable haemodynamic and grade V renal trauma but to date they represent a contra-indication in most cases. The results in these subgroups are promising, but not entirely reliable since the relevant risk of failure and the significant confounders present in the studies. Multi institutional collaborative research with control group is needed to better assess the relative role of RAE in these subgroups of patients. It is important to remind that surgical management is needed and remains a fundamental component of the trauma surgeon's armamentarium.

Abbreviations

RAE: Renal angioembolization; NOM: Non operative management; BRI: Blunt renal injuries; CT: Computed tomography.

Supplementary Information

Additional file 1. Quality assessment using the modified Newcastle-Ottawa scale of included cohort

Acknowledgements

Not applicable.

Authors' contributions

All authors have contributed to the information and material submitted for publication and all authors have read and approved the manuscript. Design of the work: GL,GR; Acquisition, analysis, interpretation of data: GR, GL, AS, AL, TC, MR, CT; Drafted the work and substantively revised it: GR. All Authors have approved the submitted version (and any substantially modified version that involves the author's contribution to the study); All authors have agreed both to be personally accountable for the author's own contributions and to ensure that questions related to the accuracy or integrity of any part of the work, even ones in which the author was not personally involved, are appropriately investigated, resolved, and the resolution documented in the literature.

Author details

[1]Azienda Sanitaria Universitaria Giuliano-Isontina, Strada di Fiume 447, 34149 Trieste, Italy. [2]Università Vita Salute San Raffaele, Milan, Italy. [3]Ospedale Santa Chiara, Trento, Italy.

References

1. Almgård LE, Fernström I, Haverling M, Ljungqvist A. Treatment of renal adenocarcinoma by embolic occlusion of the renal circulation. Br J Urol. 1973;45:474–9.
2. Wessells H, Suh D, Porter JR, Rivara F, MacKenzie EJ, Jurkovich GJ, et al. Renal injury and operative management in the United States: results of a population-based study. J Trauma. 2003;54:423–30.
3. Morey AF, Brandes S, Dugi DD, Armstrong JH, Breyer BN, Broghammer JA, et al. Urotrauma: AUA guideline. J Urol. 2014;192:327–35.
4. Santucci RA, Fisher MB. The literature increasingly supports expectant (conservative) management of renal trauma—a systematic review. J Trauma Injury Infect Crit Care. 2005;59:491–501.
5. Altman AL, Haas C, Dinchman KH, Spirnak JP. Selective nonoperative management of blunt grade 5 renal injury. J Urol. 2000;164:27–31.
6. Stewart AF, Brewer ME, Daley BJ, Klein FA, Kim ED. Intermediate-term follow-up of patients treated with percutaneous embolization for grade 5 blunt renal trauma. J Trauma Inj Infect Crit Care. 2010;69:468–70.
7. Santucci RA, McAninch JW, Safir M, Mario LA, Service S, Segal MR. Validation of the American Association for the Surgery of Trauma organ injury severity scale for the kidney. J Trauma Injury Infect Crit Care. 2001;50:195–200.
8. Rogers CG, Knight V, MacUra KJ, Ziegfeld S, Paidas CN, Mathews RI. High-grade renal injuries in children—Is conservative management possible? Urology. 2004;64:574–9.

9. McGuire J, Bultitude MF, Davis P, Koukounaras J, Royce PL, Corcoran NM. Predictors of outcome for blunt high grade renal injury treated with conservative intent. J Urol. 2011;185:187–91.
10. Chow SJD, Thompson KJ, Hartman JF, Wright ML. A 10-year review of blunt renal artery injuries at an urban level I trauma centre. Injury. 2009;40:844–50.
11. Lanchon C, Fiard G, Arnoux V, Descotes JL, Rambeaud JJ, Terrier N, et al. High grade blunt renal trauma: predictors of surgery and long-term outcomes of conservative management. A prospect Single Center Study. J Urol. 2016;195:106–11.
12. Van Der Wilden GM, Velmahos GC, Joseph DK, Jacobs L, DeBusk MG, Adams CA, et al. Successful Nonoperative management of the most severe blunt renal injuries: a multicenter study of the research consortium of new england centers for trauma. JAMA Surg. 2013;148:924–31.
13. Stewart LA, Clarke M, Rovers M, Riley RD, Simmonds M, Stewart G, et al. Preferred reporting items for a systematic review and meta-analysis of individual participant data: the PRISMA-IPD statement. J Am Med Assoc. 2015;313:1657–65.
14. Abou-Setta AM, Beaupre LA, Jones CA, Rashiq S, Hamm MP, Sadowski CA, et al. Newcastle-Ottawa Scale Assessment of Cohort Studies. 2011. https://www.ncbi.nlm.nih.gov/books/NBK56664/. Accessed 2 Apr 2021.
15. Xu H, Min X, Li Y, Yang L, Ren Y. A comparative study of conservation, endovascular embolization therapy, and surgery for blunt renal trauma. Med Sci Monit. 2020;26:1–8.
16. Vozianov S, Sabadash M, Shulyak A. Experience of renal artery embolization in patients with blunt kidney trauma. Cent Eur J Urol. 2015;68:471.
17. Desai D, Ong M, Lah K, Clouston J, Pearch B, Gianduzzo T. Outcome of angioembolization for blunt renal trauma in haemodynamically unstable patients: 10-year analysis of Queensland public hospitals. ANZ J Surg. 2020;90:1705–9. https://doi.org/10.1111/ans.16204.
18. Saour M, Charbit J, Millet I, Monnin V, Taourel P, Klouche K, et al. Effect of renal angioembolization on post-traumatic acute kidney injury after high-grade renal trauma: a comparative study of 52 consecutive cases. Injury. 2014;45:894–901.
19. Charbit J, Manzanera J, Millet I, Roustan JP, Chardon P, Taourel P, et al. What are the specific computed tomography scan criteria that can predict or exclude the need for renal angioembolization after high-grade renal trauma in a conservative management strategy? J Trauma Inj Infect Crit Care. 2011;70:1219–128.
20. Fu CY, Wu SC, Chen RJ, Chen YF, Wang YC, Chung PK, et al. Evaluation of need for angioembolization in blunt renal injury: discontinuity of Gerota's fascia has an increased probability of requiring angioembolization. Am J Surg. 2010;199:154–9.
21. Yanagi M, Suzuki Y, Hamasaki T, Mizunuma K, Arai M, Yokota H, et al. Early transcatheter arterial embolization for the American Association for the Surgery of Trauma Grade 4 Blunt renal trauma in two institutions. J Nippon Med Sch. 2018;85:204–7.
22. Breyer BN, McAninch JW, Elliott SP, Master VA. Minimally Invasive Endovascular Techniques to Treat Acute Renal Hemorrhage. J Urol. 2008;179:2248–53.
23. Baboudjian M, Gondran-Tellier B, Panayotopoulos P, Hutin M, Olivier J, Ruggiero M, et al. Factors predictive of selective angioembolization failure for moderate- to high-grade renal trauma: a French multi-institutional Study. Eur Urol Focus. 2021: 6–11.
24. Brewer ME, Strnad BT, Daley BJ, Currier RP, Klein FA, Mobley JD, et al. Percutaneous embolization for the management of grade 5 renal trauma in hemodynamically unstable patients: initial experience. J Urol. 2009;181:1737–41.
25. Muller A, Rouvière O. Renal artery embolization-indications, technical approaches and outcomes. Nat Rev Nephrol. 2015;11:288–301.
26. Sauk S, Zuckerman DA. Renal artery embolization. Semin Intervent Radiol. 2011;28:396–406.
27. Bryk DJ, Zhao LC. Guideline of guidelines: a review of urological trauma guidelines. BJU Int. 2016;117:226–34.
28. Robert M, Drianno N, Muir G, Delbos O, Guiter J. Management of major blunt renal lacerations: Surgical or nonoperative approach? Eur Urol. 1996;30:335–9.
29. Keihani S, Xu Y, Presson AP, Hotaling JM, Nirula R, Piotrowski J, et al. Contemporary management of high-grade renal trauma: results from the American Association for the Surgery of Trauma Genitourinary Trauma study. J Trauma Acute Care Surg. 2018;84:418–25. https://doi.org/10.1097/TA.0000000000001796
30. Coccolini F, Moore EE, Kluger Y, Biffl W, Leppaniemi A, Matsumura Y, et al. Kidney and uro-trauma: WSES-AAST guidelines. World J Emerg Surg. 2019;14:1–25.
31. Serafetinides E, Kitrey ND, Djakovic N, Kuehhas FE, Lumen N, Sharma DM, et al. Review of the current management of upper urinary tract injuries by the EAU trauma guidelines panel. Eur Urol. 2015;67:930–6. https://doi.org/10.1016/j.eururo.2014.12.034.
32. Petrone P, Perez-Calvo J, Brathwaite CEM, Islam S, Joseph DK. Traumatic kidney injuries: a systematic review and meta-analysis. Int J Surg. 2020;74:13–21. https://doi.org/10.1016/j.ijsu.2019.12.013.
33. Loggers SAI, Koedam TWA, Giannakopoulos GF, Vandewalle E, Erwteman M, Zuidema WP. Definition of hemodynamic stability in blunt trauma patients: a systematic review and assessment amongst Dutch trauma team members. Eur J Trauma Emerg Surg. 2017;43:823–33. https://doi.org/10.1007/s00068-016-0744-8.
34. Glass AS, Appa AA, Kenfield SA, Bagga HS, Blaschko SD, McGeady JB, et al. Selective angioembolization for traumatic renal injuries: a survey on clinician practice. World J Urol. 2014;32:821–7.
35. Hotaling JM, Sorensen MD, Smith TG, Rivara FP, Wessells H, Voelzke BB. Analysis of diagnostic angiography and angioembolization in the acute management of renal trauma using a national data set. J Urol. 2011;185:1316–20.
36. Menaker J, Joseph B, Stein DM, Scalea TM. Angiointervention: high rates of failure following blunt renal injuries. World J Surg. 2011;35(3):520–7. https://doi.org/10.1007/s00268-010-0927-0
37. Pretorius R, Vlok S, Van der Merwe A, Zarrabi AD, Du Toit K. Renal artery embolisation: indications and utilisation at Tygerberg Hospital. S Afr J Surg. 2019;57(4):33–9.
38. Chen J, Cai W, Li L. Profile of renal artery embolization (RAE) for renal trauma: a comparison of data from two major trauma center. International Braz J Urol. 2020;46(2):194–202. https://doi.org/10.1590/s1677-5538.ibju.2019.0506.
39. van der Vlies CH, Olthof DC, van Delden OM, Ponsen KJ, de la Rosette JJMCH, de Reijke TM, Goslings JC. Management of blunt renal injury in a level 1 trauma centre in view of the European guidelines. Injury. 2012;43(11):1816–20. https://doi.org/10.1016/j.injury.2011.06.034.

17

Endovascular management of a large renal artery aneurysm

Alec Zhu[1*], Peter Connolly[1] and A. Ari Hakimi[2]

Abstract

Background: A renal artery aneurysm is a rare clinical presentation that can be found incidentally on imaging or during workup for refractory hypertension. Its presentation can be similar to that of a renal artery pseudoaneurysm, but the etiologies of the two vascular lesions differ. We present a patient who had an incidental finding of a large renal artery aneurysm that was managed with endovascular embolization. We also describe the literature surrounding the etiology, presentation and management of both renal artery aneurysms and renal artery pseudoaneurysms.

Case presentation: A 62-year-old man was referred to a urologic oncologist for workup of a newly found renal mass. Initial imaging with computed tomography showed a homogenous, well-circumscribed mass arising from the right kidney. Further evaluation with Doppler ultrasonography demonstrated pulsatile flow within the renal mass that was concerning for a renal artery pseudoaneurysm. The patient initially underwent a diagnostic angiogram by interventional radiology and was found to have a true renal artery aneurysm. Interventional radiology considered placement of a covered stent or angioembolization, but treatment was deferred due to concern for compromising the patient's renal function. Patient was subsequently transferred to a neighboring hospital for management by vascular surgery. After considering both open surgical and endovascular approaches, the patient ultimately underwent angioembolization of the renal artery aneurysm. Short-term follow-up showed successful exclusion of the aneurysm with minimal adverse effects to the patient.

Conclusions: Our case report documents a unique case of an incidentally found large renal artery aneurysm that was successfully managed with endovascular embolization. Renal artery aneurysms and renal artery pseudoaneurysms, which can present similarly on imaging, are important diagnostic considerations in a patient presenting with a new renal mass. While open surgical approaches can be used to repair aneurysms, endovascular approaches using stenting or angioembolization are safe and effective options for treating renal aneurysms and renal pseudoaneurysms.

Keywords: Renal, Artery, Aneurysm, Pseudoaneurysm, Case report

Background

A renal artery aneurysm (RAA) is a rare vascular malformation that is typically found incidentally on imaging [1]. On rare occasions, RAAs can rupture and cause a life-threatening hemorrhage with a mortality rate approaching 10%, and this risk is significantly higher in pregnant women [2, 3]. The RAA is characterized by a localized defect in the internal elastic tissue that allows it

*Correspondence: aleczhu18@gmail.com
[1] NewYork-Presbyterian/Weill Cornell Medical Center, 525 E 68th St, New York, NY 10065, USA
Full list of author information is available at the end of the article

to dilate; a true aneurysm contains all three layers of the arterial wall [4]. In contrast, a renal artery pseudoaneurysm (RAP) is a hematoma that forms from an arterial defect that intermittently ruptures and clots off, forming a collection of blood products surrounded by the renal parenchyma or the renal capsule [5]. RAPs occur due to injury to the kidney following abdominal trauma or renal surgery [6, 7]. We present the case of an incidentally discovered renal artery aneurysm and review some of the literature surrounding the etiology, presentation, and management of both RAAs and RAPs.

Case presentation

A 62-year-old man with a 40-pack-year smoking history was referred to the urologic oncology clinic for workup of an incidentally discovered renal mass. After undergoing chest imaging for lung cancer screening, a right renal mass was found. Follow-up computed tomography (CT) imaging demonstrated a 7.5 × 7.4 × 7.5 cm well-circumscribed mass arising from the mid right kidney that enhanced homogenously with few calcifications (Fig. 1a, b). He did not have any recent surgeries or traumas. He was instructed to complete imaging work-up by obtaining a doppler ultrasound study. The ultrasound was completed on the same day and demonstrated a large vascular lesion with pulsatile flow concerning for a renal pseudoaneurysm (Fig. 1c). The patient was informed of the results and told to return promptly to the hospital for admission. After arriving, Interventional Radiology (IR) performed a renal angiogram which demonstrated a large aneurysm arising near the bifurcation of the right upper pole artery. IR attempted placement of a covered stent, but there was no good landing zone. A coil embolization was also considered, but it was ultimately deferred given the risk for infarction of a large portion of the right kidney.

Given the possible need for vascular reconstruction, the patient was transferred to the vascular surgery service at a neighboring hospital. The vascular team discussed options with the patient including open surgical reconstruction or endovascular intervention. Open surgery could involve auto-transplantation of the kidney after ex vivo reconstruction of the aneurysm. Another option is local repair of the aneurysm in-situ with aneurysm excision and reimplantation of the superior pole branch of the renal artery. Alternatively, endovascular approaches including placement of a covered stent or renal angioembolization could also be performed. Ultimately, the patient and the vascular team agreed to repeat an attempt for placement of a covered stent.

Selective angiogram of the right renal artery confirmed a renal artery aneurysm originating from the superior pole branch (Fig. 2a). Vascular surgery was able to pass a microwire and catheter into the superior pole artery but

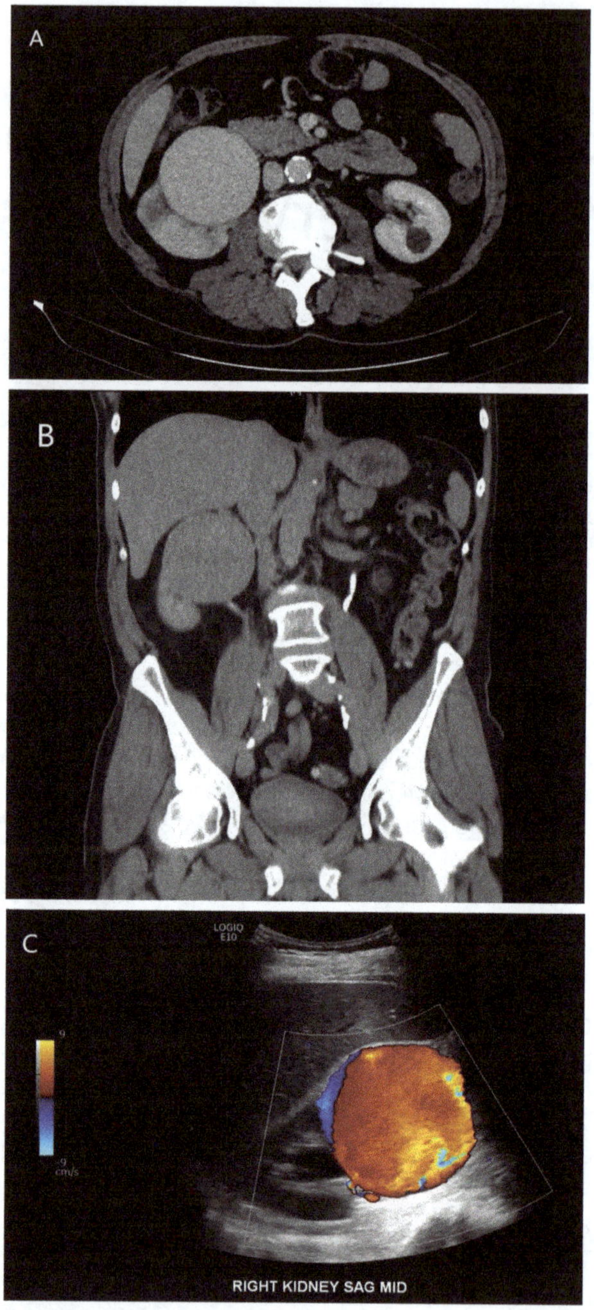

Fig. 1 CT with intravenous contrast (**a**, **b**) demonstrated a 7.5 × 7.2 cm ovoid mass that was compressing on the upper pole and interpolar regions of the right kidney. The mass had similar density to blood. Doppler ultrasound (**c**) showed pulsatile flow within the right renal mass

was unable to advance a larger wire that would facilitate the placement of a covered stent. The decision was made to proceed with coil embolization of the outflow and inflow tract. Subsequent angiography demonstrated good exclusion of flow into the aneurysm with maintained flow

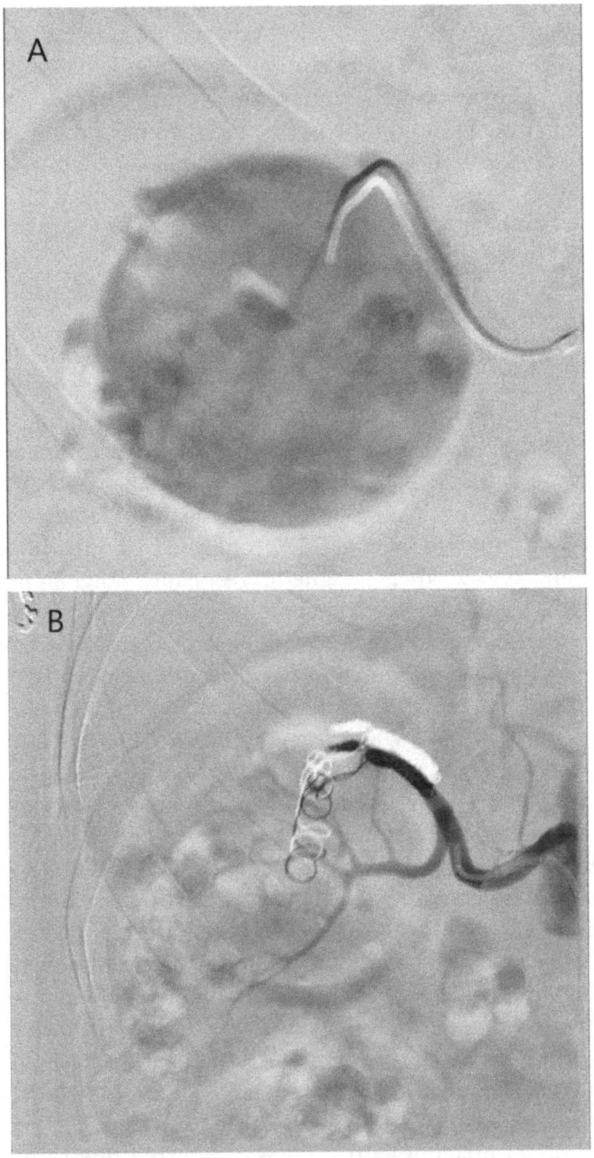

Fig. 2 Right renal angiogram (**a**) revealed a 7 cm aneurysm. A superior pole branch of the right renal artery directly fed into the aneurysm. Selective coil embolization (**b**) excluded the inflow and outflow tracts for the aneurysm within the superior pole branch of the right renal artery. The inferior pole branch of the renal artery was preserved which allowed perfusion to a majority of the right kidney

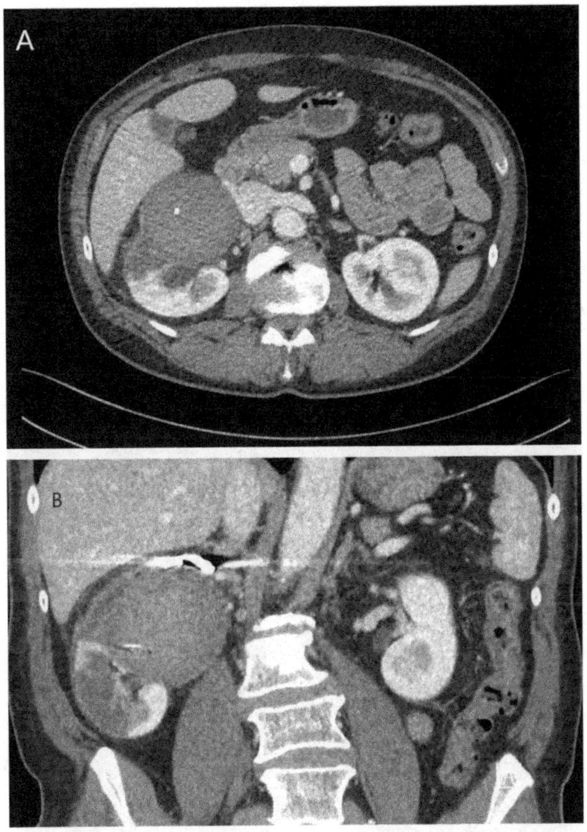

Fig. 3 CTA (**a**, **b**) performed on postoperative day 14 demonstrated a 7.5 cm aneurysm with no contrast enhancement on arterial or delayed phases of imaging. There was hypoperfusion of the superior, anterior, and lateral portions of the right kidney indicating renal infarct

into the inferior renal pole branch (Fig. 2b). The patient tolerated the procedure well and was discharged from the hospital on postoperative day 1.

The patient presented for outpatient follow-up on postoperative day 14 with new symptoms of nausea, abdominal pain, night sweats, and chills. He noted that his symptoms of nausea occurred specifically after eating fatty meals. Laboratory work showed no leukocytosis, anemia, or elevated creatinine, but there was a mild elevation in alanine aminotransferase. CT angiography (CTA) was performed and demonstrated metallic coiling in the right renal artery and a 7.5 cm aneurysm without contrast enhancement on arterial or delayed phases of imaging (Fig. 3a, b). Hypoperfusion of some areas of the kidney were also seen, consistent with infarction. At a 3-month follow-up visit, the patient reported feeling well and had resolution of prior symptoms. Repeat CTA showed stable size of the excluded renal aneurysm sac along with interval atrophy of the renal parenchyma consistent with prior renal infarct (Fig. 4a, b). Basic hematology and chemistry lab values were within normal limits. The patient is scheduled to return for additional follow-up 6 months after his procedure.

Discussion and conclusion

Our case report demonstrates a patient who presented with an incidental finding of a RAA during workup for a renal mass. Although the renal lesion was initially diagnosed as a RAP by doppler ultrasonography, the

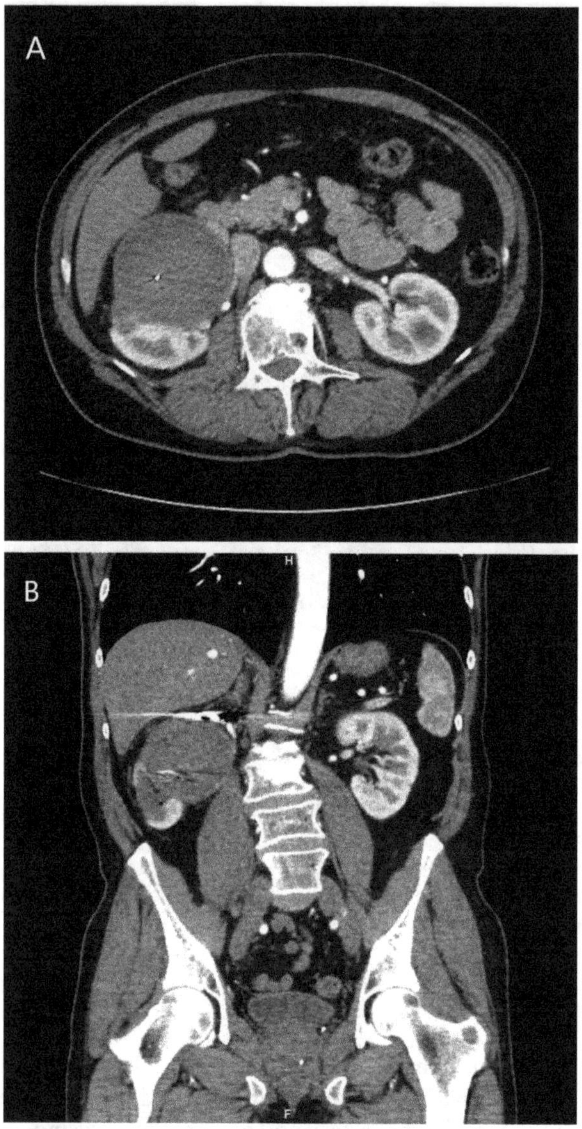

Fig. 4 CTA (**a**, **b**) performed 3 months after angioembolization showed stable size of aneurysm sac. There was interval atrophy of right renal parenchyma due to renal infarct

subsequent angiography study revealed that the patient had a true aneurysm. RAAs are a rare phenomenon with an overall incidence of 0.09% within the general population [8]. They can be classified into three different forms: type 1 consists of saccular aneurysms arising from the main renal artery or a large segmental branch, type 2 includes fusiform aneurysms, and type 3 includes intralobar artery aneurysms [9]. Our patient presented with a saccular type aneurysm, which accounts for about 94% of all aneurysms [10].

RAAs typically present without symptoms, but as they grow in size, they can lead to pain, hematuria, and hypertension due to compression of the renal parenchyma [11]. Additionally, RAAs typically present after 60 years of age, are more commonly seen in females than males, are associated with hypertension, and are predominantly found on the right side when presenting as a unilateral lesion [12]. RAAs can be diagnosed on physical exam as a pulsatile mass in the region of the renal hilum or when heard as a bruit on auscultation [13]. However, these exam findings are rare and RAAs are more commonly found incidentally on imaging [1]. Our patient was initially diagnosed with a pseudoaneurysm given the presence of a "yin-yang sign" on doppler sonography, which is depicted by the swirling motion pattern of arterial blood flow in a cystic structure. This finding on doppler ultrasound is characteristic of a pseudoaneurysm, but it can also be present in a saccular aneurysm [14]. When evaluating for RAA, the most commonly used imaging modality is CTA, followed by non-contrast enhanced CT, then magnetic resonance angiography (MRA), then catheter angiography, and lastly ultrasound [1]. Current vascular surgery guidelines recommend the use of CTA as the primary imaging modality of choice to evaluate patients with a suspected RAA [15]. Additionally, non-contrast MRA is recommended for evaluating RAA in patients who have increased radiation exposure risks (children, pregnant women) or contraindications to receiving contrast material (renal insuffiency, contrast allergy) [15]. Contrast-enhanced MRI has been shown to reliably detect renal aneurysms. However, they do not have the ability to show mural calcifications, and they have poor visualization of the external arterial wall when compared to CTA [16]. The additional use of maximum intensity projection or volume rendering reconstruction of CTA images can enhance the anatomic detail of the renal vasculature and can help identify aneurysms located at smaller branch vessels [17, 18]. In our patient, additional imaging with CTA was deferred due to high clinical suspicion for RAP, and additional imaging would not have changed the patient's plan to undergo renal angiography. Current guidelines also recommend catheter-based angiography for preoperative planning and for improving visualization of the distal arterial branches that may not be well seen on conventional cross-sectional imaging [15].

Although RAAs and RAPs are rare, it is nevertheless important to rule out its presence during the workup of a new renal mass. Our patient presented for oncologic workup of a renal mass found on CT. But if doppler ultrasonography had been performed with the CT scan, an aneurysm would have been detected sooner and the patient would not have had a delay in his care. A study by Inci et al. reported a patient who underwent laparoscopic partial nephrectomy. On interval CT scan at a three month follow-up visit, there was a hyper-vascular lesion noted at the prior resection site which was reported as a recurrence of renal cell carcinoma. The patient was asymptomatic at that time and subsequently underwent radical nephrectomy for presumed cancer recurrence. However, the pathology was negative for cancer and instead demonstrated a RAP [19]. Another study reported a similar case with an asymptomatic patient who presented with recurrent renal masses after laparoscopic partial nephrectomy. However, a renal Doppler ultrasound was performed which revealed two RAPs, and the patient subsequently underwent successful angioembolization of the two RAPs [20]. Through our case and these prior reports, we hope highlight the importance of using multiple imaging modalities in the workup of a new renal mass.

A RAP is also a rare clinical occurrence that forms after an inciting event that causes injury to the renal vasculature, such as abdominal trauma, renal biopsy, percutaneous renal surgery, partial nephrectomy, or renal transplant, [6, 7, 21–26]. While a true aneurysm is a localized dilation involving all layers of the arterial wall, a renal pseudoaneurysm is a hematoma that forms from an arterial defect and is contained by the surrounding renal parenchyma or capsule [5]. Patients with a RAP will typically present with signs and symptoms of gross hematuria, flank pain, and/or anemia, but they can also be asymptomatic [27]. Patients who developed RAP after partial nephrectomies typically presented with signs and symptoms of delayed bleeding through the urinary tract. Most patients have at least one of three signs or symptoms: gross hematuria, flank pain, or anemia. While 5% of patients will present with all three symptoms, around 87% of patients will present with gross hematuria [27]. Most patients who develop symptoms will present around two weeks after renal surgery [27, 28].

A RAP is a rare complication following percutaneous nephrolithotomy with rates reported to occur in 0.3–0.7% of cases [7, 23, 29, 30]. Despite having low reported rates, the true incidence of RAP after percutaneous procedures is unknown and may be higher if patients were asymptomatic and did not present with signs or symptoms that would lead to further diagnostic testing. RAPs also develop at low rates after partial nephrectomies. However, the risk for developing RAP after partial nephrectomies appear to be different for open and laparoscopic surgeries. Albani et al. reported 3 patients who developed RAPs out of 698 (0.43%) who had an open partial nephrectomy [24]. Conversely, Singh et al. showed that 6 patients developed RAPs out of 345 (1.7%) who had laparoscopic partial nephrectomy [21]. Similar rates were reported by Ghoneim et al. who noted that 7 out of 1,160 (0.6%) patients who underwent open partial nephrectomy and 8 out of 301 (2.7%) patients who underwent laparoscopic partial nephrectomy were diagnosed with RAPs [28]. A systematic review examined 30 published series and case reports that included 5,229 cases of open or laparoscopic partial nephrectomies and found that rates of RAP were significantly more likely to occur after laparoscopic procedures compared to open procedures (1.96% vs 1.00%, $p \leq 0.001$) [27]. While overall rates for RAP after open or laparoscopic partial nephrectomies remain low, it is unclear why RAP is more likely occur after laparoscopic surgeries. Various factors involving surgical techniques used within laparoscopic surgery may be a contributing factor: larger needles can cause greater tissue trauma, parenchymal approximation may not be as tight, and pneumoperitoneum may mask small vascular injuries that would otherwise bleed [28]. Additionally, it has been shown that laparoscopic partial nephrectomies for tumors in the central portion of the kidney are more likely to develop RAP compared to surgeries for tumors in the periphery of the kidney [31].

Treatment for a RAA or RAP is typically sought when the aneurysm is greater than 3 cm in size, in a woman of childbearing age, or in a patient with medically refractory hypertension [15]. The main reason for treatment is to reduce the risk for aneurysm rupture which can lead to life-threatening hemorrhage. Earlier reports estimated a high risk of RAA rupture ranging from 14 to 30% [32, 33]. Prior guidelines recommended repair of visceral artery aneurysms greater than 2 cm [34]. However, more recent reports suggest RAAs have a much lower risk for rupture, even in aneurysms greater than 2 cm in size. Tham et al. followed 69 patients with RAA conservatively over a mean of 4 years and found that none of these patients developed RAA ruptures [35]. A multicenter center study by Klausner et al. showed that out of a cohort of 547 patients with untreated RAA, the rupture rate was 0.55%, and ruptures only occurred in patients with aneurysms greater than 3 cm in size [1]. Pregnancy has been associated with a higher rate of aneurysm rupture, possibly due to changes in vascular flow and hormonal shifts that result in weakening of the arterial wall elastic tissue [12]. However, the true incidence of RAA within the pregnant population is unknown [12]. The presence of a RAA with renovascular hypertension is also an indication for treatment. Studies have shown that reconstruction of a RAA can improve or cure co-existing hypertension, and the benefit of repair on hypertension is more likely to occur in those with renovascular hypertension than in those without arterial stenosis [2, 36, 37].

Options for treatment of a RAA include open surgical repair or endovascular approaches. Open surgery includes ex-vivo reconstruction with auto-transplantation of the kidney or in-situ repair of the aneurysm. These open surgical approaches offer good vascular patency rates ranging 93–100% and long-term survival rates averaging 90% at 10 years [38–40]. Additionally, when these surgeries are performed in the appropriate patient, they are well tolerated with minimal morbidity and complication rates [2, 41, 42].

Endovascular treatments for RAA include deployment of a covered stent or renal angioembolization. Small series have shown that the endovascular approach is well-tolerated with reported success rates of 83–100% and variable complication rates of 13–60% [43, 44]. When comparing the endovascular approach to the open surgical approach, retrospective studies have suggested that the endovascular approach is associated with shorter hospitalizations, similar or fewer complications, and similar success rates [45, 46]. Additionally, no studies have reported a significant difference in mortality, perioperative morbidity, freedom from reintervention, or decline in renal function when comparing open and endovascular approaches to repairing RAAs [1, 45, 47].

Endovascular stenting or embolization is also the preferred approach for a RAP. In rare cases in which angioembolization is unsuccessful, open surgery with nephrectomy is necessary [27]. Angioembolization of a RAP has a high success rate ranging 93–96% in select series [27, 28]. The procedure is well tolerated with a complication rate of around 5%; most common complications include incomplete embolization, coil migration, and groin hematoma [48]. The patient in our report presented on postoperative day 14 with symptoms of nausea, abdominal pain, night sweats, and chills. These symptoms are consistent post-infarction syndrome (PIS). Around 74% of patients after renal angioembolization will experience PIS, which include symptoms of flank pain, nausea, or vomiting [48]. The vast majority of these symptoms are mild and self-limited. Loss of renal function is an additional adverse effect of angioembolization due to the devascularization of renal parenchyma and/or the use of iodinated contrast which may be nephrotoxic. However, the use of coaxial catheters and microcoils for superselective embolization can minimize the loss of renal parenchyma. The loss of renal tissue can range from 0 to 10% at 6 months post-embolization, but overall renal function is typically preserved in patients after angioembolization [49]. However, those with solitary kidneys may have increased risk for deterioration of renal function after embolization [50].

Our case report documents a unique case of an asymptomatic patient who presented for evaluation for a renal mass but was incidentally found to have a large renal artery aneurysm. A RAA is a rare clinical finding that can be managed with surveillance, open surgical reconstruction, or endovascular approaches. Given the size of the RAA and its risk for rupture, our patient underwent successful treatment with renal angioembolization and had minimal adverse effects following treatment. Although our patient presented for oncologic workup given initial imaging findings, additional testing with doppler ultrasound elucidated the presence of a renal aneurysm which allowed the patient to be directed to the proper therapy. In addition to reviewing the etiology, presentation, and management of both RAAs and RAPs, we also hope to use our case to highlight the importance of using multiple imaging modalities for the workup of renal masses.

Abbreviations

CT: Computed tomography; CTA: Computed tomography angiography; IR: Interventional radiology; MRA: Magnetic resonance angiography; PIS: Post-infarction syndrome; RAA: Renal artery aneurysm; RAP: Renal artery pseudoaneurysm.

Acknowledgements

Not applicable.

Authors' contributions

AZ performed the literature review and wrote the case report. PC and AH provided the images and edited the case report. All authors read and approved the final manuscript.

Author details

[1]NewYork-Presbyterian/Weill Cornell Medical Center, 525 E 68th St, New York, NY 10065, USA. [2]Memorial Sloan Kettering Cancer Center, 1275 York Ave, New York, NY 10065, USA.

References

1. Klausner JQ, Lawrence PF, Harlander-Locke MP, Coleman DM, Stanley JC, Fujimura N, et al. The contemporary management of renal artery aneurysms. J Vasc Surg. 2015;61(4):978–84.
2. Henke PK, Cardneau JD, Welling TH, Upchurch GR, Wakefield TW, Jacobs LA, et al. Renal artery aneurysms a 35-year clinical experience with 252 aneurysms in 168 patients. Ann Surg. 2001;234(4):454–62.
3. Cohen JR, Shamash FS. Ruptured renal artery aneurysms during pregnancy. J Vasc Surg. 1987;6(1):51–9.
4. Poutasse EF. Renal artery aneurysm: report of 12 cases, two treated by excision of the aneurysm and repair of renal artery. J Urol. 1957;77(5):697–708.
5. Dauw CA, Stuart Wolf J. Fundamentals of upper urinary tract drainage. In: Partin AW, Peters CA, Kavoussi LR, Dmochowski RR, Wein AJ, editors. Campbell Walsh Wein Urology. 12th ed. Philadelphia: Elsevier; 2020. p. 160–84.
6. Swana HS, Cohn SM, Burns GA, Egglin TK. Renal artery pseudoaneurysm after blunt abdominal trauma: case report and literature review. J Trauma. 1996;40(3):459–61.
7. Kessaris DN, Bellman GC, Pardalidis NP, Smith AG. Management of hemorrhage after percutaneous renal surgery. J Urol. 1995;153(3 Pt 1):604–8.
8. Stanley JC, Rhodes EL, Gewertz BL, Chang CY, Walter JF, Fry WJ. Renal artery aneurysms: significance of macroaneurysms exclusive of dissections and fibrodysplastic mural dilations. Arch Surg. 1975;110(11):1327–33.
9. Rundback JH, Rizvi A, Rozenblit GN, Poplausky M, Maddineni S, Crea G, et al. Percutaneous stent-graft management of renal artery aneurysms. J Vasc Interv Radiol. 2000;11(9):1189–93.
10. Zinman L, Libertino JA, et al. Uncommon disorders of the renal circula-

tion: renal artery aneurysm. In: Breslin D, Swinton N, Libertino JA, et al., editors. Renovascular hypertension. Baltimore: Williams & Wilkins; 1982. p. 110–4.
11. Sarkar R, Coran AG, Cilley RE, Lindenauer SM, Stanley JC. Arterial aneurysms in children: clinicopathologic classification. J Vasc Surg. 1991;13(1):47–56 (**discussion-7**).
12. Coleman DM, Stanley JC. Renal artery aneurysms. J Vasc Surg. 2015;62(3):779–85.
13. Silvis RS, Hughes WF, Holmes FH. Aneurysm of the renal artery. Am J Surg. 1956;91(3):339–43.
14. Mahmoud MZ, Al-Saadi M, Abuderman A, Alzimami KS, Alkhorayef M, Almagli B, et al. "To-and-fro" waveform in the diagnosis of arterial pseudoaneurysms. World J Radiol. 2015;7(5):89–99.
15. Chaer RA, Abularrage CJ, Coleman DM, Eslami MH, Kashyap VS, Rockman C, et al. The Society for Vascular Surgery clinical practice guidelines on the management of visceral aneurysms. J Vasc Surg. 2020;72(1S):3S-39S.
16. Browne RF, Riordan EO, Roberts JA, Ridgway JP, Woodrow G, Gough M, et al. Renal artery aneurysms: diagnosis and surveillance with 3D contrast-enhanced magnetic resonance angiography. Eur Radiol. 2004;14(10):1807–12.
17. Zhang LJ, Yang GF, Qi J, Shen W. Renal artery aneurysm: diagnosis and surveillance with multidetector-row computed tomography. Acta Radiol. 2007;48(3):274–9.
18. Smith PA, Fishman EK. Three-dimensional CT angiography: renal applications. Semin Ultrasound CT MR. 1998;19(5):413–24.
19. Inci K, Cil B, Yazici S, Peynircioglu B, Tan B, Sahin A, et al. Renal artery pseudoaneurysm: complication of minimally invasive kidney surgery. J Endourol. 2010;24(1):149–54.
20. Hayn MH, Jackman SV. Recurrent mass after laparoscopic partial nephrectomy. Urology. 2007;70(5):1004–5.
21. Singh D, Gill IS. Renal artery pseudoaneurysm following laparoscopic partial nephrectomy. J Urol. 2005;174(6):2256–9.
22. Jebara VA, El Rassi I, Achouh PE, Chelala D, Tabet G, Karam B. Renal artery pseudoaneurysm after blunt abdominal trauma. J Vasc Surg. 1998;27(2):362–5.
23. El-Nahas AR, Shokeir AA, El-Assmy AM, Mohsen T, Shoma AM, Eraky I, et al. Post-percutaneous nephrolithotomy extensive hemorrhage: a study of risk factors. J Urol. 2007;177(2):576–9.
24. Albani JM, Novick AC. Renal artery pseudoaneurysm after partial nephrectomy: three case reports and a literature review. Urology. 2003;62(2):227–31.
25. Dodd GD 3rd, Tublin ME, Shah A, Zajko AB. Imaging of vascular complications associated with renal transplants. AJR Am J Roentgenol. 1991;157(3):449–59.
26. Farrell TM, Sutton JE, Burchard KW. Renal artery pseudoaneurysm: a cause of delayed hematuria in blunt trauma. J Trauma. 1996;41(6):1067–8.
27. Jain S, Nyirenda T, Yates J, Munver R. Incidence of renal artery pseudoaneurysm following open and minimally invasive partial nephrectomy: a systematic review and comparative analysis. J Urol. 2013;189(5):1643–8.
28. Ghoneim TP, Thornton RH, Solomon SB, Adamy A, Favaretto RL, Russo P. Selective arterial embolization for pseudoaneurysms and arteriovenous fistula of renal artery branches following partial nephrectomy. J Urol. 2011;185(6):2061–5.
29. Srivastava A, Singh KJ, Suri A, Dubey D, Kumar A, Kapoor R, et al. Vascular complications after percutaneous nephrolithotomy: are there any predictive factors? Urology. 2005;66(1):38–40.
30. Richstone L, Reggio E, Ost MC, Seideman C, Fossett LK, Okeke Z, et al. First Prize (tie): Hemorrhage following percutaneous renal surgery: characterization of angiographic findings. J Endourol. 2008;22(6):1129–35.
31. Nadu A, Kleinmann N, Laufer M, Dotan Z, Winkler H, Ramon J. Laparoscopic partial nephrectomy for central tumors: analysis of perioperative outcomes and complications. J Urol. 2009;181(1):42–7 (**discussion 7**).
32. Cerny JC, Chang CY, Fry WJ. Renal artery aneurysms. Arch Surg. 1968;96(4):653–63.
33. Ippolito JJ, Leveen HH. Treatment of renal artery aneurysms. J Urol. 1960;83:10–6.
34. Hirsch AT, Haskal ZJ, Hertzer NR, Bakal CW, Creager MA, Halperin JL, et al. ACC/AHA 2005 Practice Guidelines for the management of patients with peripheral arterial disease (lower extremity, renal, mesenteric, and abdominal aortic): a collaborative report from the American Association for Vascular Surgery/Society for Vascular Surgery, Society for Cardiovascular Angiography and Interventions, Society for Vascular Medicine and Biology, Society of Interventional Radiology, and the ACC/AHA Task Force on Practice Guidelines (Writing Committee to Develop Guidelines for the Management of Patients With Peripheral Arterial Disease): endorsed by the American Association of Cardiovascular and Pulmonary Rehabilitation; National Heart, Lung, and Blood Institute; Society for Vascular Nursing; TransAtlantic Inter-Society Consensus; and Vascular Disease Foundation. Circulation. 2006;113(11):e463-654.
35. Tham G, Ekelund L, Herrlin K, Lindstedt EL, Olin T, Bergentz SE. Renal artery aneurysms. Natural history and prognosis Ann Surg. 1983;197(3):348–52.
36. Gonzalez J, Esteban M, Andres G, Linares E, Martinez-Salamanca JI. Renal artery aneurysms. Curr Urol Rep. 2014;15(1):376.
37. Pfeiffer T, Reiher L, Grabitz K, Grunhage B, Hafele S, Voiculescu A, et al. Reconstruction for renal artery aneurysm: operative techniques and long-term results. J Vasc Surg. 2003;37(2):293–300.
38. Robinson WP 3rd, Bafford R, Belkin M, Menard MT. Favorable outcomes with in situ techniques for surgical repair of complex renal artery aneurysms. J Vasc Surg. 2011;53(3):684–91.
39. English WP, Pearce JD, Craven TE, Wilson DB, Edwards MS, Ayerdi J, et al. Surgical management of renal artery aneurysms. J Vasc Surg. 2004;40(1):53–60.
40. Marone EM, Mascia D, Kahlberg A, Brioschi C, Tshomba Y, Chiesa R. Is open repair still the gold standard in visceral artery aneurysm management? Ann Vasc Surg. 2011;25(7):936–46.
41. Murray SP, Kent C, Salvatierra O, Stoney RJ. Complex branch renovascular disease: management options and late results. J Vasc Surg. 1994;20(3):338–45 (**discussion 46**).
42. Chandra A, O'Connell JB, Quinones-Baldrich WJ, Lawrence PF, Moore WS, Gelabert HA, et al. Aneurysmectomy with arterial reconstruction of renal artery aneurysms in the endovascular era: a safe, effective treatment for both aneurysm and associated hypertension. Ann Vasc Surg. 2010;24(4):503–10.
43. Zhang Z, Yang M, Song L, Tong X, Zou Y. Endovascular treatment of renal artery aneurysms and renal arteriovenous fistulas. J Vasc Surg. 2013;57(3):765–70.
44. Sedat J, Chau Y, Baque J. Endovascular treatment of renal aneurysms: a series of 18 cases. Eur J Radiol. 2012;81(12):3973–8.
45. Tsilimparis N, Reeves JG, Dayama A, Perez SD, Debus ES, Ricotta JJ 2nd. Endovascular vs open repair of renal artery aneurysms: outcomes of repair and long-term renal function. J Am Coll Surg. 2013;217(2):263–9.
46. Hislop SJ, Patel SA, Abt PL, Singh MJ, Illig KA. Therapy of renal artery aneurysms in New York State: outcomes of patients undergoing open and endovascular repair. Ann Vasc Surg. 2009;23(2):194–200.
47. Cochennec F, Riga CV, Allaire E, Cheshire NJ, Hamady M, Jenkins MP, et al. Contemporary management of splanchnic and renal artery aneurysms: results of endovascular compared with open surgery from two European vascular centers. Eur J Vasc Endovasc Surg. 2011;42(3):340–6.
48. Schwartz MJ, Smith EB, Trost DW, Vaughan ED Jr. Renal artery embolization: clinical indications and experience from over 100 cases. BJU Int. 2007;99(4):881–6.
49. Poulakis V, Ferakis N, Becht E, Deliveliotis C, Duex M. Treatment of renal-vascular injury by transcatheter embolization: immediate and long-term effects on renal function. J Endourol. 2006;20(6):405–9.
50. Mohsen T, El-Assmy A, El-Diasty T. Long-term functional and morphological effects of transcatheter arterial embolization of traumatic renal vascular injury. BJU Int. 2008;101(4):473–7.

18

Sequential immune-targeted surgical therapy resulted in disease-free survival in a case with advanced renal cell carcinoma

Kenichi Nishimura[1*], Noriyoshi Miura[1], Naoya Sugihara[1], Keisuke Funaki[1], Kanae Koyama[1], Yuichiro Sawada[1], Terutaka Noda[1], Tetsuya Fukumoto[1], Yuki Miyauchi[1], Tadahiko Kikugawa[1], Takashi Saika[1], Masafumi Matsumura[2], Katsuyoshi Hashine[2] and Mashio Taniwaki[3]

Abstract

Background: Currently, immunotherapy is indicated for patients with metastatic RCC or unresectable RCC, but there is no indication for immunotherapy in the neoadjuvant setting. We report a case in which the combined use of nivolumab and ipilimumab and sequential TKI therapy enabled surgical treatment.

Case presentation: A 71-year-old female was diagnosed with a metastatic clear-cell renal cell carcinoma with a level IV tumor thrombus. She was started on nivolumab-ipilimumab therapy, and was switched to pazopanib monotherapy because the tumor thrombus progressed within the right atrium. The tumor shrank to resectable status with sequential therapy. She then underwent right nephrectomy and thrombectomy. Pathological analysis showed 10–20% residual tumor in the primary tumor, but no viable cells in tumor thrombus. She remains clinically disease-free 1 year after surgery.

Conclusion: This case suggests the utility of sequential immune-targeted therapy as neoadjuvant therapy in advanced renal cell carcinoma.

Keywords: Sequential immune-targeted therapy, Advanced renal cell carcinoma, Nivolumab, Ipilimumab, Case report

Background

Renal cell carcinoma (RCC) has been reported to invade into the vena cava in 4–10% of cases [1]. Reese et al. reported the natural history of RCC patients with untreated tumor thrombus, and noted that 87% of these patients (n = 297) died of RCC with a median survival of 5 months [2]. In contrast, the 5-year survival rate after nephrectomy and tumor thrombectomy among RCC patients with tumor thrombus in the inferior vena cava (IVC) is approximately 50% [1]. Neoadjuvant therapy has been implemented in several cancer types to reduce the size of the tumor and improve surgical morbidity. However, currently no neoadjuvant systematic treatments exist for patients with advanced RCC. Multiple tyrosine kinase inhibitors (TKIs) have been evaluated in patients with locally advanced disease with the objective of downstaging to enable surgical resection. However, several studies have reported low rates of response [3]. Cost et al. reported that in 25 RCC patients with tumor thrombus, neoadjuvant TKI treatment led to a reduction of the thrombus in only 12% of patients and altered the surgical approach in only one patient [4].

Currently, immunotherapy is indicated for patients with metastatic RCC or unresectable RCC, but there are

*Correspondence: nishimura.kenichi.vx@ehime-u.ac.jp
[1] Department of Urology, Ehime University, Shitsukawa, Toon, Ehime 791-0295, Japan
Full list of author information is available at the end of the article

no indications for immunotherapy in the neoadjuvant setting. We report a case in which the combined use of neoadjuvant nivolumab and ipilimumab and sequential TKI therapy enabled surgical treatment.

Case presentation

A 71-year-old female presented with 8 kg weight loss over several months, appetite loss, and leg edema for several weeks. An enhanced computed tomography (CT) scan revealed a 94-mm right renal mass with a bulky tumor thrombus within the IVC to the junction of the IVC and the right atrium, maximum thrombus diameter of 37 mm, a few lung nodules, and para-aortic adenopathy (Fig. 1a). A transthoracic echocardiogram revealed no tumor within the right atrium. A bone scan revealed no metastasis. A core needle biopsy of the renal mass showed mostly necrotic tissue with a region of clear-cell RCC (ccRCC) (Fig. 2a). Immunohistochemical analysis revealed that PD-L1 was not expressed on tumor cells (Fig. 2b). The patient was not appropriate for radical surgery because her Karnofsky performance status (KPS) was 40. Systemic immunotherapy was administered for metastatic RCC based on International Metastatic RCC Database Consortium (IMDC) poor-risk classification including KPS < 80%, diagnosis to treatment interval < 1 year, anemia, and hyper calcemia. After 2 cycles of nivolumab and ipilimumab therapy, CT revealed that the primary tumor was stable at 94 mm in diameter and lung nodules were undetectable except for the one in the right lower lobe, but the tumor thrombus was extended within the right atrium. Nivolumab and ipilimumab therapy was changed to pazopanib monotherapy due to disease progression (Fig. 1b). She had marked improvement in Karnofsky performance status to 70 and resolution of leg edema and appetite loss.

Follow-up CT at 4 months after treatment revealed that the renal mass had decreased to 84 mm in diameter, and all lung nodules were undetectable. The tumor thrombus in the right atrium was also undetectable, but the tip of the thrombus remained at level 3. The diameter

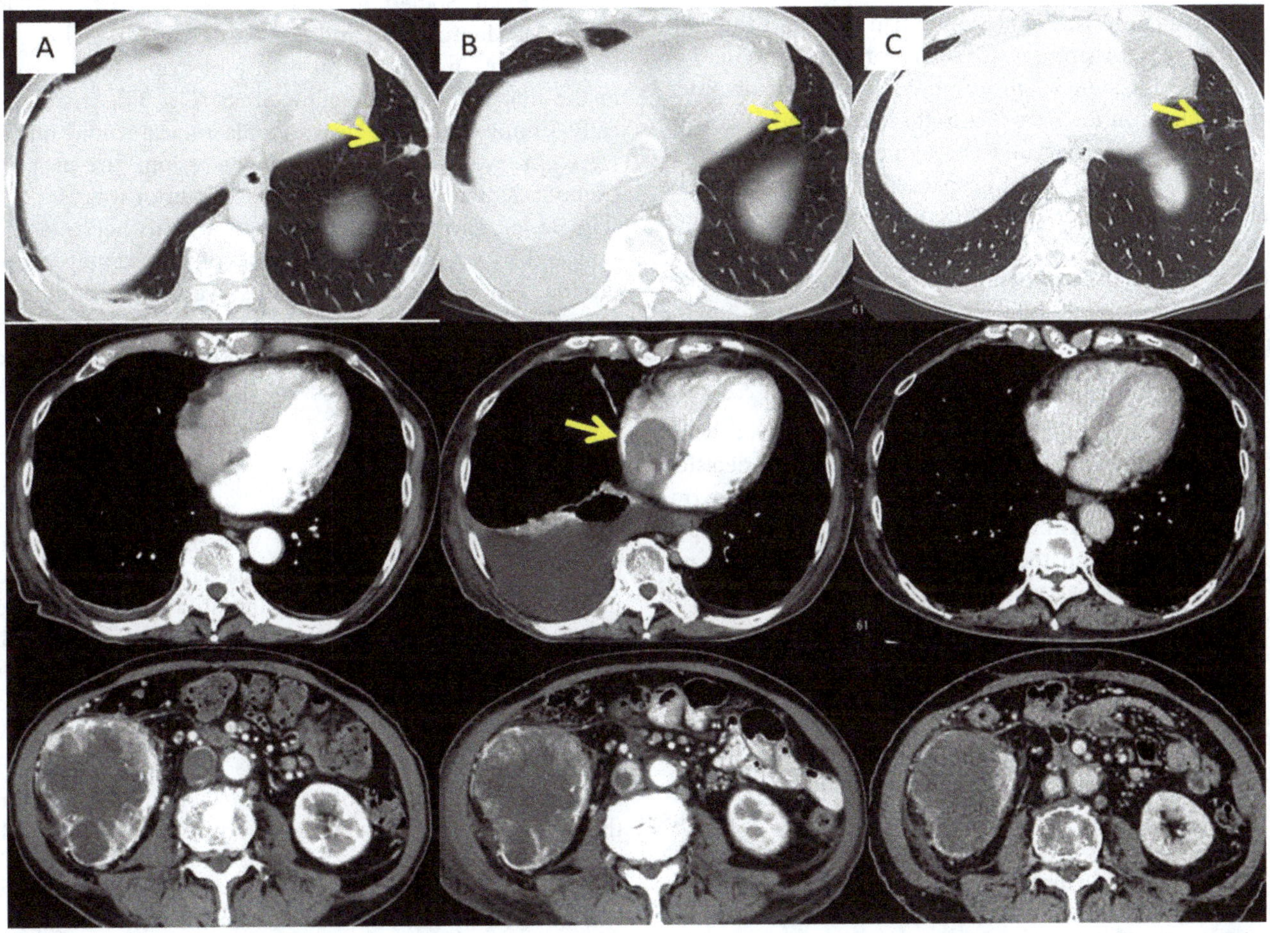

Fig. 1 CT images showing lung metastasis and the primary tumor and tumor thrombus in the right atrium. **a** Before treatment. **b** After 2 cycles of nivolumab and ipilimumab. **c** Before surgery

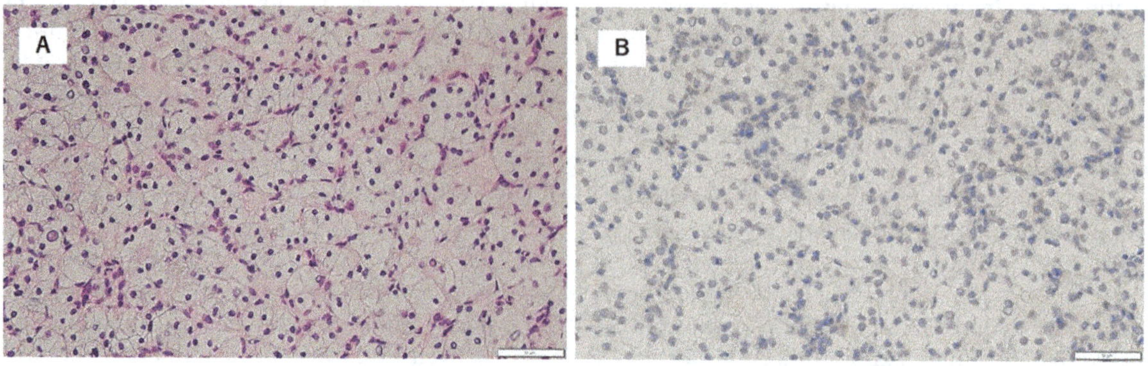

Fig. 2 Pathological findings on needle biopsy. **a** Hematoxylin–eosin (HE) staining of the primary tumor (×40). **b** Immunohistochemical analysis of the primary tumor (×40)

of the IVC at the renal vein ostium was 15.6 mm. Complete occlusion of the IVC was not observed (Figs. 1c, 4). She underwent right nephrectomy and IVC thrombectomy after 2 cycles of nivolumab and ipilimumab therapy and pazopanib therapy for 5 months.

The surgical method is described below. A cardiac surgeon secured the right upper arm vein and the right femoral vein to prepare for extracorporeal circulation. A middle incision to the xiphoid was made in addition to chevron incision. The right kidney and IVC were exposed. The area around the kidney and the IVC had strong adhesions. The right renal artery was ligated at the aortocaval. A tumor thrombus was confirmed between the common iliac vein bifurcation and the diaphragm by echoic imaging, but no tumor thrombus was observed in the right atrium. A liver surgeon secured the hepatic triad. Furthermore, an incision was made in the epicardium and the IVC was secured above the diaphragm.

Since no change in blood pressure was observed when the IVC was clamped above the diaphragm, a decision was made to perform nephrectomy without using extracorporeal circulation. The hepatic triad was clamped using a Pringle, and the IVC (above the diaphragm and on the common iliac vein bifurcation) was clamped. The vascular wall was incised at the bifurcation of the renal vein and the IVC to secure the tumor thrombus. The tumor thrombus was manually removed from the IVC wall. However, dense adhesions were revealed between the tumor thrombus and the wall of the IVC. The IVC was resectable from beneath the hepatic vein to the IVC bifurcation. Unfortunately, the tip of the thrombus could not be removed. Since the tip of the thrombus was macroscopically firm necrotic tissue, no additional excision was performed. The operative time was 9 h, and the bleeding volume was 3000 mL. No surgical complications occurred. CT and a transthoracic echocardiogram 1 week after surgery revealed no metastatic findings and only the mass within the IVC near the right atrium. Treatment for RCC after surgery was not performed because we diagnosed the mass as having no viable cells by pathological findings. 1 year after surgery, the mass has not changed and no metastatic lesions have been observed.

Finally, the pathologic diagnosis was ccRCC (7.5 cm, International Society of Urologic Pathologists [ISUP] Grade 3). Macroscopic findings showed a light yellowish-brown color in the margin area and extensive necrosis in the internal red and yellow areas (Fig. 3a). Histologically, tumor cells with clear cytoplasm and round nuclei were observed at the margin of the lesion. The proportion of residual tumor in the primary tumor was 10–20% (Fig. 3b, c). The tumor thrombus tissue was necrotic and replaced by a hemosiderin-phagocytic macrophage population. No viable cells were observed. No tumor was found in the wall of IVC. Immunohistochemical analysis revealed that PD-L1 was expressed on lymphocytes and macrophages infiltrating the tumor, but not on the tumor cells themselves (Fig. 3d).

Discussion and conclusion

We have described a patient who initially presented with invasive RCC, a level IV vena cava thrombus, and multiple lung metastases. She initiated nivolumab and ipilimumab therapy, and was switched to pazopanib monotherapy upon disease progression. Then, a smaller tumor thrombus and lack of metastases were observed on enhanced CT. She underwent right nephrectomy and tumor thrombectomy. This is the first case report describing the utility of sequential immune-targeted therapy as neoadjuvant therapy in advanced RCC (Fig. 4).

At the beginning of her treatment, ICI + ICI therapy was covered by national health care insurance in Japan, but ICI + TKI therapy was not. Therefore, nivolumab and ipilimumab therapy was selected. 3 weeks after the first cycle of nivolumab and ipilimumab therapy, a

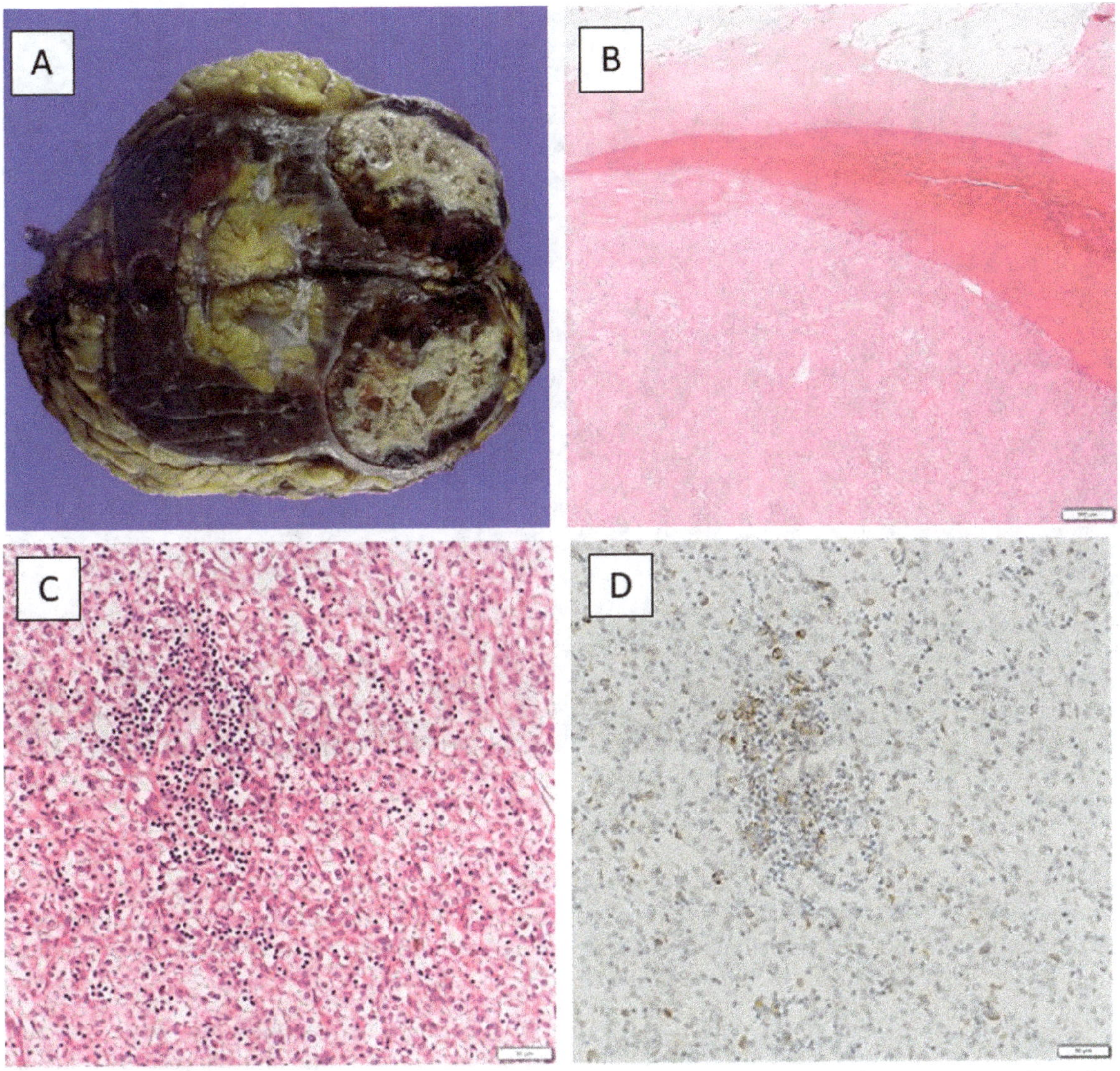

Fig. 3 Pathological findings. **a** Macroscopic findings. **b** HE staining of the primary tumor (×2). **c** HE staining of the primary tumor (×40). **d** Immunohistochemical analysis of the primary tumor using 2 FDA-approved clinical immunohistochemical makers for PD-L1 expression: Dako PD-L1 22C3 pharmDx and Dako PD-L1 28-8 pharmDx (×40)

tumor thrombus had progressed into the right atrium. We were forced to switch treatment due to an increased risk of sudden death. In patients with disease progression on immunotherapy, the possibility of pseudo-progression (PsPD) or hyper-progression must be considered. In PsPD, the tumor and/or metastatic lesions initially increase in size after immunotherapy due to infiltration of immune cells, followed by tumor shrinkage. The incidence of PsPD in RCC has been reported to be 2.9–8.8% [5, 6]. Currently, no biomarkers exist to distinguish PsPD from hyper-progression. Moreover, the use of biomarkers in patients treated with immune checkpoint inhibitors (ICIs) remains controversial and is under investigation. The neutrophil-to-lymphocyte ratio (NLR) is reported to be useful as a prognostic factor. Aly-Khan et al. investigated the utility of NLR in patients with metastatic RCC treated with ICIs. Decreases > 25 from baseline to 6 weeks after ICI therapy are associated with significantly improved outcomes in metastatic RCC patients. In addition, these authors reported that the NLR may be a helpful and available marker to diagnose PsPD [7]. In the present case, a 23% decrease in relative NLR was observed at 6 weeks after initiation of nivolumab and ipilimumab therapy (baseline NLR, 5.2; NLR at 6 weeks after treatment, [4]. No methods were available to diagnose PsPD at 3 weeks after the first cycle of nivolumab

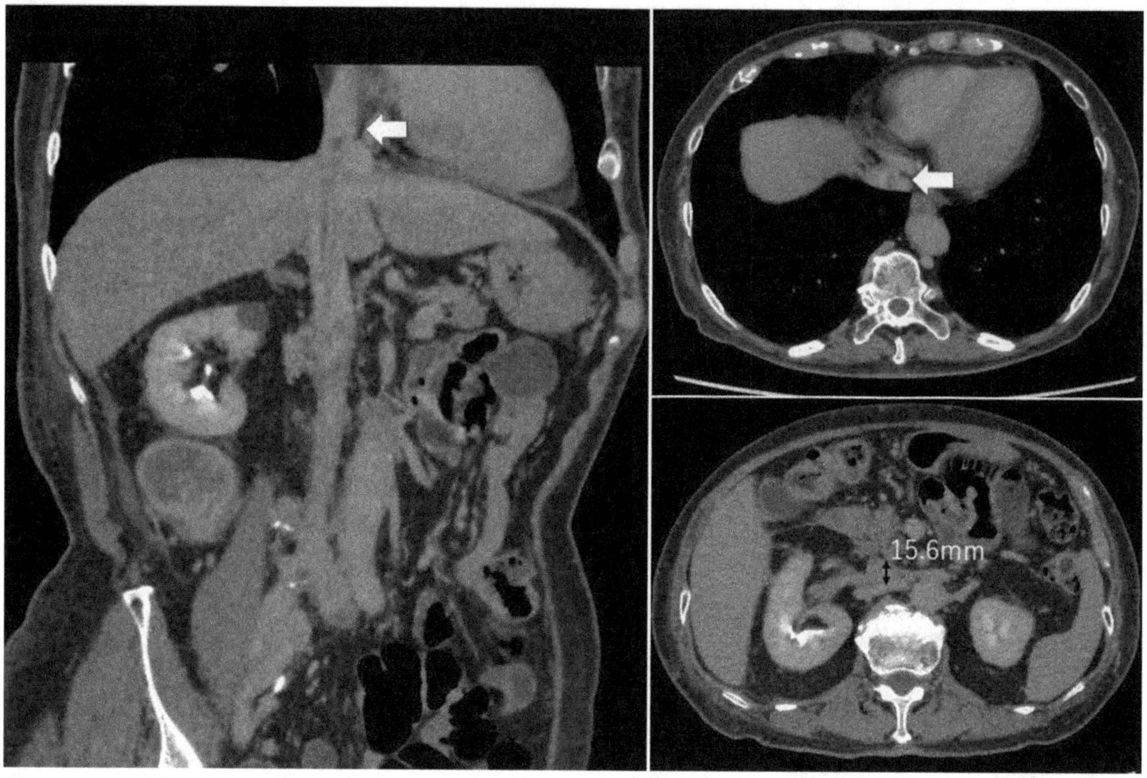

Fig. 4 Characteristics of the preoperative tumor thrombus on enhanced CT. The white arrows indicate the tip of the tumor thrombus. The black arrows indicate the diameter of the IVC at the renal vein ostium (15.6 mm)

and ipilimumab therapy. We should consider the present results in the context of other relevant clinical details to assess the risk–benefit of continuing ICIs in each individual patient.

Our surgical findings demonstrated that the tumor thrombus and IVC were firmly adhered. Psutka et al. reported that the presence of a right-sided tumor, an IVC diameter at the renal vein ostium of ≥ 24.0 mm, and radiographic identification of complete occlusion of the IVC at the renal vein ostium are related to tumor invasion of the IVC wall [8]. In the present case, the presence of a right-side tumor criterion was met, so we predicted that the possibility of IVC invasion was low.

However, the tumor thrombus had to be removed with the IVC from the hepatic vein to the bifurcation of the IVC due to the firm adhesion. The tip of the thrombus could not be removed because it was firmly adhered to the IVC near the right atrium. Adhesion of the tumor and the IVC wall was assumed to be due to inflammation, because tumor cells were not observed in the wall of the IVC on pathological findings. Labbate et al. also reported dense adhesion of the tumor and surrounding tissue after neoadjuvant immunotherapy for RCC vena cava tumor thrombus [9]. In RCC patients treated with neoadjuvant immunotherapy, we suggest a careful surgical plan that includes the removal of surrounding organs due to adhesions.

On pathological findings, the tissue of the tumor thrombus was necrotic and replaced by a hemosiderin-phagocytic macrophage population. Shinagawa et al. also reported no viable cells in the tumor thrombus but some viable cells in the primary tumor after TKI and anti–PD-1 drug therapy [10]. This pathological analysis suggested that neoadjuvant therapy is more effective for tumor thrombi. Anti–PD-1 antibodies are bound to T cells for 20 weeks or longer after ICI administration [11]. By administering TKIs immediately after the second course of ICIs, the present case received immuno-targeted therapy by ICIs and TKI prior to surgery. Immuno-targeted therapy is currently reported to be useful for mRCC patients. However, its use has not been reported in the neoadjuvant setting.

The present case is valuable in that it suggests the utility of sequential immune-targeted therapy before surgery. We recommend that clinical trials of immune-targeted therapy in the neoadjuvant setting for RCC patients are conducted.

Abbreviations

RCC: Renal cell carcinoma; IVC: Inferior vena cava; TKI: Tyrosine kinase inhibitor; CT: Computed tomography; ccRCC: Clear-cell renal cell carcinoma; PD-L1: Programmed death-ligand 1; IMDC: International Metastatic RCC Database Consortium; ISUP: International Society of Urologic Pathologists; PsPD: Pseudo-progression disease; ICIs: Immune checkpoint inhibitors; NLR: Neutrophil-to-lymphocyte ratio.

Acknowledgements

We thank the professional editing service JAM Post for excellent help in preparation of the manuscript.

Authors' contributions

KN designed the study, provided the patient data, and wrote the manuscript; YS, NS, KF, KK, TN, TF, NM, YM, TK, MM, KH, and MT provided the collection of all human material; and TS was involved in editing the manuscript. This manuscript was read and approved for submission by all coauthors. All authors read and approved the final manuscript.

Author details

[1]Department of Urology, Ehime University, Shitsukawa, Toon, Ehime 791-0295, Japan. [2]Department of Urology, National Hospital Organization Shikoku Cancer Center, Minamiumemoto, Matsuyama 791-0280, Japan. [3]Department of Pathology, Ehime University, Shitsukawa, Toon 791-0295, Japan.

References

1. Blute ML, Leibovich BC, Lohse CM, et al. The Mayo Clinic experience with surgical management, complications and outcome for patients with renal cell carcinoma and venous tumour thrombus. BJU Int. 2004;94:33–41.
2. Reese A, Whitson JM, Meng MV. Natural history of untreated renal cell carcinoma with venous tumor thrombus. Urol Oncol. 2013;31:1305–9.
3. Bindayi A, Hamilton ZA, McDonald ML, et al. Neoadjuvant therapy for localized and locally advanced renal cell carcinoma. Urol Oncol. 2018;36:31–7.
4. Cost NC, Delacroix SE, Sleeper JP, et al. The impact of targeted molecular therapies on the level of renal cell carcinoma vena caval tumor thrombus. Eur Urol. 2018;59:912–8.
5. McDermott DM, Drake CG, Sznol M, et al. Survival, durable response, and long-term safety in patients with previously treated advanced renal cell carcinoma receiving nivolumab. J Clin Oncol. 2015;33:2013–20.
6. McDermott DM, Sosman JA, Sznol M, et al. Atezolizumab, an anti-programmed death-ligand 1 antibody, in metastatic renal cell carcinoma: long-term safety, clinical activity, and immune correlates from a phase ia study. J Clin Oncol. 2016;34:833–42.
7. Lalani AA, Xie W, Martini DJ, et al. Change in neutrophil-to-lymphocyte ratio (NLR) in response to immune checkpoint blockade for metastatic renal cell carcinoma. J Immunother Cancer. 2018;22:5.
8. Psufka SP, Boorjian SA, Thompson RH, et al. Clinical and radiographic predictors of the need for inferior vena cava resection during nephrectomy for patients with renal cell carcinoma and caval tumour thrombus. BJU Int. 2015;116:388–96.
9. Labbate C, Hatogai K, Werntz R, et al. Complete response of renal cell carcinoma vena cava tumor thrombus to neoadjuvant immunotherapy. J Immunother Cancer. 2019;7:66.
10. Shinagawa T, Ito H, Sakai Y, et al. Remarkable effect of presurgical nivolumab on originally inoperable papillary renal cell carcinoma with tumor thrombus in inferior vena cava. Int Cancer Conf J. 2019;8:170–4.
11. Osa A, Uenami T, Koyama S, et al. Clinical implications of monitoring nivolumab immunokinetics in non–small cell lung cancer patients. JCI Insight. 2018;3:e59125.

Using patient feedback to adapt intervention materials based on acceptance and commitment therapy for people receiving renal dialysis

James Elander[1*], Romaana Kapadi[1], Emma Coyne[2], Maarten W. Taal[3], Nicholas M. Selby[3], Carol Stalker[1] and Kathryn Mitchell[1]

Abstract

Background: Theory-based intervention materials must be carefully adapted to meet the needs of users with specific physical conditions. Acceptance and Commitment Therapy (ACT) has been adapted successfully for cancer, chronic pain, diabetes, irritable bowel syndrome, multiple sclerosis, and a range of other conditions, but not so far for people receiving renal haemodialysis. This paper presents findings from a study to adapt ACT-based intervention materials specifically for renal dialysis.

Methods: Draft written materials consisting of four stories depicting fictitious individuals who used ACT-related techniques to help overcome different challenges and difficulties related to dialysis were adapted using a systematic patient consultation process. The participants were 18 people aged 19–80 years, with chronic kidney disease and receiving renal dialysis. Individual, semi-structured interviews were conducted to elicit participants' views about how the content of the draft materials should be adapted to make them more realistic and relevant for people receiving renal dialysis and about how the materials should be presented and delivered to people receiving renal dialysis. The interview transcripts were analysed using a qualitative adaptation of the Delphi method in which themes are used as a framework for translating feedback into proposals for modifications.

Results: The analysis of patient feedback supported the use of patient stories but suggested they should be presented by video and narrated by real dialysis patients. They also indicated specific adaptations to make the stories more credible and realistic. Participant feedback was translated into proposals for change that were considered along with clinical, ethical and theoretical factors. The outcome was a design for a video-based intervention that separated the stories about individuals from the explanations of the specific ACT techniques and provided greater structure, with material organised into smaller chunks. This intervention is adapted specifically for people receiving renal dialysis while retaining the distinctive theoretical principles of ACT.

Conclusions: The study shows the value of consulting patients in the development of intervention materials and illustrates a process for integrating patient feedback with theoretical, clinical and practical considerations in intervention design.

*Correspondence: j.elander@derby.ac.uk
[1] School of Psychology, University of Derby, Derby, UK
Full list of author information is available at the end of the article

Keywords: Acceptance and commitment therapy (ACT), Tailored intervention, Kidney failure, Haemodialysis

Introduction

Over 28,000 people with end-stage renal disease receive dialysis in the UK and over 25,000 receive hospital-based haemodialysis [1], which involves direct blood filtration by a dialysis machine for 4 h per treatment — delivered 3 times per week. Haemodialysis can extend patients' lives, but it causes significant cardiovascular morbidity and reduced quality of life [2], and is also expensive, costing over £27,000 per patient per year and consuming approximately 1.3% of all NHS spending [3]. Commencing and living with haemodialysis involves multiple losses and stressors [4, 5], and people receiving haemodialysis face significant challenges to adjust to the demands of treatment and cope with side effects and complications, which makes many dialysis patients vulnerable to impaired wellbeing and quality of life [6, 7].

It is therefore important to maximise the benefits obtained by dialysis and improve patients' experiences of treatment, as well as to help people receiving dialysis achieve and maintain the best possible quality of life. Psychological interventions can contribute to this but need to be specifically adapted to address the unique challenges of kidney failure and treatment by dialysis. For example, one study used a review of evidence about factors associated with psychological distress among people with end-stage kidney disease to guide the formulation of a cognitive behaviour therapy protocol that was specifically adapted for people undergoing dialysis [8].

Acceptance and Commitment Therapy (ACT) is a mindfulness-based behavioural therapy whose goal is to enable people to lead rich and meaningful lives while accepting the pain and suffering that inevitably go with that [9]. ACT uses metaphor, paradox, mindfulness skills and experiential exercises to promote psychological flexibility, which involves being open, aware and in contact with the present moment, and engaging in activities consistent with one's goals and values [10–12].

A review of meta-analyses including 133 randomized-controlled trials concluded that ACT is efficacious for all conditions examined [13] and ACT interventions have improved self-management, treatment adherence and adjustment among people with chronic physical conditions including cancer, cardiac disease, type 2 diabetes, epilepsy, multiple sclerosis, cerebral palsy, and paediatric brain injury [14].

ACT has considerable potential for application to people receiving renal dialysis [15], and a preliminary case study of ACT delivered individually to a person with end-stage renal disease suggested the approach had potential for improving adherence to dialysis [16]. However, ACT interventions must be carefully adapted for each condition, based on evidence about what aspects of content and delivery are most relevant for each patient group. For example, it is important to contextualise ACT-related issues and processes using realistic condition-specific examples. Factors specific to dialysis that need to be considered include the burdensome nature of dialysis, the specific ways it limits the lives of affected people, and the cognitive impact of dialysis itself on attention, thinking and memory. The present study therefore aimed to consult people with experience of receiving haemodialysis about the specific ways a prototype ACT intervention should be adapted to make it as relevant and useful as possible for people receiving haemodialysis.

Adaptations of ACT interventions need to consider both content and delivery. An adaptation of ACT content for diabetes involved incorporating behaviours relevant to diabetes adherence (mindful eating, exercising, glucose monitoring and administering insulin injections) into a generic creative hopelessness ACT exercise [17]. Other adaptations involved generating new condition-specific content; one study generated fictional people with irritable bowel syndrome who were composites of statements posted in an online forum [18].

A very common adaptation of delivery for people with chronic pain is to make the ACT intervention 'self-help,' usually by providing materials and instructions for exercises online or in book form, with little or no therapist involvement [19–21]. One study piloted a telephone-supported self-help ACT intervention for haemodialysis patients with depression, using an existing self-help manual [22]. The participants (haemodialysis patients with high depression scores) were instructed which chapters to read each week and had a weekly telephone call from the researcher to provide support in understanding the materials and encourage adherence. However, low recruitment numbers and poor adherence to the self-help manual showed that the intervention was not viable in that form; only one participant out of four completed all the chapters and health problems were the main obstacle to completion [22, 23].

Some adaptations of delivery have focused on the cognitive demands of interventions. In one study, the delivery of an ACT intervention was adapted for women with multiple sclerosis to take account of participants' cognitive difficulties. The adaptations included using a structured approach to reduce the load on working memory, and managing information with chunking and repetition, diagrams, written summaries and a cartoon drawing [24]. In an adaptation of ACT for people with psychosis, experiential exercises were kept brief and learning points were carefully paced and scaffolded to accommodate cognitive difficulties. The 'passengers on the bus' metaphor was presented first as a story and later acted out by facilitators and participants, and a scripted video was used in which a character played by an actor described the challenges in his life, to illustrate the real-world relevance of the metaphor [25].

It is vitally important to involve patients or potential end-users in the adaptation process, which can contribute to the achievement of greater personalised care, which means that "people have choice and control over the way their care is planned and delivered, based on 'what matters' to them and their individual strengths, needs and preferences" [26, p. 6, see also 27].

In one study, ACT was adapted for cancer-specific concerns by obtaining feedback from participants as well as ACT experts during the intervention development [28]. In another, a paper-based prototype of ACT for prevention of weight gain was tested in focus groups and interviews with members of the target audience, followed by expert review to ensure fidelity with the underlying theory [29]. In another, text for an ACT intervention for the partners of people with cancer was evaluated by potential users before it was further developed [30]. The present study followed good practice in adapting ACT-based materials for dialysis by conducting a systematic patient consultation exercise to obtain feedback about the content and delivery of prototype materials in order to inform the next stage of development of the intervention.

Methods

The study involved semi-structured interviews with a sample of people who were selected to take part because of their expert patient experience of treatment for chronic kidney disease with renal haemodialysis.

ACT-based draft materials

The draft materials consisted of a printed booklet of four case descriptions of fictious dialysis patients that illustrated different difficulties and challenges associated with renal disease and in-centre dialysis treatment, and ways in which the fictitious patients were helped to overcome those challenges by using techniques based on ACT (see Additional file 1). The draft materials were closely based on ACT principles and practice and were prepared in collaboration with a consultant clinical psychologist who had extensive experience of delivering ACT therapy (EC), and with clinicians who had extensive experience of haemodialysis treatment for chronic kidney disease (MWT and NMS).

Participants and recruitment

The participants were 18 people with end-stage renal disease who were aged over 18 years, had received in-centre dialysis for at least 90 days in the last two years (including patients who were presently on home haemodialysis but had previously received in-centre haemodialysis), and were able to converse in English. People with active infection or malignancy or whose medical condition made participation in an interview difficult were excluded. Key features of study participants are given in Table 1. Participants are identified by pseudonyms.

Participants were recruited from patients attending the Dialysis Unit, Royal Derby Hospital, and by posting brief invitations to participate on the Kidney Care UK and British Renal Society online support groups and Facebook groups, and on other Facebook groups including Transplant and Dialysis Support Group, Kidney Research UK, Dialysis Network UK, Kidney Care UK's Young Adult Kidney Group and Chronic Kidney Disease UK. There were twenty-eight individuals who responded initially to the invitation, who all met the inclusion criteria and were eligible to participate, of whom ten were not able to arrange an interview, so there were eighteen who took part in an interview. Recruitment and data collection took place between April and September 2020.

Procedure

All the study methods were carried out in accordance with UK National Health Service and British Psychological Society guidelines and regulations. Written informed consent was obtained from all participants. Participants recruited at the hospital were given paper copies of the participant information sheet and the booklet of draft materials at least 48 h before being asked for written informed consent, after which a convenient time was arranged to conduct a telephone or videocall interview. Participants recruited online were directed to a brief online survey hosted by Qualtrics, a secure online survey platform, where they viewed further information about the study and provided brief information about eligibility, informed consent, and availability for interview by telephone or online videocall using Microsoft Teams. The draft materials were then emailed to participants and a convenient time was arranged to conduct the interview, allowing at least 48 h between recruitment and interview. All the interviews were conducted by RK.

The interviews were up to one hour in length and followed a prepared semi-structured interview schedule. Participants were asked how the case descriptions could be adapted and improved to make them more meaningful, relevant and useful for in-centre dialysis patients, and how materials like these should be presented to dialysis

Table 1 Participant information

Participant[a]	Age	Gender	Ethnicity	Marital status	Employment status	Region	Interview method	Current type of haemodialysis	Approx. time on dialysis
1. Adam	52	Male	White	Single	Unemployed	North West England	MS Teams	In-centre	6 years
2. Albert	73	Male	White	Divorced	Retired	East Midlands	MS Teams	In-centre	25 years
3. Simon	43	Male	White	Single	Employed full-time	East of England	MS Teams	In-centre	19 years
4. Arjun	42	Male	Asian/Asian British	Married	Employed part-time	South East England	MS Teams	Home	5 years
5. George	61	Male	White	Married	Retired	North East England	Telephone	In-centre	2 years
6. Oliver	35	Male	White	Married	Unemployed	East Midlands	Telephone	Home	2 years
7. Sarah	19	Female	White	Single	Unemployed	East Midlands	MS Teams	In-centre	7 months
8. Richard	60	Male	White	Single	Retired	East Midlands	Telephone	In-centre	6 years
9. Henry	71	Male	White	Single	Retired	East Midlands	Telephone	In-centre	5 years
10. Helen	51	Female	White	Married	Retired	East Midlands	Telephone	In-centre	6 years
11. Hardeep	80	Male	Asian/Asian British	Widowed	Retired	EastMidlands	Telephone	In-centre	7 years
12. Alison	57	Female	White	Single	Unemployed	East Midlands	Telephone	In-centre	6 years
13. Steven	52	Male	White	Married	Retired	East Midlands	Telephone	In-centre	6 years
14. William	73	Male	White	Divorced	Retired	East Midlands	Telephone	In-centre	6 months
15. Diane	68	Female	White	Widowed	Retired	East Midlands	Telephone	In-centre	1 year
16. Wilfred	87	Male	White	Widowed	Retired	East Midlands	Telephone	In-centre	1 year
17. Arthur	78	Male	White	Widowed	Retired	East Midlands	Telephone	In-centre	6 years
18. Brian	79	Male	White	Widowed	Employed part-time	East Midlands	Telephone	In-centre	14 years

[a] Pseudonyms are used to identify participants

patients for the most convenient and effective use. The interviews were audio-recorded and transcribed verbatim. The transcripts were anonymised so they contained no personally identifying information and participants were given pseudonyms.

Data analysis

The interview transcripts were analysed using an adaptation of the Delphi method that employs qualitative data to elicit and summarise expert opinion [31]. The first step was to sort transcript material into pre-identified categories related to specific aspects of the draft materials, which included the overall credibility of the stories, the number and length of the stories, the structure of the stories, specific features of each individual story, suggestions for new content in the stories, suggestions about techniques and strategies portrayed in the stories, and suggestions about how the stories should be presented and delivered. Within each of these categories, participants' views were organised into themes using a descriptive thematic analysis [32]. The resulting themes were then used as a framework for translating participant feedback into proposed modifications to the materials. An ACT-trained therapist (EC) oversaw the translation of participant feedback into intervention design to ensure formally correct ACT-based psycho-educational materials with content, format and delivery methods modified to optimise benefits for patients receiving dialysis.

Results

Analysis of participant feedback

In the narrative analysis below, we present each theme together with representative statements that are extracted verbatim from the interview transcripts. A larger dataset of representative participant feedback is available in Additional file 2. In the second stage of the analysis, described afterwards, we present the ways each of those themes was translated into specific proposals for modifying the materials.

Theme 1: the stories were credible

The first theme reflected the majority view that the stories were generally credible and relatable. Eleven participants specifically commented on this aspect of the stories, for example:

"Yes, they were very good actually and some of it is spot on" (Arjun).
"I found a little bit of my situation in each of them, and when I did that I thought, oh, so, how would I react and how would I behave and would that benefit me, you know" (George).
"It's pretty much how things are I think" (Richard).
"I know they're fictional, but they probably could be real cases because people do suffer and like I say especially at the moment with things as they are um I think the mental health problems are far greater than perhaps they would've been" (Diane).
"I could relate to all of them" (Brian).

Three participants reported finding the stories artificial or unrelatable and these three provided 12 statements about this issue. The perception seemed to arise from the fact the stories were presented as fictional, and two of the participants suggested using true stories from real patients:

"I don't know why they have to be made up. I don't know why they can't just be real stories from real people" (Oliver).
"Yeah, but couldn't you get say a person like myself who wouldn't mind, get their story which is actual facts" (Steven).

Theme 2: don't sugar-coat dialysis

Four participants made eight statements describing the view that the stories should not be unrealistically positive and should reflect some of their own very difficult experiences with dialysis:

"Unfortunately, sugarcoating stories I don't think is gonna help some people because you know, some people need to be told you must do this otherwise you're gonna die ..." (Oliver).
"I found the first month or so absolutely horrific. I really did and I couldn't see anything in the stories that I could relate to, err regarding my initial start" (Arthur).

Theme 3: don't always make the first thing they try work out

Participants generally appreciated the narrative structure of the stories in which the characters encountered difficulties and then found ways to overcome them, but there were four participants and nine statements that offered the view that it seemed unrealistic that in each case the first strategy suggested worked:

"... the way that they work they sort of go down and then to a thing and then start climbing up the other side which is the way dialysis should be ..." (Albert).
"... it would be worth doing one whereby the first solution that maybe the renal psychologist or maybe the consultants suggested or maybe the nurse suggested didn't work but because they'd made that effort they were then able to go and talk to someone to find another way to try and sort it out" (Adam).

Theme 4: psychologists are not so available

There were five statements from three participants who pointed out that patients on dialysis would not have such easy access to a psychologist:

"... in my dialysis unit we have a renal counsellor but we don't really have a psychologist" (Simon).
"I was like really, really low, um and the guy in there said to me, like oh I'll refer you to a psychologist, but I never got referred to one" (Sarah).
"I've never seen a psychiatrist or psychologist" (Brian).

Theme 5: involve other people

Two of the participants commented in four statements that the stories should show people getting help and support from others:

"... what is it like to live with a dialysis patient because it's not a journey just for one person, it could be a journey for the partner, or family member that helps, or friend that helps" (Arjun).
"I think help from other people is very, very important, whether you've got a, uh, a partner or family at home, or you can see a professional" (George).

Theme 6: realism in individual stories

Participants made specific suggestions for amending details to make the stories more realistic. These included representing minority ethnic groups and depicting more positive aspects of the lives of people receiving dialysis:

"I'm a Hindu and you know when I had kidney failure for my parents it was hard to take and being an Indian is very different to being a Caucasian in all aspects of life and I think that's true whether you're a Hindu, Muslim, a Sikh or whatever. I think on general broad terms in an Asian community we have a very different way of life ..." (Arjun).
"... show that you can have local holidays in your country, you can go shopping, you can go for dinner, these things are all positive and we need to show that ..." (Arjun).
"... you have to look at other things to look forward to. Like going out for a meal or something you know or going out for a day when you're not on dialysis" (Steven).

Several participants suggested that Keiron's work situation was not very credible, although others thought it might occur sometimes and that Keiron's story had a valuable message:

> *"I think workplaces would understand that, and I don't think they would be so pushy to um, you know, call him while, call someone while they're on a session and get them to work, and especially like quite frequently" (Sarah).*
> *"... it was probably through ignorance that his bosses didn't understand what was happening to him, didn't realise that it was vital that he had treatment or else he'd die" (Diane).*
> *"...I felt it was quite sad but I've been there, done that ..." (Alison).*

Several participants identified with Joanne's story, and there were no suggestions of specific changes to make about that story:

> *"[The story] where they're struggling with the fact that they have to do this and it's not very pleasant, it's the woman who's got the two kids [...] that story rings true [...] there's a big problem with people not understanding what the treatment is, so even though you include people in the treatment they just don't get it" (Adam).*
> *"... those characters I identified with a couple of them, you know, you can you feel a bit sorry for yourself or feel down and so you seek comfort in junk food or something" (George).*

Participants also supported the story of Margaret, and suggested expanding the ways in which Margaret was portrayed doing things for herself, as well as sug gesting Margaret's family should not be so free to visit her during dialysis:

> *"I think one of the best outcomes you can have on dialysis is if you do everything yourself ... even if you're not going to needle yourself ... just coming in and lining your machine up and getting everything ready is an element of control that makes life a lot easier, so that might be worth adding into that story with her" (Adam).*
> *"... unless someone's a family member [and] is coming in to actually help to dialyse you ... I found that a very strange thing in the story that family started to pop in (George).*

Many participants identified with David because they were a similar age, but suggested it seemed incongru ous that David was previously a car mechanic but did not have a car:

> *"Yeah, well I think that and because in the early days I was very similar, like I was very impatient and very intolerant at the start. Err, I'm not now I've mellowed considerably" (Arthur).*
> *"... he was a car mechanic, retired, but he didn't seem to have a car in itself, so we went with transport. [...] in his case I just thought it was a bit strange that he was, it was, uh, it was an inappropriate choice of profession. He's a car mechanic and likes to fix peoples cars, but he doesn't drive himself" (George).*

Theme 7: focus more on the techniques

There were six participants who provided eight statements in which they identified and supported the ACT techniques that were portrayed, but also suggested the techniques should be presented carefully:

> *"I liked the one about the trains and getting on the old um, you know, I'm cross with everyone train" (Simon).*
> *"I think that was in one of their stories, you know, like gathering your thoughts and like tackling them one at a time ... Um, I think another one was set like setting goals for themselves" (Sarah).*
> *"Writing down my thoughts, I don't know, it did help me" (Hardeep).*
> *"I appreciated that because I keep a diary, that's one of the things I learnt at previous dialysis was to keep a diary" (Alison).*
> *"... a lot of the people you're dealing with in hospital, I think they would have to be shown these techniques very, very sort of gently and carefully" (Brian).*

Theme 8: use video format

Nine participants provided 12 statements commenting on the length of the stories and the time and effort needed to read them in the form of text, and suggested that video could be a better way of presenting the stories, including suggestions about using cartoons:

> *"as text it all, it was just too long. But if you are planning on doing it as a video then it wouldn't really matter ..." (Oliver).*
> *"I do think actually as well that sort of visual video or audio or whatever is a lot better than written" (Richard).*
> *"I mean you could try something humorous with animation ..." (Adam).*

Other perceived advantages of video format were that the stories could be viewed during dialysis sessions and that people could watch together:

> *"Provide a tablet and this clamp and you can just, any patient can then watch it, clamp it to the table ..." (Albert).*
>
> *"I'd watch it during dialysis definitely" (Sarah).*
>
> *"... then if they could watch something at home as well, because then if they've got, if they're living with family and stuff, wives, kids or whatever, or parents or whatever, then they can share ideas can't they" (Richard).*

Translating feedback into proposed modifications

Each of the themes was then translated into proposed changes to the intervention materials. First, we assessed the suggestions made by participants within each theme, taking account of the degree of consensus among participants and how representative participants were of the wider potential audience. Second, we identified a set of potential changes and evaluated these taking into consideration ethical constraints, practical considerations, and the need to maintain consistency with ACT theory. We also had to consider any potential impacts of modifications on the pedagogic integrity of the intervention materials, so modifications that would have reduced the integrity of the materials as psycho-educational tools were avoided. Table 2 gives an overview of the proposals for modifying the materials associated with each theme.

The translation of participant feedback into changes to the materials often involved simultaneous consideration of multiple factors. For example, although participants overwhelmingly supported the concept of using stories about individual people's experiences, several participants suggested using real stories told by real patients, possibly prompted by the fact the stories were presented as 'fictional'. We considered obtaining true stories told by real-life people receiving dialysis, but also had to consider potential ethical issues, for example to protect individuals who might potentially be identifiable, and the need to maintain consistency with ACT theory. We therefore decided to retain control over the content of the stories but present them as true stories and include examples and issues based on real patients where possible (in fact, many elements of the original stories were based loosely on real-life patients and incidents). We also decided to recruit real patients to narrate the scripted stories and to match narrators to stories as far as possible so that narrators presented stories that were close to their own personal experiences.

We also had to balance participants' feedback about presenting more of the gritty reality of dialysis against the need for the materials not to cause distress or anxiety, especially considering that potential users could include people who were new to dialysis or had not yet started dialysis. However, we could make small changes

Table 2 Proposed modifications for the draft materials

Themes	Proposed modifications
1. The stories were credible	Retain the concept of using individual stories
	Present the stories as real rather than fictitious, but still script them so that we can control the content and so that details of real-life patients are not revealed
	Have real patients narrate the stories
2. Don't sugar-coat dialysis	Include a bit more recognition of the gritty realism of dialysis (including amending the presentation of Margaret's efforts to present dialysis only in a positive way to her children)
3. Don't always make the first thing they try work out	Have some description of things that were not successful at first—possibly related to some of the gritty realism about dialysis and the non-availability of psychological support (see themes 2 and 4)
4. Psychologists are not so available	Make it more credible how people are offered help, and give renal counsellors or other staff, rather than psychologists, a bigger role in the stories
5. Involve other people	Make some of the characters' family and friends more visible in the analysis
6. Realism in individual stories	Have at least one character from a minority ethnic group
	Amend or explain some details of Keiron's work situation
	Amend the details of Margaret's family visiting her on dialysis (but keep her family visibly involved—see above)
	Give David a different occupation so his dependence on hospital transport is more credible or explain why he does not drive to dialysis
7. Focus more on the techniques	Separate out the techniques from the individual stories—giving more room within the stories for realism etc. and enabling 'technique' videos to be viewed separately and repeatedly
8. Use video format	Use video but with a cartoon format to preserve participant anonymity
	Use the Toonly© system to present scripted narratives, spoken by real patients

to alter the balance between realism and positivity, several of which were specifically suggested by participants. For example, one story described how Margaret's family "started to pop in to see her on dialysis," and a participant suggested how the wording could be changed: *"I'd certainly tweak that sentence. You know, family popped in. I would change it to something like, you know, family started to ask more questions."* (George).

There were several other points where participant feedback suggested that changes to wording and presentation would improve the realism of the stories, including the points about not everything a person tries working out first time and about the availability of psychological support. However, around two-thirds of participants were recruited from a clinical centre where there is not a clinical psychologist routinely available, and this may have influenced some of the feedback. We therefore reviewed the depiction of psychological support and gave more prominence to professionals who were not psychologists, but we did not remove the references to psychologists in two of the four stories. We also had to consider whether specific points raised by participants (for example, Keiron's work and David's driving) should be addressed by changing details of the stories or by giving more explanation of the circumstances. In some cases, we decided to explain or clarify elements of the stories rather than make the specific changes suggested.

When considering changes to the stories we also had to consider the implications of the change from written text to video, taking account of the need to preserve the integrity of the materials as educational tools. This meant that the stories needed to be shortened and simplified, so it made sense to separate the techniques from the stories, which meant that although the techniques would be mentioned in the stories, a fuller explanation of the techniques and how to use them was provided separately.

We decided to use Toonly© for both the story videos and the videos explaining the techniques. Toonly© is software to produce video recordings with cartoon animations and audio soundtrack. For the stories, this enabled us to use scripted narratives recorded by real dialysis patients but without the narrators appearing visually—they would be 'spoken' by a cartoon figure. This preserved the anonymity of the people who narrated the stories and meant that their task was simplified by not having to present themselves visually. We aimed to make the stories as realistic as possible by adjusting the content in response to participants' feedback and by choosing narrators who identified with the character they were narrating and could tell that story in an authentic way. Narrators were given the stories to read before agreeing to act as narrators so they could decide whether they felt 'right' telling that story. Using cartoon animation to present the stories

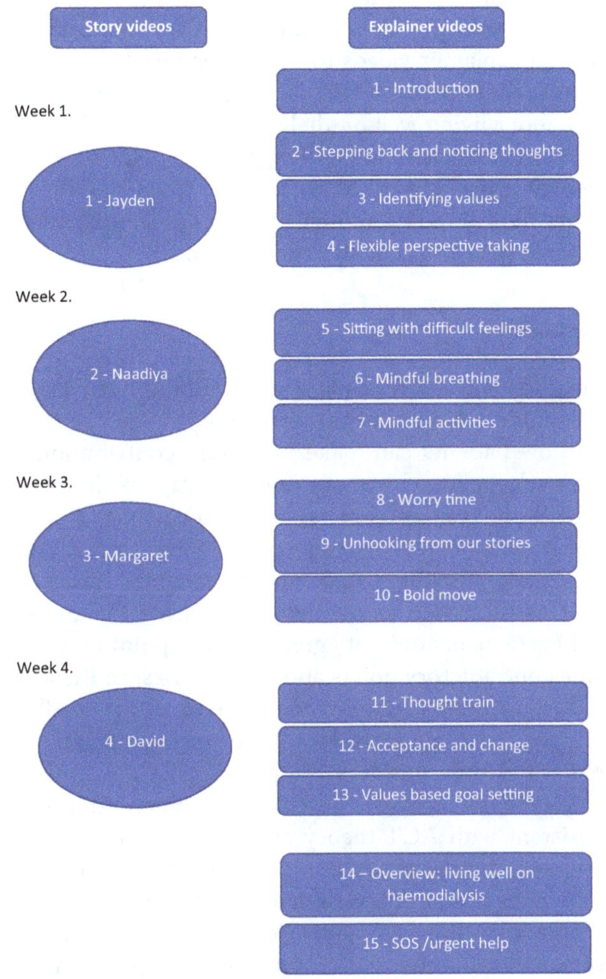

Fig. 1 Structure of the adapted ACT intervention

was also consistent with ACT theory. Using cartoon characters to present ACT-based content helps with the use of metaphor and cognitive diffusion, enabling viewers to detach more easily from the literal use of language [9, 33].

One aspect of the feedback that was important for us to implement was making the characters portrayed in the stories include minority ethnic groups. For that reason, we changed two of the characters' names, with 'Keiron' becoming 'Jayden' and 'Joanne' becoming 'Naadiya', so their names would be consistent with visual identities portraying people from minority ethnic family backgrounds.

For the techniques, using Toonly© enabled us to produce short presentations of ACT techniques with audio explanations by a clinical psychologist and ACT therapist, and the explainer videos were designed for repeated viewing. Separating the explanations of the techniques from the stories also enabled us to structure the materials into a programme of videos to be watched over four weeks, with one story video and three accompanying explainer videos to be watched each week, plus an introduction to the whole programme and an overview about living well on dialysis and advice about what to do in cases where urgent help was needed (see Fig. 1). The whole package of video materials could be delivered online and viewed on a range of different devices, including in dialysis units and in people's homes.

Discussion

The study showed how patient consultation can help to make intervention materials more credible and relatable, and how patients can make important contributions to the development of interventions in a way that is consistent with the principles of personalised care [26, 27]. Participants supported the concept of telling stories about individuals and their experiences and they recognised many of the issues and situations presented in the stories. Participants did not agree on every point and made some contradictory points about the stories, so the adaptation inevitably could not incorporate all the feedback obtained. Also, patients' views are important, but they are not the only consideration; participants' feedback had to be moderated by the need for the intervention to be consistent with ACT theory and clinically and ethically acceptable as well as psycho-educationally effective.

The consultation exercise led to a design for an ACT intervention that has many elements in common with previous adaptations of ACT for adult populations, for example the use of composite fictional characters [18], the use of scripted video depicting characters played by actors [25], and the use of stories and cartoons to help explain metaphors and encourage multiple perspective-taking [24, 34]. The resulting intervention should be more acceptable to people receiving dialysis than interventions using written material, which were shown not to be viable in that form [22, 23].

The study did have some limitations, however. It involved a purposive sample of people who were all relatively experienced with haemodialysis. Many of the participants were recruited from the same clinical centre, and minority groups and non-fluent English speakers were under-represented. When the intervention is further developed it will be useful to evaluate it with more diverse samples, including people with less experience of haemodialysis. Future evaluations might include comparing this self-paced mode of delivery with more clinically oriented applications of ACT [16] or assessing the suitability of the intervention for different groups of dialysis patients, some of whom may be depressed. A previous self-help ACT intervention that was specifically designed for haemodialysis patients with depression was not successful because of poor recruitment and adherence [22, 23], but the present intervention is not specifically designed for people with depression and aims to help dialysis patients more generally to improve their adjustment and live better with dialysis. The next step in the present programme of research is to produce the intervention presented in Fig. 1 and conduct a feasibility trial in preparation for a larger randomised trial.

Conclusions

The study showed how patient feedback can be systematically collected and analysed to inform the adaptation of ACT intervention materials for people affected by specific conditions or treatments. This is especially important for people receiving renal dialysis, which makes unique demands of patients and requires specifically adapted intervention materials, and is also especially important for ACT interventions, which are theoretically distinct and require a carefully controlled and balanced process to incorporate user feedback while ensuring theoretical consistency.

Abbreviation

ACT: Acceptance and commitment therapy.

Supplementary Information

Additional file 1. Booklet of draft materials.

Additional file 2. Dataset of participant feedback.

Acknowledgements

We are grateful to all the participants for taking part, and to the NIHR Clinical Trials Network for their support, especially Kelly White at the Renal Unit, Royal Derby Hospital, for helping to facilitate patient recruitment, and Sharon Woodward and Samantha Sharp at Kidney Care UK and Amy Robinson at the UK Renal Association, for helping with online recruitment. We are also grateful to the anonymous reviewers for their helpful comments on a previous draft.

Authors' contributions

JE conceived and designed the study, led the data analysis and wrote the manuscript. RK conducted the interviews and contributed to analysing the data and writing the manuscript. EC contributed to designing the study, led the interpretation of the data analysis and contributed to writing the manuscript. MWT, NMS, CS and KM contributed to designing the study, interpretation of the data analysis and writing the manuscript. All the authors approved the submitted manuscript.

Author details

[1]School of Psychology, University of Derby, Derby, UK. [2]Nottingham University Hospitals NHS Trust, Nottingham, UK. [3]Centre for Kidney Research and Innovation, University of Nottingham, Derby, UK.

References

1. MacNeill SJ, Ford D. UK renal registry 19th annual report: chapter 2 UK renal replacement therapy prevalence in 2015: national and centre-specific analyses. Nephron. 2017;137(Suppl. 1):45–72. https://doi.org/10.1159/000481364.
2. Yusop NB, Mun CY, Shariff ZM, Huat CB. Factors associated with quality of life among hemodialysis patients in Malaysia. PLoS ONE. 2013;8(12):e84152. https://doi.org/10.1371/journal.pone.0084152.
3. Kerr M, Bray B, Medcalf J, O'Donoghue DJ, Matthews B. Estimating the financial cost of chronic kidney disease to the NHS in England. Nephrol Dial Transplant. 2012;27:iii73-80. https://doi.org/10.1093/ndt/gfs269.
4. Cukor D, Cohen SD, Peterson RA, Kimmel PL. Psychosocial aspects of chronic disease: ESRD as a paradigmatic illness. J Am Soc Nephrol. 2007;18(12):3042–55.
5. Kaplan De-Nour A. Social adjustment of chronic dialysis patients. Am J Psychiatry. 1982. https://doi.org/10.1176/ajp.139.1.97.
6. Chilcot J, Wellsted D, Da Silva-Gane M, Farrington K. Depression on dialysis. Nephron Clin Pract. 2008;108(4):c256–64. https://doi.org/10.1159/000124749.
7. Fukuhara S, Lopes AA, Bragg-Gresham JL, Kurokawa K, Mapes DL, Akizawa T, Bommer J, Canaud BJ, Port FK, Held PJ. Health-related quality of life among dialysis patients on three continents: the Dialysis Outcomes and Practice Patterns Study. Kidney Int. 2003;64(5):1903–10. https://doi.org/10.1046/j.1523-1755.2003.00289.x.
8. Hudson JL, Moss-Morris R, Game D, Carroll A, Chilcot J. Improving Distress in Dialysis (iDiD): A tailored CBT self-management treatment for patients undergoing dialysis. J Ren Care. 2016;42(4):223–38. https://doi.org/10.1111/jorc.12168.
9. Harris R. Embracing your demons: An overview of acceptance and commitment therapy. Psychotherapy in Australia. 2006 Aug;12(4): 70–76. https://contextualscience.org/files/article%20psychOz.pdf
10. Bond FW, Hayes SC, Barnes-Holmes D. Psychological flexibility, ACT, and organizational behavior. J Organ Behav Manage. 2006;26(1–2):25–54. https://doi.org/10.1300/J075v26n01_02.
11. Hayes SC, Luoma JB, Bond FW, Masuda A, Lillis J. Acceptance and commitment therapy: model, processes and outcomes. Behav Res Ther. 2006;44(1):1–25. https://doi.org/10.1016/j.brat.2005.06.006.
12. Levin ME, Herbert JD, Forman EM. Acceptance and commitment therapy: a critical review to guide clinical decision making. In: McKay D, Abramowitz JS, Storch EA, editors. Treatments for psychological problems and syndromes. London: Wiley; 2017. p. 413–32. https://doi.org/10.1002/9781118877142.
13. Gloster AT, Walder N, Levin M, Twohig M, Karekla M. The empirical status of acceptance and commitment therapy: a review of meta-analyses. J Contextual Behav Sci. 2020. https://doi.org/10.1016/j.jcbs.2020.09.009.
14. Graham CD, Gouick J, Krahe C, Gillanders D. A systematic review of the use of Acceptance and Commitment Therapy (ACT) in chronic disease and long-term conditions. Clin Psychol Rev. 2016;46:46–58. https://doi.org/10.1016/j.cpr.2016.04.009.
15. Stalker C, Elander J, Mitchell K, Taal MW, Selby N, Stewart P. What is acceptance, and how could it affect health outcomes for people receiving renal dialysis? Health Psychol Update. 2018;27(2):17–23.
16. Rzeszut ME. The application of acceptance and commitment therapy with hemodialysis treatment adherence: a case study. J Nephrol Soc Work. 2011;35:17–25.
17. Hadlandsmyth K, White KS, Nesin AE, Greco LA. Proposing an Acceptance and Commitment Therapy intervention to promote improved diabetes management in adolescents: a treatment conceptualization. Int J Behav Consult Ther. 2013;7(4):12. https://doi.org/10.1037/h0100960.
18. Ferreira NM. Investigating the role of psychological flexibility and the use of an acceptance and commitment therapy based intervention in irritable bowel syndrome. University of Edinburgh; PhD Thesis. 2011. https://era.ed.ac.uk/handle/1842/6312.
19. Dahl J, Lundgren T. Living beyond your pain: using acceptance and commitment therapy to ease chronic pain. New Harbinger Publications; 2006.
20. Johnston M, Foster M, Shennan J, Starkey NJ, Johnson A. The effectiveness of an acceptance and commitment therapy self-help intervention for chronic pain. Clin J Pain. 2010;26(5):393–402. https://doi.org/10.1097/AJP.0b013e3181cf59ce
21. Trompetter HR, Bohlmeijer ET, Veehof MM, Schreurs KM. Internet-based guided self-help intervention for chronic pain based on Acceptance and Commitment Therapy: a randomized controlled trial. J Behav Med. 2015;38(1):66–80. https://doi.org/10.1016/j.brat.2009.01.010.
22. Vogt W. Acceptance and Commitment Therapy self-help intervention for depression in haemodialysis patients: a feasibility randomised controlled *trial* (Doctoral dissertation, University of Lincoln). http://eprints.lincoln.ac.uk/id/eprint/29714/.
23. Vogt W, das Nair R, Moghaddam NG, Proctor B, Coyne E. Acceptance and commitment therapy self-help for depression in haemodialysis: a feasibility randomised controlled trial. Poster presented at the British Renal Society Conference 2016.
24. Gillanders S, Gillanders D. An acceptance and commitment therapy intervention for a woman with secondary progressive multiple sclerosis and a history of childhood trauma. Neuro Disabil Psychother. 2014;2(1–2):19–40.
25. Johns LC, Oliver JE, Khondoker M, Byrne M, Jolley S, Wykes T, Joseph C, Butler L, Craig T, Morris EM. The feasibility and acceptability of a brief Acceptance and Commitment Therapy (ACT) group intervention for people with psychosis: the 'ACT for life' study. J Behav Ther Exp Psychiatry. 2016;50:257–63. https://doi.org/10.1016/j.jbtep.2015.10.001.
26. Sanderson J, Kay N, Watts R. Universal personalised care: implementing the comprehensive model. London: NHS England. 2019. https://www.england.nhs.uk/publication/universal-personalised-care-implementing-the-comprehensive-model/.
27. Coulter A, Entwistle VA, Eccles A, Ryan S, Shepperd S, Perera R. Personalised care planning for adults with chronic or long-term health conditions. Cochrane Database Syst Rev. 2015. https://doi.org/10.1002/14651858.CD010523.pub2.
28. Arch JJ, Mitchell JL. An Acceptance and Commitment Therapy (ACT) group intervention for cancer survivors experiencing anxiety at re-entry. Psychooncology. 2016;25(5):610–5. https://doi.org/10.1002/pon.3890.
29. Boucher S, Edwards O, Gray A, Nada-Raja S, Lillis J, Tylka TL, Horwath CC. Teaching intuitive eating and acceptance and commitment therapy skills via a web-based intervention: a pilot single-arm intervention study. JMIR Res Protocols. 2016;5(4):e5861. https://doi.org/10.2196/resprot.5861.
30. Köhle N, Drossaert CH, Schreurs KM, Hagedoorn M, Verdonck-de Leeuw IM, Bohlmeijer ET. A web-based self-help intervention for partners of cancer patients based on Acceptance and Commitment Therapy: a protocol of a randomized controlled trial. BMC Public Health. 2015;15(1):1–3. https://doi.org/10.1186/s12889-015-1656-y.
31. Brady SR. Utilizing and adapting the Delphi method for use in qualitative research. Int J Qual Methods. 2015;14(5):1609406915621381. https://doi.org/10.1177/1609406915621381.
32. Braun V, Clarke V. Using thematic analysis in psychology. Qual Res Psychol. 2006;3(2):77–101. https://doi.org/10.1191/1478088706qp063oa.
33. Gaudiano BA, Busch AM. Engaging people with psychosis in acceptance and commitment therapy and mindfulness: acceptance and commitment therapy and mindfulness for psychosis. In: Morris EMJ, Johns LC, Oliver JE (eds), Acceptance and commitment therapy and mindfulness for psychosis, Wiley and Sons, New York, 2013; 76–94. https://doi.org/10.1002/9781118499184.ch6.
34. Vilardaga R, Davies PS, Vowles KE, Sullivan MD. Theoretical grounds of Pain tracker self manager: an acceptance and commitment therapy digital intervention for patients with chronic pain. J Contextual Behav Sci. 2020;15:172–80. https://doi.org/10.1016/j.jcbs.2020.01.001.

20

Feasibility of single position laparoscopic radical nephrectomy and tumor thrombectomy for left renal cell carcinoma with high-risk Mayo grade 0 and 1 tumor thrombus

Adili Keranmu[1,2†], Mingshuai Wang[1,2,3†], Yajian Li[1,2], Feiya Yang[1,2], Wasilijiang Wahafu[1,2], Dong Chen[1,2], Jing Liang[4], Kaopeng Guan[1,2] and Nianzeng Xing[1,2*]

Abstract

Background: To explore the feasibility of single-position laparoscopic radical nephrectomy (LRN) and tumor thrombectomy for left renal cell carcinoma with high-risk Mayo 0 and 1 tumor thrombus (TT).

Methods: All patients with left renal cell carcinoma and venous TT (high-risk Mayo grade 0 and 1) who were performed single-position LRN and tumor thrombectomy were involved. After the renal artery was controlled by Hem-o-lok, the left renal vein was dissected through descending colon mesentery. The left renal vein was divided by EndoGIA for high-risk Mayo grade 0 TT. For Mayo grade 1 TT, part of the inferior vena cava was blocked by a bulldog clamp after milking the TT into the left renal vein and the inferior vena cava was sutured after complete excision of the TT.

Results: 3 patients were involved and operations were performed successfully without conversion to open surgery. The mean operation time was 136 min and the mean estimated blood loss was 60 mL. No postoperative complications occurred.

Conclusions: It is feasible to control left renal vein and partial inferior vena cava through descending colon mesentery in a single position during LRN and tumor thrombectomy for the treatment of high-risk Mayo grade 0 and 1 TT.

Keywords: Renal cell carcinoma, Laparoscopy, Tumor thrombus, Nephrectomy

Introduction

Invasion of the venous system is one of the clinical features of locally advanced kidney cancer. Approximately 4–10% of locally advanced renal cell carcinomas have venous tumor thrombus (TT) [1]. Studies have shown that radical nephrectomy and inferior vena cava TT removal for patients with locally advanced renal cancer can effectively improve the prognosis, and the 5-year tumor-specific survival rate is 40–65% [2]. In recent years, robot-assisted/laparoscopic surgery has become the first choice for the treatment of kidney cancer with venous TT for minimal invasion. For patients with renal cell carcinoma and Mayo grade 0–2 TT, minimally invasive surgery can achieve long-term tumor control similar to open surgery and has better perioperative outcomes [3]. Left renal vein TT is more complicated than right renal vein TT and the length of Mayo grade 0 TT determines the complexity of the surgery. If it is a low-risk

*Correspondence: xingnianzeng@126.com

†Adili Keranmu and Mingshuai Wang contributed equally to this work

[2] Present Address: Department of Urology, National Cancer Center/National Clinical Research Center for Cancer/Cancer Hospital, Chinese Academy of Medical Sciences and Peking Union Medical College, No. 17, Panjiayuan South Li, Chaoyang District, Beijing 100021, People's Republic of China

Full list of author information is available at the end of the article

Mayo grade 0 TT, the end of the TT is on the left side of the mesenteric artery, the left renal vein can be fully controlled by traditional approach. If it is a high-risk Mayo grade 0 TT or even grade 1 TT, traditionally two steps were utilized including management of the inferior vena cava and removement of the TT, and then nephrectomy after changing the surgical position. In order to simplify the procedure, we explored the trans-mesocolon approach to fully dissect the left renal vein to the inferior vena cava in single position to treat high-risk Mayo 0-grade and grade 1 TT.

The aim of the study was to explore the feasibility of single position transperitoneal laparoscopic radical nephrectomy (LRN) and high-risk Mayo 0 and 1 tumor thrombectomy and the surgical techniques were described in detail.

Methods

General information

All patients with left renal cell carcinoma and venous TT (Mayo grade 0–1) who were performed single-position LRN and tumor thrombectomy were involved. The 3 enrolled patients were males, aged 54–57 years old, with a median age of 57 years old. Urinary tract ultrasound, enhanced MRI, MRA, chest CT and bone scan were performed before surgery to determine the location, size and metastasis of the tumor. The clinicopathological data are outlined in Table 1.

Case 1 imaging examination revealed a left kidney tumor with venous TT (Mayo stage 1) and multiple lung metastases. The kidney biopsy confirmed clear renal cell carcinoma with poorly differentiated and accompanied by necrosis. Two cycles of axitinib combined with PD-1 inhibitor were provided for neoadjuvant treatment.

The imaging examinations of case 2 showed a left kidney tumor with venous TT (Mayo grade 1), accompanied by left adrenal gland metastasis. The pathology from kidney biopsy demonstrated clear renal cell carcinoma and the patient received 2 cycles of axitinib for neoadjuvant treatment.

The imaging examination of case 3 showed left kidney tumor with retroperitoneal lymphadenopathy, left renal vein TT (Mayo grade 0) and multiple lung metastases. The kidney biopsy showed clear renal clear cell carcinoma. The TT shrunk to high-risk Mayo grade 0 after 3 months neoadjuvant treatment of sintilimab and axitinib.

Position and trocar placement

After successful anesthesia, the patient was placed in a supine position obliquely 70° on the right side, fixed with a lumbar pillow, and raised the lumbar bridge. The position of the trocar was shown in Fig. 1: The 5 mm trocar A, located 1 cm below the costal margin of the left clavicle midline, was used to puncture into the abdominal cavity and then the pneumoperitoneum was established. The pressure is maintained at 12 mmHg. The 10 mm trocar B was used for laparoscopic lens, locating on the outer edge of the affected rectus abdominis muscle. The

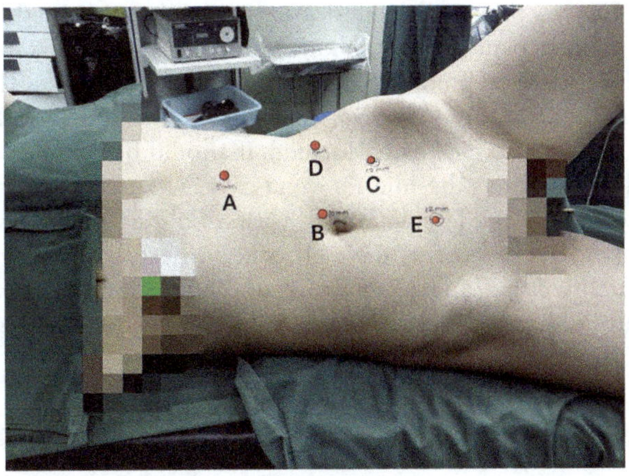

Fig. 1 The position and trocar placement

Table 1 The patient's clinicopathological characteristics

Case	Age (year)/sex	BMI (kg/m^2),	ECOG score standard	ASA grades	Tumor thrombus level	Other organs with metastasis	Kidney puncture	Preoperative treatment
1	57/M	20.18	1	II	Mayo 1	Multiple lung metastases	Renal cell-derived carcinoma	Targeted therapy + immunotherapy
2	54/M	25.95	1	I	Mayo 1	Left adrenal gland metastasis	Renal cell carcinoma	Targeted therapy
3	57/M	22.53	1	II	Mayo 0	Multiple lung metastases + Retroperitoneal lymphadenopathy	Renal clear cell carcinoma	Targeted therapy + immunotherapy

M male, *BMI* body mass index, *ECOG* Eastern Cooperative Oncology Group, *ASA* the American Society of Anesthesiologists

12 mm trocar C is placed at the midpoint of the connection between the left anterior superior iliac spine and the belly button. The 5 mm trocar D is located at the flat umbilicus of the anterior axillary line. The 12 mm trocar E is established at the midpoint of the connection between the umbilical cord and the pubic symphysis.

Techniques of nephrectomy and tumor thrombectomy

The operation is performed according to the principle of treating the artery first and then treating the vein. The specific method is as follows after the left descending colon and part of the sigmoid colon lateral ligament were incised, the small intestine was pulled to the mid-abdomen. It's worth noting that to avoid the loss of mesangial blood vessels during dissociation. A dense connective tissue can be seen in the middle of the dorsal medial side of the kidney, and the arterial pulsation can be seen under it. After open the connective tissue and the left renal vein could be seen. At the same time, the adrenal vein and reproductive vein are disconnected when separating the renal vein. The laparoscopic interventional ultrasound was used to detect the end of the TT, then the left renal vein was divided by EndoGIA for Mayo grade 0 TT and part of the inferior vena cava was blocked by a bulldog clamp after milking the thrombus into renal vein for Mayo grade 1 TT. After completely remove the TT, the inferior vena cava was sutured and finally radical nephrectomy was performed. It should be noted that when handling the inferior vena cava, we usually clamp the root of the left renal vein with a bulldog clamp. We only clamp a part of the wall of the inferior vena cava, which will not affect the return of the inferior vena cava and lumbar vein. Therefore, there is no need to deliberately isolate the lumbar vein and cut it off.

Results

All operations were successfully completed without transfer to open surgery, and no postoperative compli cations occurred. The mean operation time was 136 min (45–196) min and the mean estimated blood loss was 60 ml (30–100) mL. The normal diet was restored on postoperative two.

No complications such as fever, intestinal obstruction, intestinal fistula, and urine leakage occurred. The wound recovered well when the patient was discharged from the hospital, and there was no wound infection. There were no complications such as bleeding and pulmonary embo lism during the perioperative period.

The postoperative pathology of two cases showed the tumors were clear renal cell carcinoma (postoperative pathological gross specimen was shown in Fig. 2). The postoperative specimen of another patient showed large necrotic foci, and no residual tumor was seen under the microscope. Combined with the medical history, it was consistent with pathological complete remission (pCR) (Fig. 3). The median follow-up period of 3 patients was 14 months, and there was no tumor recurrence or metastasis (Table 2).

Discussion

Invasion of the venous system is one of the clinical features of locally advanced renal cancer, including invasion of the renal vein and inferior vena cava. The aim of the study was exploring the feasibility and safety of single-position LRN and tumor thrombectomy for left renal cell carcinoma with high-risk Mayo 0 and 1 TT. In short, the operation in our study was completed in a single position without changing the position. The surgical procedures were reasonable and the techniques could be quickly mastered, saving anesthesia and operation time. The surgical outcomes were encouraging including small trauma, quick postoperative recovery, short hospital stay, and few postoperative complications.

For the left renal cell carcinoma with high-risk Mayo 0 and 1 TT, the traditional robot-assisted/laparoscopic surgical method is to remove the affected kidney, then change the position and remove the TT. Another method is performing embolization of the left renal artery before the operation and treating the inferior vena cava and TT during the operation time, then change the position to remove the left kidney. Using traditional method increases the risk of surgery such as damaging the mesangial blood vessels. At the same time, anesthesia and operation time are prolonged. Open surgery, the standard approach for treating inferior vena cava thrombus, is technically complex, has high complication rates, and requires multidisciplinary cooperation [4]. Furthermore, these methods are failed to fully reflect the advantages of minimally invasive surgery. In recent years, scholars at home and abroad have explored single-position LRN and tumor thrombectomy for left renal cell carcinoma with high-risk Mayo 0 and 1 TT, but there are few related reports [5]. In our study, the operation was completed in a single position and a single way without changing the position. The surgical procedures were reasonable and standardized.

In 2009, our team took the lead in completing and reporting retroperitoneal LRN and tumor thrombectomy and summing up experience. In 2012, we completed the first complete LRN and grade II vena cava tumor thrombectomy in China. In view of the fact that the transperitoneal route has a greater impact on the gastrointestinal tract and the patient's recovery is slow after surgery, in 2014, the retroperitoneal route of radical nephrectomy plus the removal of grade II inferior vena cava TT was completed for the first time in the world

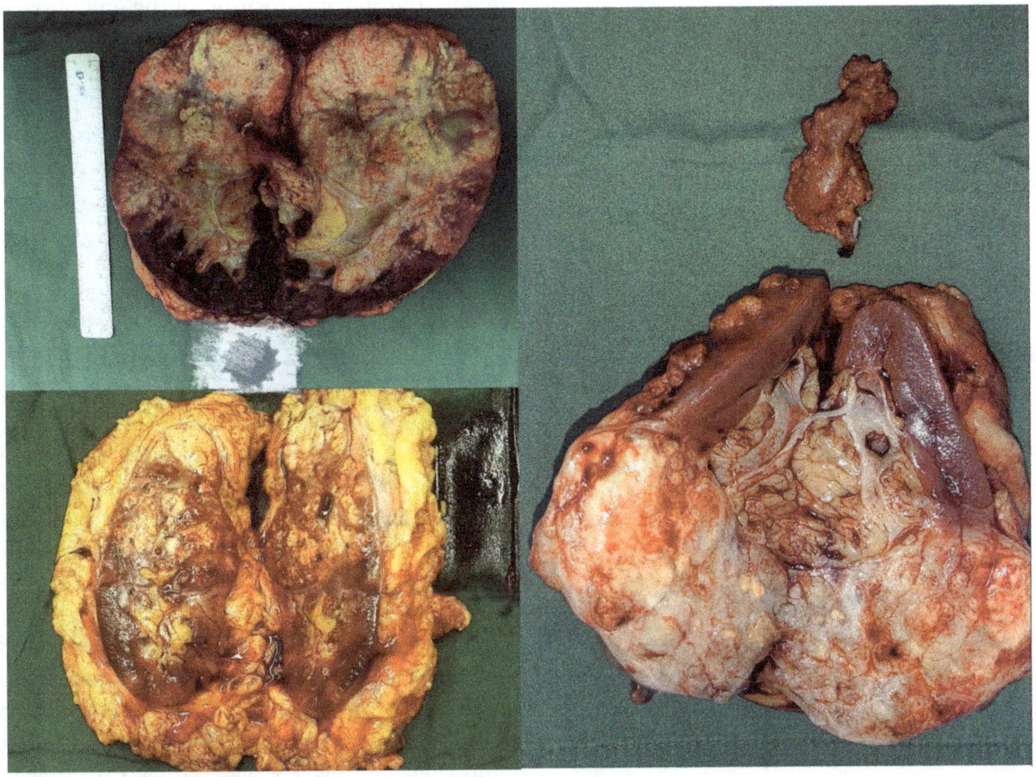

Fig. 2 Postoperative pathological gross specimen

[6]. Based on years of attempts, our center has accumulated rich experience in renal cancer surgery with venous tumor thrombi. Therefore, we are more confident to explore single-position LRN and tumor thrombectomy for left renal cell carcinoma with high-risk Mayo 0 and 1 TT.

The key points and techniques of this study are as follows: 1. Reasonably design the patient's position and scientifically place the Trocar position to facilitate the operation and cooperation of the surgeon and assistant. The patient's position and Trocar position are the key to the success or failure of a single-position operation; 2. The method of finding and processing the renal pedicles using laparoscopic procedures: For the left renal pedicle, the kidney can be pushed to the ventral side with a vascular clamp. A dense connective tissue can be seen in the middle of the dorsal medial side of the kidney, and arterial pulses can be seen below to open the connective tissue. The left renal artery can be seen [7]. After the renal artery is found, the hem-o-lok clamp is used to block the renal blood flow, but not cut off. After the renal vein is processed, then cut off the renal artery in order to reduce blood oozing; 3. Determine the corresponding surgical strategy according to the height of the TT; 4. Using the laparoscopic ultrasonography in this operation to detect the location of the TT in the vein, determine the size of the TT, and detect the specific position of the end of the TT to determine how to block the vein [8–10]; 5. Strictly follow the principle of tumor free and sterile; 6. Before the specimen is taken out, suture the peritoneum of the incised paracolonic sulcus with an absorbable thread to Reduce the risk of intestinal adhesions and intestinal obstruction which is conducive to the recovery of intestinal function; 7. The specimens must be taken out in the specimen bag, which can reduce the risk of tumor implantation and the length of the incision. Female patients can use the NOSES procedure to remove the specimens from the vagina, which can achieve less trauma, fast recovery, good cosmetic effects, and short hospital stay and many other advantages.

The height of the TT determines the specific treatment strategy, especially the surgical strategy, so a grading system based on the height of the TT came into being. Mayo Clinic's five-level classification of tumor thrombi has been widely used in clinical work [1]. The 3 cases in this study are high-risk Mayo 0 and 1 TT patients. Based on conventional knowledge and traditional diagnosis and treatment methods, for grade 0 or I tumor thrombosis, and TT that hardly extends to the inferior vena cava, the thrombus can be removed. Squeeze the renal vein back,

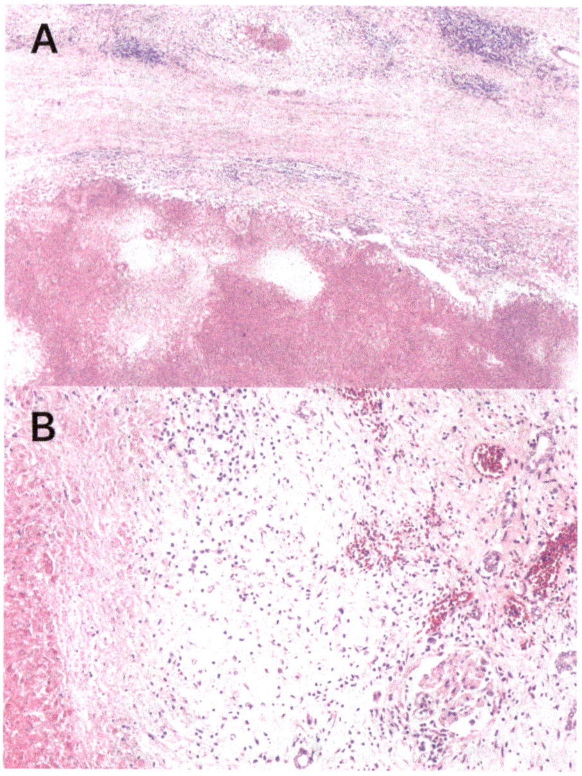

Fig. 3 Microphotograph of renal cell cancer (hematoxylin and eosin stain, **A** magnification × 4, **B** magnification × 10)

and then place it in the renal vein orifice with a vascular clip to isolate it to avoid complete blockage of the inferior vena cava [11]. For patients with left renal tumor with venous tumor thrombosis, we have confirmed through this study that it can be done under single position laparoscopy.

In laparoscopic renal vein/inferior vena cava TT removal surgery, because we cannot accurately determine the position of the end of the TT with the naked eye, it is very dangerous to blindly test before blocking the renal vein or inferior vena cava which increasing the risk of TT shedding. As mentioned earlier, laparoscopic ultrasonography is used in this operation to detect the location of the TT in the vein, determine the size of the TT, and detect the specific position of the end of the TT to determine how to block the vein [8–10]. After the inferior vena cava is incised and the thrombus is removed, check again to prevent residual tumor thrombi. It can prevent the TT from remaining or falling off due to insufficient blocking range, and it can also avoid damage to the inferior vena cava due to excessive dissociation, making the operation more accurate and greatly reducing the risk of surgery [9, 10, 12]. Therefore, hospitals that perform such operations recommend routine preparations for Laparoscopic ultrasonography before surgery [10].

The use of neoadjuvant systemic therapy to reduce locally advanced tumors to promote surgical resection and improve survival is used in various malignant tumors [13]. The rapid development and approval of anti-angiogenesis targeted therapy for metastatic renal cell carcinoma since 2006 has aroused people's interest in the potential application of these drugs in reducing tumor thrombosis levels [14]. For example, in a study by Cost, the median height of venous TT decreased by 1.5 cm, and one patient was successfully reduced from Mayo Clinic grade 4 to grade 3 [15]. All 3 patients in this study received targeted and immunotherapy before surgery. One patient received Sintilimab and axitinib for 3 months and then Venous TT was reduced from Mayo 1 to high grade 0. Another patient received axitinib combined with PD-1 treatment for 2 cycles and Postoperative pathology suggests pCR. However, the results of these studies are diverse. It has been reported that 5–44% of cases have reduced TT height, 28–91% of cases have stable disease, and 5–28% of cases have advanced tumor thrombi [16–18]. So far, there is no first-level evidence to support the use of targeted drugs before venous TT resection.

In summary, compared with traditional surgical methods, the single-position LRN and tumor thrombectomy for left renal cell carcinoma with high-risk Mayo 0 and 1 TT through abdominal cavity has the advantages like standardized methods, simple steps, less trauma, less bleeding, and quick postoperative recovery. It is a safe and effective minimally invasive technique for the treatment of renal cell carcinoma with venous TT. We initially discussed the safety and feasibility of this surgical method. However, due to the small number of clinical samples, patients and operations involved are summarized by a

Table 2 The patient's perioperative clinical data

Case	Operation time	Intraoperative blood loss	Postoperative drainage volume	Drainage tube placement time (days)	Catheter placement time (days)	Postoperative hospital stay (days)	Major complications in 90 days
1	166	100	5421	4	1	4	None
2	196	50	82	2	1	4	None
3	45	30	2760	12	1	11	None

single center, its technology promotion, clinical efficacy and prognostic evaluation need to be further verified by multi-center, large sample size and long-term follow-up. Therefore, it is recommended to carry out a comparative study with classic laparoscopic procedures to explore the advantages of different procedures.

Abbreviations

LRN: Laparoscopic radical nephrectomy; TT: Tumor thrombus; MRI: Magnetic resonance imaging; MRA: Magnetic resonance angiography; CT: Computed tomography; BMI: Body mass index; pCR: Pathologic complete response; IVC: Inferior vena cava.

Acknowledgements

We thank all the people who willingly participated in this study.

Authors' contributions

NX conceived the task. AK, MW, YL, FY, WW and DC performed the manuscript and collected original studies. AK, MW, YL, FY, WW and KG wrote the first draft of the manuscript. YJ, JL and KG prepared figures. All authors revised the manuscript. NZ contributed to language editing and final revision. All data were generated in-house, and no paper mill was used. All authors agree to be accountable for all aspects of work ensuring integrity and accuracy. All authors read and approved the final manuscript.

Author details

[1]State Key Laboratory of Molecular Oncology, National Cancer Center/National Clinical Research Center for Cancer/Cancer Hospital, Chinese Academy of Medical Sciences and Peking Union Medical College, Beijing 100021, People's Republic of China. [2]Present Address: Department of Urology, National Cancer Center/National Clinical Research Center for Cancer/Cancer Hospital, Chinese Academy of Medical Sciences and Peking Union Medical College, No. 17, Panjiayuan South Li, Chaoyang District, Beijing 100021, People's Republic of China. [3]Department of Urology, Institute of Urology, Beijing Chaoyang Hospital, Capital Medical University, Beijing 100020, People's Republic of China. [4]Department of Pathology, National Cancer Center/National Clinical Research Center for Cancer/Cancer Hospital, Chinese Academy of Medical Sciences and Peking Union Medical College, Beijing 100021, People's Republic of China.

References

1. Blute ML, Leibovich BC, Lohse CM, Cheville JC, Zincke H. The Mayo Clinic experience with surgical management, complications and outcome for patients with renal cell carcinoma and venous tumour thrombus. BJU Int. 2004;94(1):33–41.
2. Al Otaibi M, Abou Youssif T, Alkhaldi A, Sircar K, Kassouf W, Aprikian A, Mulder D, Tanguay S. Renal cell carcinoma with inferior vena caval extention: impact of tumour extent on surgical outcome. BJU Int. 2009;104(10):1467–70.
3. Gu L, Ma X, Gao Y, Li H, Li X, Chen L, Wang B, Xie Y, Fan Y, Zhang X. Robotic versus open level I-II inferior vena cava thrombectomy: a matched group comparative analysis. J Urol. 2017;198(6):1241–6.
4. Shao P, Li J, Qin C, Lv Q, Ju X, Li P, Shao Y, Ni B, Yin C. Laparoscopic radical nephrectomy and inferior vena cava thrombectomy in the treatment of renal cell carcinoma. Eur Urol. 2015;68(1):115–22.
5. Crisan N, Andras I, Grad DL, Telecan T, Coman RT, de Cobelli O, Matei DV, Coman I. Dual combined laparoscopic approach for renal-cell carcinoma with renal vein and level I-II inferior vena cava thrombus: our technique and initial results. J Endourol. 2018;32(9):837–42.
6. Wang M, Ping H, Niu Y, Zhang J, Xing N. Pure conventional laparoscopic radical nephrectomy with level II vena cava tumor thrombectomy. Int Braz J Urol Off J Braz Soc Urol. 2014;40(2):266–73.
7. Yang F, Zhou Q, Li X, Xing N. The methods and techniques of identifying renal pedicle vessels during retroperitoneal laparoscopic radical and partial nephrectomy. World J Surg Oncol. 2019;17(1):38.
8. Liu B, Zhan Y, Chen X, Xie Q, Wu B. Laparoscopic ultrasonography: the wave of the future in renal cell carcinoma? Endosc Ultrasound. 2018;7(3):161–7.
9. Yang F, Liu S, Mou L, Wu L, Li X, Xing N. Application of intraoperative ultrasonography in retroperitoneal laparoscopic partial nephrectomy: a single-center experience of recent 199 cases. Endosc Ultrasound. 2019;8(2):118–24.
10. Kang N, Niu Y, Zhang J, Wang J, Tian X, Yan Y, Yu Z, Xing N. Intraoperative ultrasonography: a useful tool in retrolaparoscopic nephron-sparing surgery. Urol Int. 2012;88(3):338–42.
11. Psutka SP, Leibovich BC. Management of inferior vena cava tumor thrombus in locally advanced renal cell carcinoma. Ther Adv Urol. 2015;7(4):216–29.
12. Fergany AF, Gill IS, Schweizer DK, Kaouk JH, ElFettouh HA, Cherullo EE, Meraney AM, Sung GT. Laparoscopic radical nephrectomy with level II vena caval thrombectomy: survival porcine study. J Urol. 2002;168(6):2629–31.
13. Keranmu A, Zheng H, Wu Y, Zhao J, Xu X, Liu F, Cai S, Wang Y, Xu Y. Comparative study of single-center patients with thyroid metastases from colorectal cancer and previously reported cases in the literature. World J Surg Oncol. 2017;15(1):88.
14. Bukowski R, Cella D, Gondek K, Escudier B. Effects of sorafenib on symptoms and quality of life: results from a large randomized placebo-controlled study in renal cancer. Am J Clin Oncol. 2007;30(3):220–7.
15. Cost NG, Delacroix SE Jr, Sleeper JP, Smith PJ, Youssef RF, Chapin BF, Karam JA, Culp S, Abel EJ, Brugarolas J, et al. The impact of targeted molecular therapies on the level of renal cell carcinoma vena caval tumor thrombus. Eur Urol. 2011;59(6):912–8.
16. Bex A, Kroon BK, de Bruijn R. Is there a role for neoadjuvant targeted therapy to downsize primary tumors for organ sparing strategies in renal cell carcinoma? Int J Surg Oncol. 2012;2012:250479.
17. Bigot P, Fardoun T, Bernhard JC, Xylinas E, Berger J, Roupret M, Beauval JB, Lagabrielle S, Lebdai S, Ammi M, et al. Neoadjuvant targeted molecular therapies in patients undergoing nephrectomy and inferior vena cava thrombectomy: is it useful? World J Urol. 2014;32(1):109–14.
18. Peters I, Winkler M, Juttner B, Teebken OE, Herrmann TR, von Klot C, Kramer M, Reichelt A, Abbas M, Kuczyk MA, et al. Neoadjuvant targeted therapy in a primary metastasized renal cell cancer patient leads to down-staging of inferior vena cava thrombus (IVC) enabling a cardio-pulmonary bypass-free tumor nephrectomy: a case report. World J Urol. 2014;32(1):245–8.

21

Modified vein clamping technique for renal cell carcinoma complicated with level I–II IVC thrombi

Jiaxing Ma, Wei Sun, Weiwei Qian, Jie Min, Tao Zhang and Dexin Yu*

Abstract

Objectives: To share our initial experience with the modified vein clamping technique for the treatment of renal cell carcinoma complicated with level I–II IVC thrombi.

Methods: From March 2018 to April 2021, 11 patients with renal cell carcinoma (RCC) involving an IVC tumour thrombus were admitted to our hospital. They all underwent laparoscopic radical nephrectomy and IVC thrombectomy (LRN-IVCTE) using a modified vein clamping technique.

Results: All procedures were successfully completed without conversion to open surgery. The median operative time was 185.00 min (145.00–216.00 min); the median estimated blood loss was 200.00 ml (155.00–300.00 ml), and four patients received an intraoperative transfusion. In addition, the median IVC clamping time was 18.00 min (12.00–20.00 min); the median postoperative hospital stay was 6.00 days (4.00–7.00 days), while the median follow-up period was 28.00 months (4.00–34.00 months).

Conclusions: The modified vein clamping technique for the treatment of renal cell carcinoma complicated with level I–II IVC thrombi may be a safe and technically feasible alternative technique.

Keywords: Renal cell carcinoma, Tumor thrombus, Laparoscopy, Modified vein clamping technique

Introduction

Tumour thrombi can be found in many cases of renal cell carcinoma (RCC). Most tumour thrombi are located in the renal vein and inferior vena cava, accounting for approximately 10%, while a few are located in the heart, accounting for approximately 1% [1]. Compared with other treatments, nephrectomy with IVC thrombectomy is becoming a more popular option because it provides a better prognosis [2]. For the treatment of RCC, patients who underwent radical nephrectomy with any level of IVC thrombectomy had a satisfactory 5-year survival rate of 64% [3]. In fact, with the introduction of novel therapeutic agents, the survival rate has significantly improved recently. Regardless of the thrombus level, early surgical resection is still the classic treatment in nonmetastatic RCC patients with an IVC thrombus [4]. In addition, in metastatic RCC patients, treatment of the primary tumour may be indicated in the cytoreductive setting, as it ensures a lower level of circulating tumour-derived immunosuppressive factors and a better prognosis [5]. Furthermore, the open approach has previously been considered the standard when performing radical nephrectomy with IVC thrombectomy. More recently, the focus has shifted towards minimally invasive techniques (laparoscopy and robotic assistance), whose feasibility for performing extremely complex surgeries has been proven [6]. In this case, ensuring maximal oncologic control with minimal morbidity for the patient

*Correspondence: yudx_urology@126.com
Department of Urology, The Second Affiliated Hospital of Anhui Medical University, 678 Furong Rd, Hefei 230032, Anhui, People's Republic of China

is the current challenge for the surgical treatment of RCC with an IVC thrombus. Since Varkarakis et al. [7] first reported their experience with LRN-VCTE in 2004, several reports have been published [6, 8–10]. Recently, robot-assisted surgery has also been reported [11–13]. All these reports have only described their major surgical procedure and oncologic results, whereas there is no relevant research on the technique of vein clamping.

In this paper, we present our initial experience with a modified vein clamping technique for the treatment of renal cell carcinoma with a level I–II IVC thrombus at our single medical centre.

Patients and methods

Patients

We retrospectively evaluated the records of 11 patients with RCC involving an IVC tumour thrombus (level I–II) who underwent laparoscopic radical nephrectomy and IVC thrombectomy (LRN-IVCTE) at our hospital from March 2018 to April 2021. However, patients in whom the primary tumour was invading adjacent organs, who had multiple distant metastases, or in whom the IVC was extensively infiltrated by the thrombus were excluded from laparoscopic IVC thrombectomy, except for the single metastatic lesion. Moreover, patients with a history of upper abdominal surgery and those with an unacceptable anaesthetic risk and cardiopulmonary insufficiency were also not included. Patient characteristics (age, sex, body mass index, KPS score, ASA score, clinical stage, renal tumour size, IVC thrombus classification, and thrombus length) were assessed. In total, eight cases had RCC on the right side, and three had RCC on the left. All patients underwent abdominal magnetic resonance imaging (MRI), abdominal enhanced computed tomography (CT), and chest CT before the operation so that the tumour size (cm) and thrombus length (cm) were measured from CT or MRI. In addition, through renal emission computed tomography (ECT), it was determined that all patients had a normal kidney on the contralateral side, whereas the Mayo classification was used to evaluate the position of the IVC thrombus [14], with the levels defined as follows: level 0, a thrombus limited to the renal vein; level I, a tumour thrombus extending ≤ 2 cm above the renal vein; level II, an extension of > 2 cm above the renal vein, but below the hepatic vein; level III, a thrombus at the level of or above the hepatic vein but below the diaphragm; and level IV, extension above the diaphragm or into the right atrium. Here, it should be mentioned that two patients with single metastasis in the lung were administered preoperative neoadjuvant targeted therapy for 3 months. RCC was classified according to the American Joint Committee on Cancer 2010 TNM staging criteria [15].

Perioperative data (median operative time, estimated blood loss, IVC clamping time, lymphadenectomy surgical time, blood transfusion, preoperative and postoperative serum creatinine, preoperative and postoperative alanine aminotransferase (ALT) and aspartate aminotransferase (AST), preoperative and postoperative haemoglobin, and perioperative complications) were assessed. In addition, perioperative complications were graded according to the Clavien–Dindo classification [16].

All procedures were performed by a single surgeon (Dexin Yu) with LRN-IVCTE using a modified vein clamping technique.

This study was carried out in accordance with the Helsinki Declaration and was approved by the Research Ethics Committee at the Second Affiliated Hospital of Anhui Medical University. In addition, written informed consent was obtained from all participants prior to their inclusion within this study.

Preoperative preparation

Following the enhanced recovery after surgery (ERAS) protocol, general preoperative preparation included preoperative skin preparation, fasting for 6 h and water deprivation for 2 h, except for a water enema and placement of an indwelling gastric tube. The anticoagulation therapy used in these patients was 1 mg/kg enoxaparin administered subcutaneously twice a day from the moment of diagnosis and paused 12 h before surgery. Then, twelve hours after the procedure, anticoagulation therapy was resumed and continued for up to 21 days [17, 18]. Moreover, special preoperative preparation included renal artery embolization on the related side 1–2 h before the operation in 3 patients who were diagnosed with RCC on the left side with an IVC tumour thrombus.

Surgical procedure

The pure LRN-IVCTE was performed in all cases. All procedures were followed by a single surgical team with experience in open surgery and laparoscopic surgery, and the transperitoneal approach was adopted in all patients. Furthermore, transoesophageal echocardiography was used to monitor the extent and stability of the thrombus and to ensure that the tumour thrombus was removed completely during surgical manipulation. Extension of lymphadenectomy should involve the lymph nodes surrounding the ipsilateral great vessel and the inter-aortocaval region from the crus of the diaphragm to the inferior mesenteric artery.

For right RCC, no patient accepted preoperative right renal artery embolization. After general anaesthesia and Foley catheter placement, patients were placed in the 70° flank position on a flat bed, when four laparoscopic ports were in the right lumbar area (Fig. 1). In addition, insufflation with CO_2 at a pressure of 15 mmHg was conducted, the hepatocolic ligament was incised, and the liver was retracted cephalically. After mobilization of the colon and duodenum, the IVC was frontally exposed. Then, the surfaces of the right and left renal veins were isolated. The IVC was mobilized above and below the renal vein for a distance of 3–5 cm along the length of the thrombus, and the lumbar veins were transected. For level II IVC thrombi, the gonadal vein and accessory hepatic veins were also clipped and divided for circumferential dissection of the IVC. Next, the right artery was exposed and ligated between the IVC and aorta ventralis. Then, the vessel loops were placed under the IVC above and below the thrombus and around the left renal vein, which was secured with a Hem-o-lok clip prepared for clamping, followed by sequential clamping of the caudal IVC, left renal vein, and cephalic IVC with laparoscopic bulldog clamps. Here, it should be noted that laparoscopic bulldog clamps rather than the vessel loops directly with Hem-o-lok clips were used to clamp the veins by moderately pulling the vessel loops and narrowing the venous wall. After occlusion of the above vessels, the IVC wall was incised at the right renal vein ostium to avoid stenosis after suturing the inferior vena cava (Fig. 2). Then, the thrombus was removed and fully covered with a specimen bag to prevent tumour dissemination. After the IVC lumen was irrigated with heparinized saline, the IVC was repaired with a continuous suture using the 5–0 polypropylene suture. Before the IVC was closed, the IVC tourniquet was loosened to remove any clot in the IVC. After that, the right kidney was subsequently mobilized, excised, and placed with the main body of the thrombus into the specimen bag, followed by removal through the abdominal incision. In addition, for the level I IVC thrombus, first, the caudal IVC was clamped; then, only one laparoscopic bulldog clamp was employed to clamp the left renal vein and the cephalic IVC simultaneously (Fig. 3).

For left RCC, all three patients underwent preoperative left renal artery embolization so that the IVC thrombus

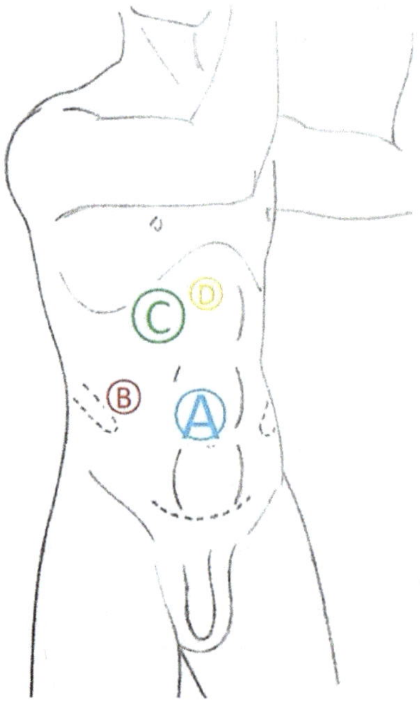

Fig. 1 The positioning of the trocars for the transperitoneal approach: the optic trocar (10 mm) lateral to the umbilicus, at the lateral border of the abdominal rectus muscle (**A**); the trocar for the left-hand instrument on the axillary line parallel to the navel (**B**); the trocar for the right-hand instrument (12 mm) on the perpendicular line from the umbilicus to the costal margin, 2 cm below the costal margin (**C**); a 4th trocar (5 mm) for the assistant to use for liver retraction and suction in the epigastric region (**D**)

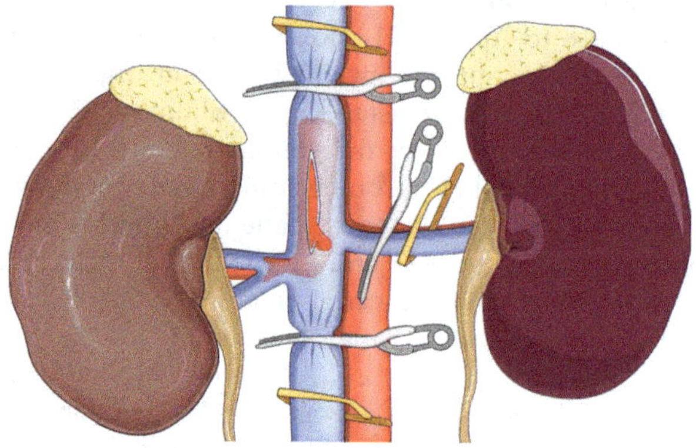

Fig. 2 The caudal IVC, left renal vein, and cephalic IVC were sequentially clamped using laparoscopic bulldog clamps. We used laparoscopic bulldog clamps to clamp the veins by moderately pulling the vessel loops and narrowing the venous wall

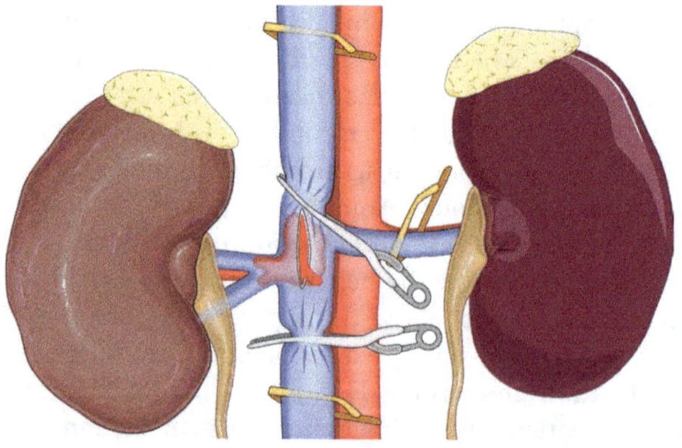

Fig. 3 For level I IVC thrombi, the caudal IVC was clamped first, and then we used just one laparoscopic bulldog clamp to clamp the left renal vein and cephalic IVC at the same time

could be directly handled when the position and placement of ports were the same as those for right RCC (Fig. 1). The IVC combined with the right and left renal veins was isolated sequentially. Beyond that, the caudal IVC, right renal vein, and cephalic IVC were sequentially clamped using laparoscopic bulldog clamps, while the IVC wall was incised at the left renal vein ostium. In the same way, a specimen bag was used to cover the thrombus to avoid tumour dissemination. In general, the specimen bag was seamed with silk thread. After this procedure, the patients were converted to a right lateral decubitus position, and left LRN was performed.

Result

As shown in Table 1, the median age was 57.00 years (54.00–71.00 years); ten of eleven patients were men; the median tumour size was 7.20 cm (6.00–10.50 cm), and eight of eleven patients were on the right side; the median thrombus length was 3.00 cm (2.00–4.00 cm). Six patients had a level I thrombus, while five had a level II thrombus. We identified two patients with a single metastasis in the lung who were administered preoperative neoadjuvant targeted therapy. One patient did not experience tumour or thrombus shrinkage before nephrectomy. One patient experienced tumour shrinkage (shrinkage from 15.1 cm to 13.2 cm) and thrombus shrinkage (shrinkage from 6.0 cm to 4.5 cm) preoperatively. The IMDC scores for the two metastatic patients were both 2. No patient was converted to open surgery.

The perioperative data are shown in Table 2. The median operative time was 185.00 min (145.00–216.00 min); the median estimated blood loss was 200.00 ml (155.00–300.00 ml). Four patients received an intraoperative transfusion. The transfusion was due to preoperative anaemia in three of the patients. The fourth patient's case was complicated with coronary heart disease, while intraoperative arterial blood gas analysis of haemoglobin was 88 g/l. Considering that blood loss would affect the heart blood supply, blood transfusion was given to improve the heart blood supply and avoid increasing the burden on the heart after discussion with the anaesthesiologist. The median IVC clamping time was 18.00 min (12.00–20.00 min), while the lymphadenectomy surgical time was 22.00 min (20.00–24.00 min). The median postoperative hospital stay was 6.00 days (4.00–7.00 days). Moreover, histological analysis revealed clear cell carcinoma in all patients. Surgical margins were negative in all cases, and no major complications were noted (Clavien–Dindo grade ≥ 3). All cases were pathologically confirmed to be renal clear cell carcinoma without regional lymph node metastasis.

Preoperative and postoperative data are shown in Table 3. The median and interquartile range for all

Table 1 Baseline characteristics of all 11 patients

Characteristics	Value
Patients, n	11
Gender, n (%)	
Male	10 (90.9)
Female	1 (9.1)
Median age, years (IQR)	57.00 (54.00–71.00)
Median BMI, kg/m^2 (IQR)	21.36 (20.42–25.21)
Median KPS score (IQR)	90.00 (80.00–90.00)
ASA score, n (%)	
II	7 (63.6)
III	4 (36.4)
Affected side, n (%)	
Left	3 (27.3)
Right	8 (72.7)
Median tumor size, cm (IQR)	7.20 (6.00–10.50)
Clinical stage, n (%)	
T3bN0M0	9 (81.8)
T3bN1M0	0 (0)
T3bN0M1	2 (18.2)
IVC thrombus level, n (%)	
I	6
II	5
Median IVC thrombus length, cm (IQR)	3.00 (2.00–4.00)
Preoperative embolization, n (%)	
Yes	3 (27.3)
No	8 (72.7)

Continuous data are reported as median (IQR)

BMI body mass index, *KPS* Karnofsky Performance Status, *ASA* American Society of Anesthesiologists, *IVC* inferior vena cava, *IQR* interquartile range

Table 2 Perioperative data

Characteristics	Value
Median operative time, min (IQR)	185.00 (145.00–216.00)
Median IVC clamping time, min (IQR)	18.00 (12.00–20.00)
Median lymphadenectomy surgical time, min (IQR)	22.00 (20.00–24.00)
Median estimated blood loss, ml (IQR)	200.00 (155.00–300.00)
Patients receiving transfusion, n (%)	4 (36.4)
Median day to surgical drain removal, day (IQR)	5.00 (3.00–6.00)
Median day to full ambulation, day (IQR)	2.00 (1.00–2.00)
Median day to oral feeding, day (IQR)	2.00 (1.00–2.00)
Median postoperative hospital stay, day (IQR)	6.00 (4.00–7.00)
Perioperative complications, n (%)	
Low grade Clavien I–II	4 (36.4)
High grade Clavien III–IV	0 (0)
Median follow-up, month (IQR)	28.00 (4.00–34.00)

Continuous data are reported as median (IQR)

IVC inferior vena cava, *IQR* interquartile range

Table 3 Preoperative and postoperative data

Characteristics	Preoperative	Postoperative	Z value	P value
Median SCr, μmol/l (IQR)	79.00 (75.00–91.00)	110.00 (79.00–148.00)	−2.578	0.010
Median hemoglobin, g/l (IQR)	123.00 (96.00–134.00)	100.00 (93.00–110.00)	−2.492	0.013
Median AST, μ/l (IQR)	23.00 (17.00–32.00)	25.00 (21.00–31.00)	−1.946	0.052
Median ALT, μ/l (IQR)	18.00 (12.00–29.00)	25.00 (15.00–29.00)	−2.492	0.005

Continuous data are reported as median (IQR)

SCr serum creatinine, *AST* aspartate aminotransferase, *ALT* alanine aminotransferase, *IQR* interquartile range

continuous variables were used, while we used the Wilcoxon signed ranks test to compare preoperative and postoperative data. All patients exhibited mild renal insufficiency. No significant difference was found in AST between preoperation and postoperation measurements. Significant differences were found in haemoglobin and ALT between preoperation and postoperation measurements. However, the value of postoperative ALT was within the normal range. The median follow-up period was 28.00 months (4.00–34.00 months). In addition, pulmonary metastasis was identified before surgery in two patients who survived and were treated with targeted therapy (pazopanib), whereas the remaining nine patients had no local recurrence or distant metastasis during follow-up.

Discussion

Traditionally, the classic surgical approach of radical nephrectomy and IVC thrombectomy is open surgery. For RCC patients with an IVC thrombus, radical nephrectomy with thrombectomy can provide a better prognosis than nonaggressive surgical treatment [2]. Therefore, surgery is a priority for patients with suitable physical conditions. Moreover, with the development of surgical techniques and perioperative management, pure laparoscopic and robotic-assisted thrombectomy has become safe and feasible [8]. Currently, in most reports, vessel loops are used to clamp veins [19, 20], but we believe vein injury would occur if the vessel loops are pulled tautly, and this procedure cannot ensure successful clamping of the vein on one attempt. In addition, the vessel should be wrapped twice, which may prolong the operation time. Furthermore, surgeons have used a Hem-O-lok to tighten the vessel loops, indicating that they need to cut off the Hem-O-lok when loosening the block, which is less convenient than the laparoscopic bulldog clamp. Shao et al. [8] reported their experience in using open bulldog clamps to clamp renal veins and the IVC successfully in laparoscopic surgery, but it is known that using a laparoscopic instrument to control open bulldog clamps is not convenient and that the bulldog clamps can slide out of the laparoscopic instrument during the clamping procedure. In our single medical centre, the vessel loops were combined with laparoscopic bulldog clamps to clamp veins as described.

During minimal access surgery, small tricks may yield important gains. In this report, the application of laparoscopic bulldog clamps in laparoscopic urologic surgery was presented. In fact, the use of bulldog clamps during laparoscopic or robotic procedures, especially in urology surgery, is common (such as in laparoscopic or robotic partial nephrectomy). Specifically, bulldog clamps were used to clamp the renal artery before excising the renal mass. Then, it was proven that the clamps can thoroughly clasp the renal artery. In this report, laparoscopic bulldog clamps combined with vessel loops were used to clamp the caudal IVC, left renal vein and cephalic IVC. By moderately pulling the vessel loops and narrowing the venous wall, the veins could be clamped using laparoscopic bulldog clamps easily and conveniently. After early control of the renal artery and the lumbar veins to reduce haemorrhagic complications, it is believed that the use of laparoscopic bulldog clamps for the occlusion of the vessels during IVC thrombectomy may be preferable to the tourniquets or vessel loops, since slow retrograde bleeding up to the end of IVC suturing was experienced. Using only vessel loops is time-consuming, and cases may be complicated with caval injury if force is inequitably applied to block veins. However, laparoscopic bulldog clamps are easy to use with the aid of an applicator. In addition, this approach is safe, quick and reproducible while providing good surgical exposure in a limited surgical field without interfering with the laparoscopic instrument and blocking any trocar access during the operation. Moreover, the bulldog clip always exerts the same defined pressure, minimizing the damage to the veins. Otherwise, in cases of a level I IVC thrombus, the thrombus was milked down, followed by clamping of the caudal IVC. Then, the vessel loops combined with contralateral renal veins and the cephalic IVC were moderately pulled to narrow the venous wall. To make the next clamping step easy, the direction in which vessel loops are pulled should be adjusted properly. The angle between the inferior vena cava and the left renal vein should be narrowed to an acute angle as far as possible by proper pulling of the vessel loops to reduce the distance between the inferior vena cava and the left renal vein. In particular, attention should be given to the force exerted in pulling the vessel loops in order to avoid vein injury. Next, one laparoscopic bulldog clamp is adopted to clamp the left renal vein and cephalic IVC at the same time, thus saving operative time. Laparoscopic bulldog forceps are easy to use with the aid of a companion applicator. This set of instruments has been routinely used in laparoscopic partial nephrectomy.

The reported operative time when performing IVC thrombectomy ranged between 100 and 275 min, the IVC clamping time varied between 12 and 25 min, and the mean blood loss measured between 150 and 320 ml [8, 19], which was similar to our experience. In addition, none of the authors pointed out significant intraoperative or postoperative complications or conversions to open surgery, and the patients were discharged 9 days after the operation [8], which is similar to our figures to some extent. All of the cases we reported successfully completed surgery without serious complications. All the instruments used in our operation are conventional laparoscopic instruments, which are easily available in all centres. It has good feasibility and popularity.

In addition, to ensure that laparoscopic thrombectomy can be performed safely, patients need to be carefully selected. The criteria for a qualified patient are as follows: 1. the primary tumour is localized; 2. the intraluminal thrombus is free floating, without extensive involvement of the peripheral tissue or vascular wall [8]. Open surgery may be considered if the thrombus appears to be fixed or if the IVC wall is extensively involved [21].

Early control of the renal artery before renal vein manipulation and kidney mobilization is essential to minimize surgical risks, as this helps to decrease intraoperative bleeding and prevent thrombus detachment caused by venous blood flow. In addition, it can also reduce blood flow, with the kidney shrinking, allowing for easier handling, while the thrombus may also shrink. Wang et al. [19] reported that they underwent special preoperative preparation including renal artery embolization on the related side 1–2 h before the operation. However, we think renal artery embolization is unnecessary for right RCC because the right artery can be easily exposed and ligated between the IVC and aorta ventralis. As the surgical procedure was described, when the IVC and the left renal vein were exposed, the right renal artery in the interaortocaval space could be easily found before clamping the IVC. For left RCC, it is believed here that renal artery embolization is necessary. Chopra et al. carried out renal artery embolism before surgery in 80.3% of their patients [13]. It is difficult to expose the left renal artery when the IVC thrombus is handled in the left decubitus position. For left-side tumour cases, the procedures for pedicle control and kidney mobilization require operation from the left side, while major vessel control and thrombectomy should be operated on from the right side, which is more complex than right-side cases. Thus, left renal artery embolization before surgery leads to decompression of venous collaterals and decreased blood loss [22]. In this case, this technology can reduce the difficulty of surgery.

Preventing the risk of pulmonary embolism as a result of thrombosis during the procedures is one of the most important tips. Chopra et al. proposed the "IVC-first, kidney-last" technique for robot-assisted IVC thrombectomy [13]. He detached the tumour thrombus using a stapler to separate the part of the tumour thrombus from that of nephrectomy, but the tumour thrombus may shatter toward the cephalad side at the moment when pressure with the stapler is applied to the renal vein. In addition, the vein wall might collapse, and the tumour thrombus might be seeded into the peritoneal cavity. Yoichiro T et al. adopted a method of "en bloc" nephrectomy with IVC thrombectomy, where detaching the tumour thrombus is unnecessary [23]. However, that method also features two main disadvantages. Specifically, one is that a twisting force is applied to the renal vein (containing the tumour) during kidney mobilization, which may cause the tumour thrombus to unexpectedly break and scatter, while the other is difficulty in mobilizing the kidney in cases where the tumour is large, particularly when the renal vein is not detached and adheres to the IVC. In our single centre, for right RCC, the modified "IVC-first, kidney-last" technique was proposed. After artery control, the IVC tumour thrombus still attached to the renal vein was removed, and then, the tumour thrombus was placed in a specimen bag that was closed immediately by using 2–0 silk. After kidney mobilization, the kidney combined with the tumour thrombus was placed in a larger specimen bag.

The present study has several limitations. First, it was a single-centre study with a small patient population. Second, there are few reports on long-term oncological outcomes, and further research is required. Third, further animal studies are required to verify the difference between laparoscopic bulldog clamps and vessel loops that block veins. However, given the lack of studies on using laparoscopic bulldog clamps in IVC tumour thrombi, it is believed that the present study has clinical significance.

Conclusions

The modified vein clamping technique for the treatment of renal cell carcinoma complicated with a level I–II IVC thrombus is a valid alternative. However, larger patient samples and longer follow-up times are required to further define the role of modified laparoscopic surgery for high-level IVC thrombi in RCC patients.

Acknowledgements

Not applicable.

Authors' contributions

Each author has participated sufficiently in the work and takes public responsibility for appropriate portions of the content. The authors have agreed to be accountable for all aspects of the work and to ensure that questions related to the accuracy or integrity of any part of the work are appropriately investigated and resolved. Dexin Yu created the design and concept of the study together with Jiaxing Ma and Tao Zhang. Supported by Tao Zhang and Jie Min, they acquired the data and implemented the clinical trial. Literature research was conducted by Wei Sun and Weiwei Qian. The manuscript was prepared by Jiaxing Ma. Statistical analysis was carried out by Jiaxing Ma and Tao Zhang. All authors read and approved the final manuscript.

References

1. Blute ML, Leibovich BC, Lohse CM, Cheville JC, Zincke H. The Mayo Clinic experience with surgical management, complications and outcome for patients with renal cell carcinoma and venous tumour thrombus. BJU Int. 2004;94:33–41.
2. Skinner DG, Pritchett TR, Lieskovsky G, et al. Vena caval involvement by renal cell carcinoma.Surgical resection provides meaningful long-term survival. Ann Surg. 1989;210:387–92.
3. Ciancio G, Manoharan M, Katkoori D, De Los Santos R, Soloway MS. Long-term survival in patients undergoing radical nephrectomy and inferior vena cava thrombectomy: single-center experience. Eur Urol. 2010;57:667–72.
4. Ljungberg B, Albiges L, Abu-Ghanem Y, Bensalah K, Dabestani S, Fernández-Pello S, et al. European Association of Urology Guidelines on renal cell carcinoma: the 2019 update. Eur Urol. 2019;75:799–810.
5. Russo P. Multi-modal treatment for metastatic renal cancer: the role of surgery. World J Urol. 2010;28:295–301.
6. Bansal RK, Tu HY, Drachenberg D, et al. Laparoscopic management of advanced renal cell carcinoma with renal vein and inferior vena cava thrombus. Urology. 2014;83:812–6.
7. Varkarakis IM, Bhayani SB, Allaf ME, Inagaki T, Gonzalgo ML, Jarrett TW. Laparoscopic-assisted nephrectomy with inferior vena cava tumor thrombectomy: preliminary results. Urology. 2004;64:925–9.
8. Shao P, Li J, Qin C, et al. Laparoscopic radical nephrectomy and inferior vena cava thrombectomy in the treatment of renal cell carcinoma. Eur Urol. 2015;68:115–22.
9. Wang W, Wang L, Xu J, Adams TS, Tian Y, Lv W. Pure retroperitoneal laparoscopic radical nephrectomy for right renal masses with renal vein and inferior vena cava thrombus. J Endurol. 2014;28:819–24.
10. Ghareeb GM, Kenleigh DA, Brown JA. Left hand-assisted laparoscopic nephrectomy with renal vein thrombectomy for stage T3b renal cell carcinoma. Urology. 2016;90:e3-4.
11. Abaza R, Shabsigh A, Castle E, et al. Multi-institutional experience with robotic nephrectomy with inferior vena cava tumor thrombectomy. J Urol. 2016;195(4 Pt 1):865–71.
12. Kundavaram C, Abreu AL, Chopra S, et al. Advances in robotic vena cava tumor thrombectomy: Intracaval balloon occlusion, patch grafting, and vena cavoscopy. Eur Urol. 2016;70(5):884–90.
13. Chopra S, Simone G, Metcalfe C, et al. Robot-assisted level II–III inferior vena cava tumor thrombectomy: step-by-step technique and 1-year outcomes. Eur Urol. 2017;72(2):267–74.
14. Neves RJ, Zincke H. Surgical treatment of renal cancer with vena cava extension. Br J Urol. 1987;59:390–5.
15. Edge SB, Compton CC. The American Joint Committee on Cancer: the 7th edition of the AJCC cancer staging manual and the future of TNM. Ann Surg Oncol. 2010;17:1471–4.
16. Dindo D, Demartines N, Clavien PA. Classification of surgical complications:a new proposal with evaluation in a cohort of 6336 patients and results of a survey. Ann Surg. 2004;240:205–13.
17. Tang B, Dong HY, Shao PF, et al. The clinical application of enhanced recovery after surgery protocol in perioperative period of laparoscopic nephron sparing surgery. Transl Androl Urol. 2020;9(4):1566–71.
18. Nicolae C, Lulia A, Doru-Lucian G, et al. dual combined laparoscopic approach for renal-cell carcinoma with renal vein and level I–II inferior vena cava thrombus: our technique and initial results. J Endourol. 2018;32(9):837–42.
19. Wang B, Li H, Ma X, et al. Robot-assisted laparoscopic inferior vena cava thrombectomy: different sides require different techniques. Eur Urol. 2016;69(6):1112–9.
20. Christopher M, Ronney A. Complex robotic nephrectomy and inferior vena cava tumor thrombectomy: an evolving landscape. Robot Surg Urol. 2019;30(1):83–9.
21. Pouliot F, Shuch B, LaRochelle JC, et al. Contemporary management of renal tumors with venous tumor thrombus. J Urol. 2010;184:833–41.
22. Chopra S, Simone G, Metcalfe C, et al. Robot-assisted level II–III inferior vena cava tumor thrombectomy: step-by-step technique and 1-year outcomes. Eur Urol. 2017;72:267–74.
23. Yoichiro T, Noriyuki M, Issei S, et al. En bloc laparoscopic radical nephrectomy with inferior vena cava thrombectomy: a single-institution experience. Int J Urol. 2019;26(3):363–8.

22

Symptomatic renal papillary varicosities and medullary nephrocalcinosis

Brent Cleveland* and Michael Borofsky

Abstract

Background: Nephrocalcinosis is often asymptomatic but can manifest with renal colic or hematuria. There is no reported association between nephrocalcinosis and renal vascular malformations, which may also be a source of hematuria. We herein present a case of a patient with hematuria related to nephrocalcinosis and renal papillary varicosities. These varicosities were diagnosed and successfully treated with flexible ureteroscopy and laser fulguration.

Case presentation: A 24-year-old female with a history of epilepsy (on zonisamide), recent uncomplicated pregnancy, and new diagnosis of nephrocalcinosis presented with right flank pain and intermittent gross hematuria. Imaging revealed intermittent right sided hydronephrosis. A cystoscopy identified hematuria from the right ureteral orifice. Diagnostic flexible ureteroscopy revealed numerous intrapapillary renal stones and varicose veins of several renal papillae. A 200 μm holmium laser fiber was used to unroof these stones and fulgurate the varicosities with resolution of her symptoms for several months. She later presented with left-sided symptoms and underwent left ureteroscopy with similar findings and identical successful treatment.

Conclusion: Unilateral hematuria from discrete vascular lesions of the renal collecting system may be obscured by other benign co-existing conditions, such as nephrocalcinosis and nephrolithiasis. Although a simultaneous presentation is rare, flexible ureteroscopy with laser fulguration offers an ideal diagnostic and therapeutic modality for these concurrent conditions if symptoms arise.

Keywords: Renal papillary varicosity, Renal vascular malformation, Nephrocalcinosis, Essential hematuria, Laser fulguration, Case report

Background

Nephrocalcinosis describes a condition in which calcium oxalate or calcium phosphate deposition occurs within the renal parenchyma. It is often asymptomatic and discovered incidentally on radiographic imaging. When symptoms do occur, they often include renal colic from associated nephrolithiasis or extrusion of calcium deposits into the collecting system, both of which can result in hematuria [1].

There is no reported association between nephrocalcinosis and renal vascular malformations. Although rare bilateral cases have been reported, generally these malformations are unilateral sources of hematuria. When diagnosed endoscopically, these vascular abnormalities have been classified as either discrete or diffuse lesions. Benign discrete lesions include renal hemangioma, minute venous rupture, or previously unidentified renal calculi. Although varices of the renal papillae have been categorized with MVR, there is a paucity of literature describing this unique clinical entity and its management. After obtaining informed voluntary consent from the patient, herein we describe a case of the incidental diagnosis and successful treatment of symptomatic varicosities of renal papillae in the setting of medullary nephrocalcinosis and recent pregnancy.

*Correspondence: cleve169@umn.edu
University of Minnesota, 420 Delaware St. S. E., MMC 394, Minneapolis, MN 55455, USA

Case presentation

A 24-year-old female with a history of epilepsy (on zonisamide) and an uncomplicated pregnancy with spontaneous vaginal delivery 1 week prior presented with right flank pain and intermittent gross hematuria. Her work-up was concerning for pyelonephritis, and CT imaging revealed right hydronephrosis as well as findings consistent with medullary nephrocalcinosis. The hydronephrosis was suspected to be secondary to her recent pregnancy; however, due to concern for possible urosepsis she underwent multiple attempts at renal decompression, including placement of 2 ureteral stents and a percutaneous nephrostomy tube, all which were dislodged. Of note, during the second ureteral stent placement, right distal ureteroscopy was performed and identified blood clot within the right ureter. She was treated with culture directed antibiotics but re-presented to a tertiary center with recurrent fevers. Repeat CT imaging demonstrated persistent right hydronephrosis. Ultimately, she declined another surgical intervention and elected for conservative management with additional antibiotics.

She was later seen on an outpatient basis at which time she reported intermittent right flank pain and gross hematuria, including string-like clots suspicious for upper tract bleeding. Physical exam revealed inconsistent right CVA tenderness. Initially, a renal ultrasound demonstrated resolution of her right hydronephrosis. Over the course of several months she visited the hospital several times for these symptoms. During one such visit, repeat CT imaging showed recurrent right hydronephrosis and proximal hydroureter suggesting new obstruction. It also demonstrated stable bilateral focal nephrocalcinosis in the right upper and mid poles as well as the left lower pole (Fig. 1). Laboratory work-up included normal serum creatinine (1.02 mg/dL), bicarbonate (25 mmol/L), calcium (8.7 mmol/L), and intact parathyroid hormone (22 pg/mL). Urinalysis confirmed gross hematuria with > 182 RBC per high power field. A urine culture was negative for significant pathogenic bacterial growth. A 24-h urine collection revealed borderline low urine volume (1.89 L), normocalciuria (154 mg/day), hypocitraturia (103 mg/day), hyperoxaluria (48 mg/day), hypernatriuria (253 mmol/day), and elevated urine pH (6.9). Her zonisamide was identified as a potential contributing factor to her nephrocalcinosis, as it has been known to be associated with pharmacologically induced renal tubular acidosis, a pathophysiology capable of causing nephrocalcinosis and stone formation. The patient's Neurologist therefore transitioned her to lamotrigine for her history of epilepsy.

After discussion of further diagnostic and management options, the patient elected for diagnostic right ureteroscopy. Her cystoscopy was unremarkable. Right retrograde pyelogram confirmed mild right hydronephrosis but showed no filling defects. Right ureteroscopy identified no ureteral lesions but did reveal numerous intrapapillary renal stones in the upper and mid poles of the right kidney with associated varicose veins of the renal papillae (Fig. 2). A 11/13 Fr 36 cm ureteral access sheath was placed under fluoroscopic guidance. A 200 μm holmium laser fiber was introduced and on the settings of 0.8 J and 8 Hz several embedded stones estimated to be < 2 mm in size were unroofed from the papillae. Next, using the laser settings of 0.4 J and 40 Hz on a long pulse mode the varicose veins were laser fulgurated (Fig. 2). Finally, a 6 Fr × 26 cm double J ureteral stent was placed on the right. She was observed overnight to monitor for hematuria. Her ureteral stent was dislodged overnight. She experienced no clinically significant bleeding. Her preoperative and post-operative hemoglobin values were 12.7 and 12.2, respectively. She was discharged home the day after her surgery.

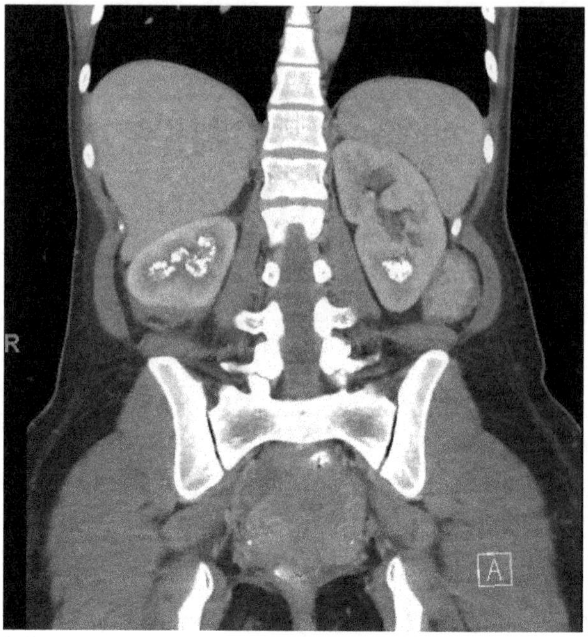

Fig. 1 Coronal CT image demonstrating patient's focal nephrocalcinosis prior to treatment

The patient was seen virtually for follow up 6 weeks later at which point she reported intermittent passage of tiny stones and complete resolution of her hematuria. A repeat renal ultrasound 9 weeks post-operatively demonstrated no hydronephrosis. A stone composition analysis revealed her renal stones were 10% calcium oxalate and 90% calcium phosphate.

She returned with left flank pain and gross hematuria about 10 weeks after her right sided treatment. CT imaging revealed a left ureteral stone and nonobstructing left

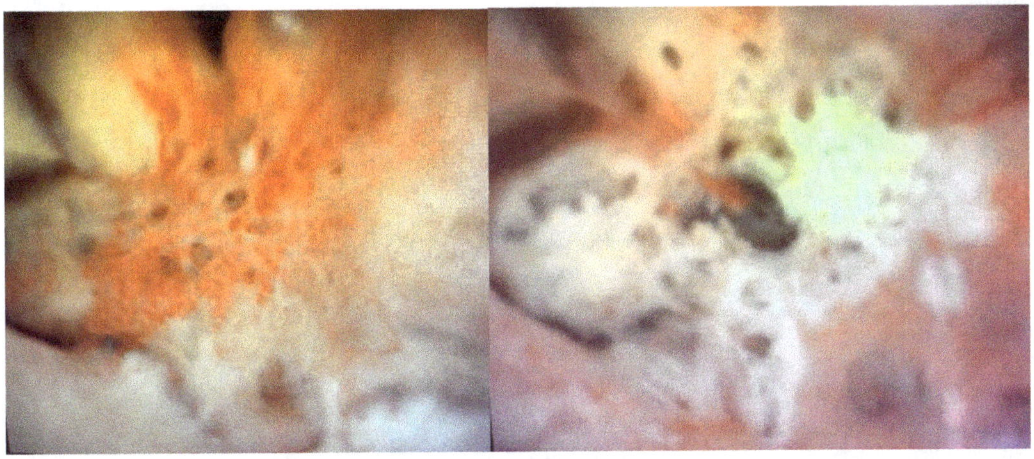

Fig. 2 Intra-operative photo renal papillary varices before (left) and after (right) laser fulguration

renal calculi. Cystoscopy revealed isolated hematuria from the left ureteral orifice and a left sided ureteral stent was placed. She was transferred to a tertiary center where she underwent left diagnostic ureteroscopy. Nearly identical findings of embedded stones and papillary varices were discovered on the left. These were treated with laser unroofing and fulguration, respectively, with resolution of her symptoms once again.

Discussion and conclusion

Varicose veins of the renal papillae have previously been described as the underlying etiology of chronic unilateral hematuria. Historically, diagnosis of such entities required radical or partial nephrectomy with subsequent pathologic examination. With the advent of endoscopic urology techniques, namely ureteroscopy, both the diagnosis and treatment of chronic unilateral hematuria was advanced such that the urologist might identify the source of bleeding in vivo. Thus, the categorization of diffuse and discrete lesions could be made more easily. Amongst the discrete lesions are MVR, which has been used as a catch-all term encompassing renal papillary varicosities. Not only was diagnosis advanced with modern endourologic techniques, but treatment was also revolutionized as surgical resection gave way to electrode fulguration and most recently laser ablation. Endoscopic techniques, predominantly flexible ureteroscopy with fulguration or laser ablation, have been shown to resolve 93% of cases of chronic unilateral hematuria with only a 10% rate of recurrence [2].

No prior case reports have demonstrated an association between nephrocalcinosis and renal papillary varicosities. Unique to this patient are the use of zonisamide and recent pregnancy prior to symptom onset. The underlying cause of renal stone formation related to zonisamide use is the inhibition of carbonic anhydrase, which leads to a renal tubular acidosis; however, rates of renal calculi formation with zonisamide are lower compared to those of other anti-epileptics, like topiramate and acetazolamide [3]. Pregnancy is known to cause renal physiologic changes that both promote renal calculi formation, such as hypercalciuria, but also counter-act it, like an increase in total urinary volume. But pregnancy also leads to systemic and renal vasodilatory changes. During pregnancy hormones such as RAAS, relaxin, and progesterone are all upregulated leading to vasodilatory effects and increased circulating blood volume [4]. This vasodilation could conceivably promote the development of renal papillary varices. The combination of these dilated blood vessels and inflammation from eroding renal calculi may explain the new onset and continuation of gross hematuria following her pregnancy.

Renal papillary varicose veins are an underlying cause of chronic unilateral hematuria. On one hand, work-up for discrete vascular lesions of the renal collecting system such as varices may be obscured by other benign co-existing conditions, such as nephrocalcinosis and nephrolithiasis in this case. On the other hand, a confluence of these conditions may in fact be the source of the patient's symptoms. Regardless, flexible ureteroscopy with laser fulguration offers an ideal diagnostic and therapeutic modality for symptomatic renal papillary varicosities.

Abbreviations

CVA: Costovertebral angle; CT: Computed tomography; Fr: French; MVR: Minute venous rupture; RAAS: Renin-angiotensin-aldosterone system; RBC: Red blood cells.

Acknowledgements

Not applicable.

Authors' contributions

BC and MB conceived of the case report, performed the operation, and drafted the manuscript. MB was involved in postoperative follow-up. Both authors read and approved the final manuscript.

References

1. Oliveira B, Kleta R, Bockenhauer D, et al. Genetic, pathophysiological, and clinical aspects of nephrocalcinosis. Am J Physiol Renal Physiol. 2016;311:1243–52.
2. Tanimoto R, Kumon H, Bagley DH. Development of endoscopic diagnosis and treatment for chronic unilateral hematuria: 35 years experience. J Endourol. 2017;31(1):76–80.
3. Jion YI, Raff A, Grosberg BM, et al. The risk and management of kidney stones from the use of topiramate and zonisamide in migraine and idiopathic intracranial hypertension. Headache. 2015;55:161–6.
4. Cheung KL, Lafayette RA. Renal physiology of pregnancy. Adv Chronic Kidney Dis. 2013;20(3):209–14.

23

Multiple drug resistance bacterial isolates and associated factors among urinary stone patients at the University of Gondar Comprehensive Specialized Hospital, Northwest Ethiopia

Desie Kasew[1*], Setegn Eshetie[1], Abeje Diress[2], Zerubabiel Tegegne[2] and Feleke Moges[1]

Abstract

Background: The urinary stone and urinary tract infection (UTI) are invariably associated and are frequent causes of morbidity. Date on burden of UTI among urinary stone patients is lacking in Ethiopia. This study was aimed to assess bacterial profile, antimicrobial susceptibility and associated factors among urinary stone patients at the University of Gondar Comprehensive Specialized Hospital.

Methods: An institution based cross sectional study was conducted. Basic sociodemographic data were collected using a structured questionnaire. Bacterial identification of uropathogens and drug susceptibility testing were done following standard microbiological techniques. The data were entered and analyzed using SPSS version-23. Bivariate and multivariate logistic regressions were used to identify possible associated risk factors. Results with P value <0.05 was considered statistically significant.

Result: A total of 300 urinary stone patients were enrolled. Of these, 153 (51%) were male and 261(87%) were urban residents. The overall prevalence of urinary tract infection was 49 (16.3%) (95% CI 12–21%). A high level of resistance was observed to ampicillin, penicillin and trimethoprim-sulfamethoxazole while majority of isolates were most sensitive to nitrofurantoin and ciprofloxacin. Multi-drug resistant isolates were 16/49 (32.7%), 75% of them being Enterobacteriaceae isolates. More than one-third 9/26 (34.6%) of Gram-negative isolates were Extended Spectrum Beta-Lactamase (ESBL) producing *E. coli* and *K. pneumoniae*. Being female, history of urinary tract infection and history of drug use were the independent risk factors.

Conclusion: Most of the bacterial isolates from urinary stone patients were resistant to ampicillin, penicillin and trimethoprim-sulfamethoxazole. *E. coli* and *K. pneumoniae* were the most common extended spectrum beta-lactamase producing isolates. Sex, history of urinary tract infection and previous drug use were found to be risk factors. Routine diagnosis of urinary stone patients for urinary tract infection should be promoted and further researches are encouraged.

*Correspondence: dessalegnkassaw83@gmail.com; Desie.Kasaw@uog.edu.et
[1] Department of Medical Microbiology, School of Biomedical and Laboratory Sciences, College of Medicine and Health Sciences, University of Gondar, P.O. Box 196, Gondar, Ethiopia
Full list of author information is available at the end of the article

Keywords: Urinary stone, Multiple drug resistance, Urinary tract infection

Background

Urinary stone and urinary tract infections (UTI) are constantly associated complaints of the urinary system [1]. Urinary stones also known as urolithiasis [2] are hard masses produced in the urinary tract and cause infection, pain, bleeding or obstruction. Multiple types of stones such as oxalate, uric acid, cysteine, or struvite stone can be produced in the urinary tract [3]. Infection stones include magnesium ammonium phosphate or struvite (which accounts to 10–15% of urinary stone), carbonate apatite and ammonium urate. Urease producing bacteria such as *Proteus* are responsible for production of urease enzyme which alkalinizes urine and produce these stones [4, 5]. Moreover, ammonia and oxalate stones damage the urothelial layer facilitating microbial invasion [6].

E. coli, a urease negative bacterium is the most common cause of UTI and dominant isolate in urinary stones and urine cultures. Its existence in stone indicates either urease negative bacteria have a role in stone formation or urease producing bacteria transiently infect and lost after stone formation [7]. Urease producing bacteria include *Proteus, Morganella, Pseudomonas, Providencia, Klebsiella* and *S. aureus* and are common causes of UTI [8]. *P. mirabilis* is the prominent urease producing species and cause of struvite calculi [9]. Bacteria incrusted in or attached on the surface of stone forming biofilm and cause recurrent and multidrug resistant (MDR) UTI [10]. The rate of UTI among urolithiasis patients ranges from 7 to 60% [11] with the coincidence of these comorbidities results in complications such as renal failure and death [12].

Urinary stone disease is one of the worldwide threats which has been increasing particularly in the last 15 years [13, 14]. Factors such as sex, previous history of UTI, condom use, vaginal infection, extremes of age, anatomical abnormalities like congenital urinary tract malformations, urinary obstruction, catheterization, resent sexual activity, comorbidities like urinary stone, diabetes and obesity [8, 15, 16], hospitalization, antibiotic use are risks factors to UTI [17]. Information about the burden of UTI among patients with urinary calculi is lacking in Ethiopia. This study is aimed to investigate bacterial uropathogens, antimicrobial resistance and associated factors among Urinary stone patients at the University of Gondar Comprehensive Specialized Hospital, Gondar Ethiopia.

Materials and methods

Study area, design, and period

A prospective cross-sectional study was conducted from January to April, 2019, at the University of Gondar Comprehensive Specialized Hospital. The hospital is located in Gondar town, Amhara regional state, Northwest Ethiopia, situated at 742 km from the capital city of Ethiopia, Addis Ababa. The hospital is a tertiary level teaching and referral hospital catering more than 500 beds for inpatients and rendering referral health services for over 5 million inhabitants in Northwest Ethiopia.

Population All patients who have visited the hospital during the study period and clinically suspected of urinary stone disease were the source population while patients with ultrasound confirmed urinary stone were study population. All the study participants were enrolled from the outpatient department.

Exclusion criteria Patients with history of antibiotic use in the last 2 weeks prior to diagnosis and during the data collection period were excluded or denied from the study because those who have been taking antibiotics may have culture negative due to their resent drug use. All patients who had urinary system complains, were confirmed to have urinary stone with ultrasound and not on antibiotics treatment in the last 2 weeks as well as during the study period and willing to be included were eligible to this study.

Sample size and sampling methods

The sample size was calculated by a single population proportion formula taking 50% prevalence since previous study involving urinary stone patients was not available.

$$n = \frac{z^2_{\alpha/2}p(1-p)}{d^2}$$

$$= \frac{1.96^2 * 0.5(1-0.5)}{(0.05)^2} = 384$$

Using reduction formula as the total population based on the same period of the last year's record, estimated population was 1350, the final sample size was

$$n_f = \frac{n * N}{n + N}$$

$$n_f = \frac{384 * 1350}{384 + 1350} = 299$$

where N is the total population, n_f—the final sample size, $Z_{\alpha/2}$—the standard normal deviation, at 95% confidence level = 1.96, p—The prevalence = 0.5; 1 − p = 0.5 and d—The desired degree of accuracy = 0.05.

Data collection and laboratory methods

A total of 300 study participants with urinary stone were enrolled in the study using convenient sampling technique. Sociodemographic and clinical features of study participants such as age, gender, residence, history of UTI and drug use, stone size and its position, presence of stone at multiple sites, condom use, catheterization and presence of comorbidites like history of diabetes, HIV were colleceted using structured questionaire. Clean catch mid-stream urine was collected in a sterile wide mouthed urine cup with prior adiquate instruction of the participant (Additional file 1).

Culture and microbiological identification

Early morning mid-stream urine sample was collected and transported to medical bacteriology laboratory; inoculated in Cysteine lactose electrolyte deficient (CLED) agar (BIOMARK^R Laboratories, India) within two hours and incubated for 18–24 h at 35–37 °C. A 0.001 mL inoculating loop was used to inoculate the urine specimen. Colonies with significant bacteriuria ($\geq 10^5$ CFU/mL) were subcultured on blood agar plate (BAP) and MacConkey agar for isolation of a single species and further characterization by hemolysis on BAP, lactose fermentation on MacConkey agar. Gram staining and biochemical tests such TSI, motility test, indole test, citrate test, urease test, Lysine decarboxylase, catalase, coagulase tests, novobiocin sensitivity, and Bile Esculin (BIOMARK^R Laboratories, India) hydrolysis test were used for species identification [18].

Antimicrobial susceptibility testing

Antimicrobial susceptibility testing (AST) was performed using Kirby-Bauer disc diffusion method on Muller-Hinton agar (BIOMARK^R Laboratories, India). Selected antimicrobial agents such as Ampicillin (10 µg), Amoxicillin-clavulanate (20/10 µg), Ciprofloxacin (5 µg), Tobramycin (10 µg), Gentamicin (10 µg), Cefixime (5 µg), Cefoxitin (30 µg), Cefuroxime (30 µg), Nitrofurantoin (300 µg), Rifampin (5 µg), Tetracycline (30 µg), Penicillin 10 units, Norfloxacin (10 µg), Vancomycin (30 µg), Trimethoprim-sulphamethoxzole (1.25/23.75 µg) (Abtek Biologicals Ltd, United Kingdom) and Cefotaxime (30 µg), Ceftazidime (30 µg), Cefotaxime-Clavulanate (30/10 µg), Ceftazidime-Clavulanate (30/10 µg) (HiMedia Laboratories Pvt Ltd India) were used for antimicrobial susceptibility test [19]. Zones of inhibition were measured after 16–18 h of incubation at 37 °C and classified as susceptible or resistant. Isolates intermediate between susceptible and resistant were considered as resistant [20]. Isolates resistant to three or more classes of antibiotics were considered as MDR [21].

Extended spectrum beta lactamase detection

First screening for ESBL production was done for Cefotaxime and Ceftazidime 30 µg each. Isolates with zone of inhibition ≤ 27 mm for cefotaxime and ≤ 22 mm for ceftazidime were phenotypically confirmed for ESBL production by using Ceftazidime-clavulanic acid (30 µg/10 µg), Cefotaxime-clavulanic acid (30 µg/10 µg) with their respective single disks using combined disk test. The suspension of screened isolates was prepared and inoculated on MHA. The target antibiotics were then placed at least 25 mm apart from each other followed by 16–18 h of incubation at 35 °C ± 2 °C and zone of inhibition was measured. At least 5 mm difference to either of the combined drugs and their respective single disks was considered as ESBL producing species [19].

Quality control The questionnaire was pretested for standardization and clearity. The culture media were checked for sterility and performance prior to inoculation by incubating 5% of the newly prepared media overnight. The reagents for Gram's stain were also assured for their expiry date and staining. The control strains *E. coli* ATCC25922 and *S. aureus* ATCC25923 were used to control performance of media and antibiotic disks. Furthermore, *K. pneumoniae* ATCC 700603 and *E. coli* ATCC25922 were used as a positive and negative control for ESBL production respectively. The suspension was standardized against 0.5 McFarland standards [19].

Data processing and analysis Data were entered and analyzed using SPSS version 23 software. Discriptive statistics such as frequency and percentage were determined. The binary mogistic regression model was used. The assumption Hosmer–Lemeshow goodness of fit as well as cox and snell and Nagelkerke R squire valus were checked and the model was fit. Bivariate and multivariate logistic regression analysis were carried out with enter method to determine statistically significant association and odds ratio at 95% confidence interval was computed. Variables with a *P* value < 0.2 in bivariate logistic regression analysis were entered to multivariate logestic regression analysis [22, 23]. Variables with *P* value < 0.05 in multivariate logistic regression analysis were considered as statistically significant.

Table 1 Sociodemographic characteristics of urinary stone patients at the University of Gondar Comprehensive Specialized Hospital, January to April 2019

Variables	Frequency (%)
Sex	
Male	153(51)
Female	147(49)
Age	
< 20 years	23(7.7)
20–29	123(41)
30–39	97(32.3)
40–49	32(10.7)
≥ 50	25(8.3)
Residence	
Urban	261(87)
Rural	39(13)
Educational level	
Cannot read and write	35(11.7)
Elementary	71(23.7)
High school and preparatory	60(20)
College and above	134(44.7)
Family monthly income (ETB)	
< 1000	54(18)
1001–2000	70(23.3)
> 2000	176(58.7)
Sexual activity	
Within 2 days	43(14.3)
Within 7 days	84(28)
Pregnancy (for females)	
Yes	6(2)
No	141(47)
Use of birth control mechanisms	
Condom	6(2)
No	141(46.3)
Body mass index	
< 18.5	40(13.3)
18.5–24.5	211(70.3)
> 24.5	49(16.3)

Table 2 Clinical characteristics of urinary stone patients at the University of Gondar Comprehensive Specialized Hospital, January to April 2019

Variable	Frequency (%)
History of UTI	
Yes	33(11)
No	267(89)
Urinary blockage	
Yes	9(3)
No	291(97)
History of catheterization	
Yes	4(1.3)
No	296(98.7)
Stone size	
< 5 mm	275(91.7)
≥ 5 mm	25(8.3)
Stones at multiple locations	
Yes	75(25)
No	225(75)
Location of stone	
Renal	282(94)
Renal and/or extra renal	18(6)
History of chronic disease	
Yes	21(7)
No	279(93)
History of drug use	
Yes	172(57.3)
No	128(42.7)
Drug type used	
Antibiotics	166(55.3)
Antibiotics, steroids and HAART	7(2.3)
Antibiotic use	
Within the past one month	70(23.3)
Within the past 3 months	41(13.7)
History of hospitalization	
Yes	17(5.7)
No	283(94.3)

Extra renal-(Kidney and ureter, Kidney and bladder, or Kidney and urethra)

Result

Sociodemographic and clinical characteristics of patients with urinary stone

Of the 300 urinary stone patients enrolled in the present study, 153(51%) were male, 123(41%) were in age group 20–29 years, 261(87%) were urban dwellers and 134(44.7%) were patients with educational level of college and above. More than half, 176(58.7%) of participants had family monthly income 2000 Ethiopian birr and above (Table 1). Thirty-three (11%) of study participants had history of UTI, 25(8.3%) of them had stone size of 5 mm and above. Nine (3%) of the participants had history of urinary blockage and 166(55.3%) of them had history of antibiotic use while 17(5.7%) were hospitalized previously (Table 2).

The prevalence of bacterial uropathogens among patients with urinary stone

Forty-nine 49/300(16.3%) (95% CI 12–21%) of the urinary stone patients had UTI. The most common cause of UTI was *E. coli* 14/49(28.6%) followed by *S. saprophyticus* and *Enterococcus* species 8/49(16.3%) each, *K. pneumoniae* and *S. aureus* 7/49(14.3%) each (Fig. 1).

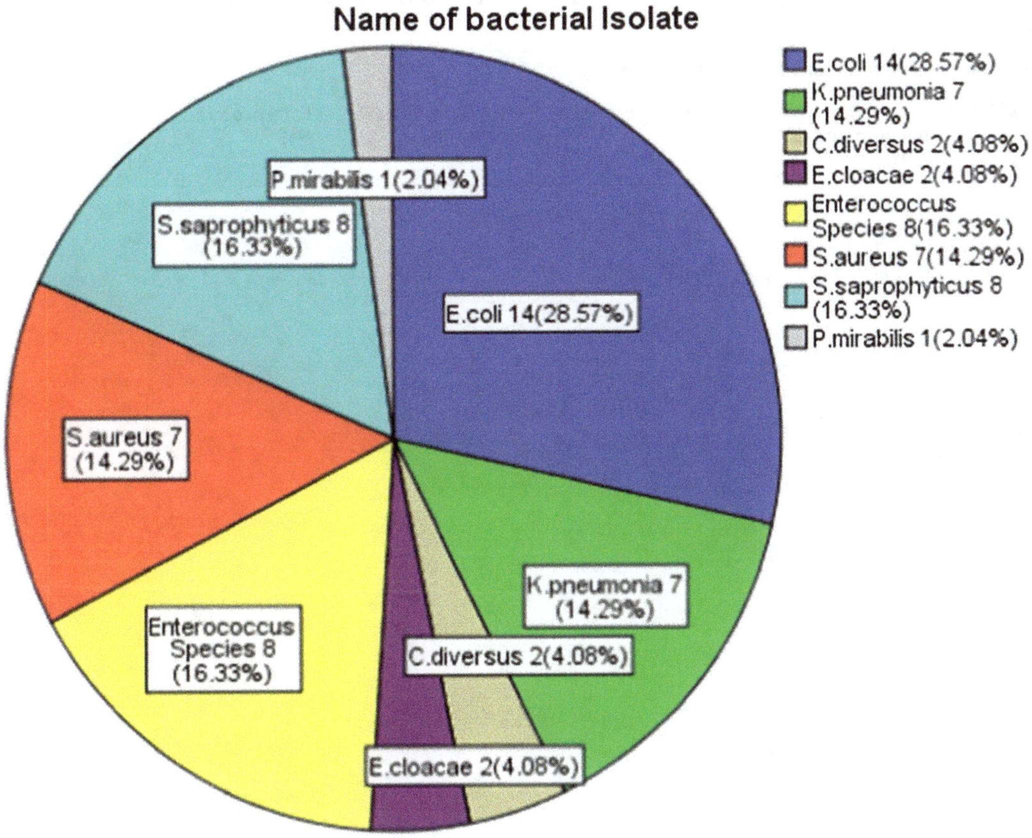

Fig. 1 The proportion of bacterial uropathogens isolated from Urinary stone patients at the University of Gondar Comprehensive Specialized Hospital, January to April 2019

Antimicrobial susceptibility of bacterial uropathogens among patients with urinary stone

Majority of Gram-negative isolates were resistant to ampicillin 25/26 (96.2%), amoxicillin-clavulanate 18/26 (69.2%) while 46/49 (94%) and 44/49(90%) of the Gram-negative isolates were susceptible to nitrofurantoin and ciprofloxacin respectively. All *S. saprophyticus* 8(100%) and 6/7 (85.7%) of *S. aureus* were susceptible to gentamycin. Two 2/8(25%) *S. saprophyticus* and 1/7 (14.3%) of *S. aureus* isolates were resistant to cefoxitin (surrogate marker for methicillin resistance), and one vancomycin resistant *Enterococcus* was isolated (Table 3).

MDR and ESBL producing uropathogenic isolates among patients with urinary stone

Of the total uropathogens, 16/49(32.7%) were MDR and 75% of which were Enterobacteriaceae. The most common MDR species were *E. coli* 7/49(14.3%), followed by *K. pneumoniae* 3/49(6.12%). Furthermore, from a total of 26 Enterobacteriaceae 9/26(34.6%) isolates were confirmed ESBL producing species. These confirmed ESBL producing isolates were *E. coli* 6/26 (23.1%) and *K. pneumoniae* 3/26(11.5%) (Table 4).

Factors associated with urinary tract infection among patients with urinary stone

Among the variables, sex, age, education, monthly income, history of UTI, blockage of urinary system, stone size, stone location in the urinary system, history of chronic disease and drug use, sexual activity, history of hospitalization, and body mass index had P value < 0.2 in bivariate analysis and were computed by multivariate logistic regression analysis to check statistically significant association by controlling possible confounders. The result of multivariate logistic regression showed that being female, history of UTI, drug use had a P value of < 0.05; which indicates statistically significant association with patients having urinary stone diseases (Table 5).

Discussion

The overall prevalence of UTI among patients with urinary stone was 49/300 (16.3%) (95% CI 12–21%). This result is similar to reports by Gutierrez et al. 16.2%

Table 3 Antimicrobial Susceptibility Pattern of Bacterial Isolates from Urinary stone Patients at the UOGCSH, January to April 2019

Antibiotic used	Species of isolate with their antibiotic susceptibility							
	E. coli N (%)	*K. pneumoniae* N(%)	*C. diversus* N (%)	*E. cloacae* N (%)	*P. mirabilis* N (%)	*Enterococci* N (%)	*S. saprophyticus* N (%)	*S. aureus* N (%)
AMP								
S		1(14.3)				2(25)		
R	14(100)	6(85.7)	2(100)	2(100%)	1(100)	6(75)		
AMC								
S	2(14.3)	4(57.1)		1(50)	1(100)			
R	12(85.7)	3(42.9)	2(100)	1(50)				
CTX								
S	7(50)	6(85.7)	1(50)	2(100)	1(100)			
R	7(50)	1(14.3)	1(50)					
CAZ								
S	14(100)	6(85.7)	1(50)	2(100%)	1(100)			
R		1(14.3)	1(50)					
FOX								
S	13(92.9)	6(85.7)	2(100)	2(100%)	1(100)		5(62.5)	6(85.7)
R	1(7.1)	1(14.3)					3(37.3)	1(14.3)
CFM								
S	12(85.7)	4(57.1)	1(50)	2(100)	1(100)			
R	2(14.3)	3(42.9)	1(50)					
CRX								
S	13(92.9)	6(85.7)	1(50)	2(100)	1(100)			
R	1(7.1)	1(14.3)	1(50)					
CPR								
S	12(85.7)	6(85.7)	1(50)	2(100)	1(100)	8(100)	7(87.5)	7(100)
R	2(14.3)	1(14.3)	1(50)				1(12.5)	
GEN								
S	13(92.9)	7(100)	1(50)	2(100)	1(100)		8(100)	6(85.7)
R	1(7.1)		1(50)					1(14.3)
TOB								
S	10(71.4)	7(100)	1(50)	2(100)	1(100)			
R	4(28.6)		1(50)					
TET								
S	7(50)	4(57.1)		2(100)		3(37.5)	3(37.5)	5(71.4)
R	7(50)	3(42.9)	2(100)		1(100)	5(62.5)	5(62.5)	2(28.3)
SXT								
S	6(42.9)	4(57.1)		2(100%)	1(100)		6(75)	5(71.4)
R	8(57.1)	3(42.9)	2(100)				2(25)	2(28.6)
NIT								
S	14(100)	6(85.7)	2(100)	2(100%)	1(100)	8(100)	6(75)	7(100)
R		1(14.3)					2(25)	
NOR								
S	11(78.6)	6(85.7)	1(50)	2(100%)	1(100)	5(62.5)	7(87.5)	6(85.7)
R	3(21.4)	1(14.3)	1(50)			3(37.5)	1(12.5)	1(14.3)
PEN								
S						3(37.5)	2(25)	4(57.1)
R						5(62.5)	6(75)	3(42.9)

Table 3 (continued)

Antibiotic used	Species of isolate with their antibiotic susceptibility							
	E. coli N (%)	*K. pneumoniae* N(%)	*C. diversus* N (%)	*E. cloacae* N (%)	*P. mirabilis* N (%)	*Enterococci* N (%)	*S. saprophyticus* N (%)	*S. aureus* N (%)
RIF								
S						6(75)		
R						2(25)		
VAN								
S						7(87.5)		
R						1(12.5)		

AMP Ampicillin, *AMC* Amoxicillin-clavulanate, *FOX* Cefoxitin, *CFM* Cefixime, *CRX* Cefuroxime, *CPR* Ciprofloxacin, *GEN* Gentamycin, *CAZ* Ceftazidime, *CTX* Cefotaxime, *RIF* Rifampin, *NOR* Norfloxacin, *NIT* Nitrofurantoin, *PEN* Penicillin, *RIF* Rifampin, *SXT* Trimethoprim-Sulfamethoxazole, *TET* Tetracycline, *TOB* Tobramycin, *VAN* Vancomycin

Table 4 The prevalence of MDR isolates from urinary stone patients at the University of Gondar Comprehensive Specialized Hospital, January to April 2019

Antibiotics	Species of bacteria					Total
	E. coli	*K. pneumoniae*	*C. diversus*	*Enterococci*	*S. saprophyticus*	
AMP, TET, NOR				2		2
AMP, TET, SXT		1				1
AMP, AMC, TOB, SXT	1					1
AMP, TET, TOB, SXT	1					1
AMP, AMC, TET, SXT			1			1
AMP, AMC, CTX, SXT	1					1
CXT, TET, SXT, PEN					1	1
CXT, TET, NOR, PEN					1	1
AMP, AMC, CTX, SXT, TET	1					1
AMP, AMC, CTX, CFM, SXT	1					1
AMP, FOX, CFM, CPR, NIT		1				1
AMP, AMC, CRX, TET, SXT		1				1
AMP, AMC, SXT, GEN, NOR, TET, TOB	1					1
AMP, AMC, CTX, CFM, GEN, TOB, TET, CPR, SXT, NOR			1			1
AMP, AMC, CTX, FOX, CFM, CRX, CPR, TOB, TET, NOR	1					1
Total	7	3	2	2	2	16
ESBL positive	6	3				9

AMP Ampicillin, *AMC* Amoxicillin-clavulanate, *CTX* cefotaxime, *FOX* Cefoxitin, *TET* Tetracycline, *CPR* Ciprofloxacin, *CTX* Cefotaxime, *PEN* Penicillin, *TOB* Tobramycin, *SXT* Trimethoprim-Sulfamethoxazole, *CRX* Cefuroxime, *GEN* Gentamycin, *NOR* Norfloxacin

[24] and lower than a study done in china 22.0% [25], Iran 35.5% [26], Romania 25.8% [27] and India 45% [11] among urinary stone patients. However, this result was higher than 7.8% prevalence of UTI reported from Los Angeles, United States [28]. The variation might be because of the socioeconomic, geographical and population difference. The predominant species isolated in this study were *E. coli*, 14/49(28.6%) followed by *S. saprophyticus* and *Enterococcus* species 8/49 (16.3%) each. The result was comparable to other reports 33% *E.coli* and 18.5% *Enterococci* isolated from patients with urinary stone [29]. On the other hand the result was higher than 6.5% prevalence of *E.coli* reported by Gutierrez et al. [24].

The resistance to antibiotics such as ampicillin, amoxicillin-clavulanate and Trimethoprim-sulphamethoxzole in this study was 31/33(94%), 18/26(69.23%) and 17(41.5%) respectively which was slightly lower than a report in India ampicillin 96% and amoxicillin-clavulanate 87% [30]. The result of this study was higher than resistance to Ampicillin 70%, and Amoxicillin-clavulanic acid 30% reported in Romania [27]. The high rate of resistance might be due to easy access and

Table 5 Factors associated with UTI among urinary stone patients at the UOGCSH, January to April 2019

Variable	Significant bacteriuria		COR 95% CI	*P* value	AOR 95% CI	*P* value
	Yes (%)	No (%)				
Sex						
Male	13(26.5)	140(55.8)	1			
Female	36(73.5)	111(44.2)	3.5(1.77–6.90)	0.00	5.76(2.23–13.32)	0.00
Age						
< 20 years	3(6)	20(8)	1		1	
20–29	21(42.9)	102(40.6)	1.37(0.37–5.04)	0.63	2.00(0.43–9.26)	0.38
30–39	12(24.5)	85(33.9)	0.94(0.24–3.65)	0.93	1.05(0.25–6.57)	0.77
40–49	9(18.4)	23(9.16)	2.6(0.62–10.98)	0.19	2.04(0.38–14.92)	0.36
≥ 50 years	4(8.2)	21(8.4)	1.27(0.25–6.40)	0.77	1.25(0.16–12.16)	0.77
Residence						
Urban	42(85.7)	219(87.3)	1		1	
Rural	7(14.3)	32(12.7)	1.14(0.47–2.76)	0.77	1	
Education						
Cannot read and write	10(20.4)	25(10)	2.15(0.90–5.13)	0.08	1.80(0.54–4.5.95)	0.34
Elementary	13(28.3)	58(23.1)	1.21(0.56–2.58)	0.63	1.42(0.50–4.07)	0.51
High school	5(10.2)	55(21.9)	0.49(0.18–1.37)	0.17	0.31(0.09–1.02)	0.05
College and above	21(42.9)	113(45)	1		1	
Family monthly income (ETB)						
≤ 1000	16(32.7)	38(15.1)	2.95(1.413–6.15)	0.004	2.40(0.84–6.88)	0.104
1001–2000	11(22.4)	59(23.5)	1.31(.596–2.857)	0.50	1.60(0.61–4.20)	0.34
> 2000	22(44.9)	154(61.4)	1		1	
History of UTI						
Yes	15(30.6)	18(7.2)	5.71(2.63–12.38)	0.00	4.66(1.76–12.30)	0.002
No	34(69.4)	233(92.8)	1		1	
Urinary blockage						
Yes	3(6.1)	6(2.4)	2.66(0.64–11.03)	0.18	0.26(0.03–2.20)	0.22
No	46(93.9)	245(97.6)	1		1	
Stone size						
< 5 mm	43(87.8)	232(92.4)	1			
≥ 5	6(12.2)	19(7.6)	1.7(0.64–4.5)	0.28		
Stone location						
Renal	46(93.9)	236(94)	1			
Renal and/or extra renal	3(6)	15(6)	1.03(0.29–3.7)	0.97		
Chronic disease						
Yes	6(12.2)	15(6)	2.2(0.81–1.5.97)	0.12	1.17(0.24–5.65)	0.85
No	43(87.8)	236(94)	1		1	
Drug use						
Yes	36(73.5)	136(54.2)	1		1	
No	13(26.5)	115(45.8)	0.43(0.22–0.84)	0.014	0.33(0.14–0.77)	0.01
Hospitalization						
Yes	7(14.3)	10(4)	4.02(1.45–11.14)	0.008	3.85(0.92–16.07)	0.065
No	42(85.7)	241(96)	1		1	
Sexual activity						
Within 2 days	6(12.2)	37(14.7)	0.55(0.21–1.45)	0.23	0.61(0.20–1.92)	0.40
Within 7 days	11(22.4)	73(29.1)	0.51(0.24–1.10)	0.09	0.48(0.19–1.21)	0.12
Within a month	5(10.2)	49(19.5)	0.35(0.13–0.96)	0.041	0.30(0.086–1.02)	0.054
Never	27(55.1)	92(36.7)	1		1	
BMI						
18.5–24.5	32(65.3)	179(71.3)	1		1	
> 24.5	7(14.3)	42(16.7)	0.536(0.24–1.20)	0.13	1.24(0.41–3.79)	0.71
< 18.5	10(20.4)	30(12)	0.5(0.17–1.46)	0.21	2.89(0.98–8.50)	0.053

Table 5 (continued)

AOR adjusted odds ratio, *COR* crude odds ratio, *CI* confidence interval, *ETB* Ethiopian Birr

self-medication, weak adherence of patients to prescribed antimicrobial agents, wider availability of empirical treatment in health care settings [12, 31, 32]. Most of the isolates identified were susceptible to nitrofurantoin 46/49(94%) and ciprofloxacin 44/49(90%). There were two methicillin resistant *S. saprophyticus* and one methicillin resistant *S. aureus* (MRSA) which was nearly similar to a case of methicillin resistant coagulase negative staphylococcus report in Romania [27].

From a total of 16 MDR isolates, *E. coli* 7/16(43.75%) and *K. pneumoniae* 3/16(18.75%) were the most common MDR species. The MDR isolates in this study were higher than 29.3% MDR *E. coli*, 6.8% *K. pneumoniae* but lower compared to 12.0% MDR *E. faecalis*. The difference could be due to sample size variation [33]. Furthermore, 9/26(34.6%) of the total 26 Enterobacteriaceae, were ESBL producing species. These ESBL producing species were *E. coli* 6/26(23%) and *K. pneumoniae* 3/26(11.5%) species. This result was lower than 51.8% of the overall prevalence of ESBL producing Enterobacteriaceae [12]. The prevalence of ESBL producing Enterobacteriaceae from the total *E.coli* isolates was higher than 8.7% result by Bianca et al. [31]. This might be due to variation in the management and use of antibiotics.

In the present study the prevalence of UTI was higher among female participants 36/49 (73.5%). This corresponds to a study done by Bianca et al. [31] 74.2% in females and 25.8% in males. The result was slightly higher than a 67% prevalence in females as compared to 33% in males [11]. The likelihood of acquiring UTI in females was 5.76 times higher compared to males (AOR 5.76, 95% CI 2.23–13.32). This could be due to the physio-anatomical variations between males and females including anal and genital proximity, short urethra as well as sexual activity in females which ease the access of intestinal flora to the urinary tract in females. On the other hand antimicrobial activity of the prostate secretions in males could contribute to the reduced infection rate among males than female participants [25, 27].

The finding of this study showed that 15/49(31%) of patients with significant bacteriuria had previous history of UTI. Having history of UTI increases the risk of UTI by 4.7 times (AOR 4.66, 95% CI 1.76–12.30) than those who had not. This might be due to the release of bacteria from the inside of stone or from its matrix protected surface resulting in persistence or recurrence of the UTI. Previous history of UTI is among the factors that predisposes to the occurrence of the infection [15]. The treatment might not have completely removed the etiologic agent of UTI in patients. Because the bacteria can be incrusted in the stone or extracellular matrix and escape from the treatment [34].

In addition, 36/49(73.5%) patients with significant bacteriuria had previous history of drug use and showed a statistically significant association with UTI. The risk of UTI among patients who had not history of drug use reduces by 67% compared to those who had history of drug use (AOR 0.33, 95% CI 0.14–0.77). This could be due to the fact that steroidal drugs are immunosuppressive and patients could be immunocompromised [30]. The increased antimicrobial resistance in drug users and the recurrence or persistence of drug resistant UTI might also contribute.

As a limitation only urine specimen was taken for culture and stone culture was not performed to which could help to know the agreement of stone and urine culture strain characterization was not performed due to lack of resources.

Conclusion

The commonest bacterial species isolated from patients with urinary stone disease was *E. coli*. The most common MDR and ESBL producing isolates were *E. coli* and *K. pneumoniae*. Being female, previous history of UTI and drug use were the independent risk factors. Isolated uropathogens were most susceptible to nitrofurantoin, ciprofloxacin and gentamycin. However, most of the isolates were resistant to ampicillin, penicillin and trimethoprim-Sulfamethoxazole. Routine diagnosis of urinary stone patients for urinary tract infection should be promoted. Antimicrobial stewardship program should be implemented to reduce drug resistance.

Supplementary Information

Additional file 1. English version of the questionnaire.

Abbreviations

AST: Antimicrobial susceptibility test; ATCC: American Type Culture Collection; BAP: Blood agar plate; CLSI: Clinical Laboratory Standards Institute; CLED: Cysteine lactose electrolyte deficient agar; ESBL: Extended spectrum beta lactamase; HAART: Highly active antiretroviral therapy; MAC: MacConkey agar; MDR: Multidrug resistance; TSI: Triple sugar iron agar; USD: Urinary stone disease; UTI: Urinary tract infection.

Acknowledgements

We would like to acknowledge study participants for their cooperation and the University of Gondar for financial and material support.

Authors' contributions

DK: Conception of the research idea, study design, data collection, data analysis, interpretation, write up of the research. ZT, FM and SE: supervision and review of the manuscript: AD: Data collection and review of the manuscript. All authors read and approved the final manuscript.

Author details

[1] Department of Medical Microbiology, School of Biomedical and Laboratory Sciences, College of Medicine and Health Sciences, University of Gondar, P.O. Box 196, Gondar, Ethiopia. [2] Department of Radiology, School of Medicine, College of Medicine and Health Sciences, University of Gondar, P.O. Box 196, Gondar, Ethiopia.

References

1. Schwaderer AL, Wolfe AJ. The association between bacteria and urinary stones. Ann Transl Med. 2017;5(2):32.
2. Kirkali Z, Rasooly R, Star RA, Rodgers GP. Urinary stone disease: progress, status, and needs. Urology. 2015;86(4):651–3.
3. Sakhaee K, Maalouf NM, Sinnott B. Kidney stones 2012: pathogenesis, diagnosis, and management. J Clin Endocrinol Metab. 2012;97(6):1847–60.
4. Miano R, Germani S, Vespasiani G. Stones and urinary tract infections. Urologia Int. 2007;79(Suppl. 1):32–6.
5. Thomas B, Tolley D. Concurrent urinary tract infection and stone disease: pathogenesis, diagnosis and management. Nat Rev Urol. 2008;5(12):668–75.
6. Hassan JK. Crystalluria types and incidence in Basra City; southern of Iraq. J Basrah Res (Sciences). 2011;37(5A):72–81.
7. Shojaeian A, Rostamian M, Noroozi J, Pakzad P. The identification of chemical and bacterial composition and determination of FimH gene frequency of kidney stones of Iranian patients. J Res Med Sci. 2016;18(6):e7363.
8. Flannigan R, Choy WH, Chew B, Lange D. Renal struvite stones—pathogenesis, microbiology, and management strategies. Nat rev Urol. 2014;11(6):333–41.
9. Norsworthy AN, Pearson MM. From catheter to kidney stone: the uropathogenic lifestyle of *P. mirabilis*. Trends Microbiol. 2017;25(4):304–15.
10. Romanova YM, Mulabaev N, Tolordava E, Seregin A, Seregin I, Alexeeva N, et al. Microbial communities on kidney stones. Mol Gen Microbiol Virol. 2015;30(2):78–84.
11. Songra M, Damor M, Namdev RK, Patbamniya NK, Nawalakhe P, Jain R. A study on positive stone culture and its association with rate of sepsis after urological procedures. Int Surg J. 2016;2(2):239–46.
12. Chen D, Zhang Y, Huang J, Liang X, Zeng T, Lan C, et al. The analysis of microbial spectrum and antibiotic resistance of uropathogens isolated from patients with urinary stones. Int J Clin Pract. 2018;72(6):e13205.
13. Raheem OA, Khandwala YS, Sur RL, Ghani KR, Denstedt JD. Burden of urolithiasis: trends in prevalence, treatments, and costs. Eur Urol Focus. 2017;3(1):18–26.
14. Scales CD Jr, Smith AC, Hanley JM, Saigal CS. Prevalence of kidney stones in the United States. Eur Urol. 2012;62(1):160–5.
15. Foxman B. Urinary tract infection syndromes: occurrence, recurrence, bacteriology, risk factors, and disease burden. Infect Dis Clin North Am. 2014;28(1):1–13.
16. Tandogdu Z, Wagenlehner FM. Global epidemiology of urinary tract infections. Curr Opin Infect Dis. 2016;29(1):73–9.
17. Eshetie S, Unakal C, Gelaw A, Ayelign B, Endris M, Moges F. Multidrug resistant and carbapenemase producing Enterobacteriaceae among patients with urinary tract infection at referral Hospital, Northwest Ethiopia. Antimicrob Resist Infect Control. 2015;4(1):12.
18. Cheesbrough M. District laboratory practice in tropical countries. Cambridge: Cambridge University Press; 2006.
19. CLSI. Performance Standards for Antimicrobial Susceptibility Testing. 28th ed. CLSI supplement M100. 2018.
20. Tellevik MG, Blomberg B, Kommedal Ø, Maselle SY, Langeland N, Moyo SJ. High prevalence of faecal carriage of ESBL-producing Enterobacteriaceae among children in Dar es Salaam, Tanzania. PLoS ONE. 2016;11(12):e0168024.
21. Goyal D, Dean N, Neill S, Jones P, Dascomb K, editors. Risk Factors for Community-Acquired Extended-Spectrum Beta-Lactamase–Producing Enterobacteriaceae Infections—A Retrospective Study of Symptomatic Urinary Tract Infections. In: Open forum Infect Dis; 2019; 6(12):ofz517. Oxford University Press.
22. Pasricha J, Koessler T, Harbarth S, Schrenzel J, Camus V, Cohen G, et al. Carriage of extended-spectrum beta-lactamase-producing enterobacteriacae among internal medicine patients in Switzerland. Antimicrob Resist Infect Control. 2013;2(1):20.
23. Kin-On K, Emily C, Chung P-H, Arthur T, Wan-In W, Chendi Z, et al. Prevalence and associated factors for carriage of Enterobacteriaceae producing ESBLs or carbapenemase and Methicillin-resistant Staphylococcus aureus in Hong Kong Community. J Infect. 2020;81(2):242–7.
24. Gutierrez J, Smith A, Geavlete P, Shah H, Kural AR, de Sio M, et al. Urinary tract infections and post-operative fever in percutaneous nephrolithotomy. World J Urol. 2013;31(5):1135–40.
25. Yongzhi L, Shi Y, Jia L, Yili L, Xingwang Z, Xue GJ. Risk factors for urinary tract infection in patients with urolithiasis primary report of a single center cohort. BMC Urol. 2018;18(1):45.
26. Shafi H, Shahandeh Z, Heidari B, Sedigiani F, Ramaji AA, Pasha YRY, et al. Bacteriological study and structural composition of staghorn stones removed by the anatrophic nephrolithotomic procedure. Saudi J Kidney Dis Transpl. 2013;24(2):418–23.
27. Maier A, Man A, Chibelean C, Cighir T, Nemes-Nagy E, Maier I, et al. Bacteriological evaluation of the non-struvite nephrolithiasis and its association with urinary tract infections. Rev Rom Med Lab. 2015;23(4):457–68.
28. Abrahamian FM, Krishnadasan A, Mower WR, Moran GJ, Talan DA. Association of pyuria and clinical characteristics with the presence of urinary tract infection among patients with acute nephrolithiasis. Ann Emerg Med. 2013;62(5):526–33.
29. Tavichakorntrakool R, Prasongwattana V, Sungkeeree S, Saisud P, Sribenjalux P, Pimratana C, et al. Extensive characterizations of bacteria isolated from catheterized urine and stone matrices in patients with nephrolithiasis. Nephrol Dial Transplant. 2012;27(11):4125–30.
30. Bora DI, Lyngdoh DW, Khyriem DB. Bacteriological profile of rena. Int J Curr Res. 2015;7(6):16898–901.
31. Bianca T, Adrian M, Emil M, Adrian T. Microbiological study of urinary calculi in patients with urinary infections. Acta Medica Transilv. 2013;2(2):245–9.
32. Bell BG, Schellevis F, Stobberingh E, Goossens H, Pringle M. A systematic review and meta-analysis of the effects of antibiotic consumption on antibiotic resistance. BMC Infect Dis. 2014;14(1):13.
33. Wang S, Zhang Y, Zhang X, Li J. An evaluation of multidrug-resistant (MDR) bacteria in patients with urinary stone disease: data from a high-volume stone management center. World J Urol. 2020;38(2):425–32.
34. Hedelin H. Uropathogens and urinary tract concretion formation and catheter encrustations. Int J Antimicrob Agents. 2002;19(6):484–7.

24

Let-7i-5p enhances cell proliferation, migration and invasion of ccRCC by targeting HABP4

Yujie Liu[1†], Xing Hu[2†], Liang Hu[3], Changjing Xu[4] and Xuemei Liang[1*]

Abstract

Background: Clear cell renal cell carcinoma (ccRCC) is one of the best-characterized and most pervasive renal cancers. The present study aimed to explore the effects and potential mechanisms of let-7i-5p in ccRCC cells.

Methods: Using bioinformatics analyses, we investigated the expression of let-7i-5p in The Cancer Genome Atlas (TCGA) database and predicted biological functions and possible target genes of let-7i-5p in ccRCC cells. Cell proliferation assay, wound healing assay and transwell invasion assay were conducted to characterize the effects of let-7i-5p in ccRCC cells. To verify the interactions between let-7i-5p and HABP4, dual-luciferase reporter assay, quantitative real-time polymerase chain reaction, and western blotting were conducted. Rescue experiments were used to investigate the relationship between let-7i-5p and HABP4.

Results: TCGA data analysis revealed that ccRCC tissues had significantly increased let-7i-5p expression, which was robustly associated with poor overall survival. Further verification showed that ccRCC cell proliferation, migration and invasion were inhibited by let-7i-5p inhibitor but enhanced by let-7i-5p mimics. Subsequently, HABP4 was predicted to be the target gene of let-7i-5p. TCGA data showed that ccRCC tissues had decreased expression of HABP4 and that HABP4 expression was negatively correlated with let-7i-5p. Further verification showed that downregulation of HABP4 expression promoted cell proliferation, migration and invasion. The dual-luciferase reporter gene assay suggested that the let-7i-5p/HABP4 axis was responsible for the development of ccRCC.

Conclusion: Our results provide evidence that let-7i-5p functions as a tumor promoter in ccRCC and facilitates cell proliferation, migration and invasion by targeting HABP4. These results clarify the pathogenesis of ccRCC and offer a potential target for its treatment.

Keywords: Clear cell renal cell carcinoma, Let-7i-5p, HABP4, Cell proliferation, Cell migration, Cell invasion

Background

Renal cell carcinoma (RCC), one of the most common urological tumors, can be categorized into non-clear cell renal cell carcinoma (nccRCC) and clear cell renal cell carcinoma (ccRCC) based on cytogenetic and histological signatures [1, 2]. ccRCC is the most common type of RCC, accounting for 70% of cases [3]. The early signs and symptoms of ccRCC are challenging to distinguish, with most patients already having middle-to-late stage ccRCC upon diagnosis [4].

Given that most patients with ccRCC are not sensitive to chemotherapy or radiation, surgical treatment has remained most effective [5, 6]. Thus, exploring the molecular mechanisms underlying the development of ccRCC and identifying effective treatment strategies to

*Correspondence: xuemei_liang@163.com
†Yujie Liu and Xing Hu contributed equally to this work
[1] Department of Geriatric Medicine, The Affiliated Hospital of Southwest Medical University, Luzhou 646000, China
Full list of author information is available at the end of the article

improve the survival rate of patients with ccRCC hold considerable clinical value.

MicroRNAs (miRNAs) are a class of endogenous, small non-protein coding single-stranded RNA molecules that regulate gene expression by binding to messenger RNA (mRNA) and inhibiting mRNA translation or promoting its degradation [7, 8]. Let-7, one of the first miRNAs to be discovered, has been found to be highly conserved and widely expressed among species [9, 10]. As a member of the let-7 family, let-7i-5p has been shown to play an important role in the proliferation and metastasis of various tumors [11–13]. However, the role of let-7i-5p in ccRCC has yet to be studied.

Hyaluronan-binding protein 4 (HABP4, also named Ki-1/57), an intracellular cross-reactant of the monoclonal antibody Ki-1, has been the first protein used to specifically detect malignant cells in Hodgkin's lymphoma [14]. It is involved in gene expression regulation at both the transcriptional and mRNA metabolism levels. Studies in transcriptome data have suggested that HABP4 can function as a tumor suppressor gene by affecting the expression of genes involved in cell proliferation, cell cycle, and apoptosis [15]. However, the biological effects of HABP4 in ccRCC have yet to be elucidated.

The present study utilized The Cancer Genome Atlas (TCGA) database to study the prognostic significance of let-7i-5p expression levels in ccRCC, as well as investigate the effects of let-7i-5p on ccRCC proliferation and metastasis. Furthermore, this study explored the function of HABP4 in ccRCC and the negative regulatory relationship between let-7i-5p and HABP4 to further our understanding of the molecular mechanism underlying ccRCC tumorigenesis and offer a potential target for ccRCC therapies.

Methods

Retrieving ccRCC data from TCGA

The level 3 data on ccRCC were obtained from in TCGA using the UCSC Xena Browser (https://xenabrowser.net/). Using RNAseq (IlluminaHiseq), let-7i-5p expression was measured in 70 normal samples and 494 primary ccRCC tumor samples, whereas HABP4 expression was measured in 72 normal samples and 533 primary ccRCC tumors. The clinicopathological data of the patients with intact survival information, including age at initial pathologic diagnosis, histology, tumor grade, clinical stage, recurrence status, and living status, were downloaded for survival-related analysis.

Bioinformatics analysis of possible let-7i-5p targets and genes negatively related to let-7 expression in ccRCC

Possible targets of miR-361-3p were predicted using DIANA (http://www.microrna.gr/microT-CDS), miRanda (http://www.microrna.org/microrna/home.do), TargetScan (http://www.targetscan.org/vert_72/), and miRmap (https://mirmap.ezlab.org/app/). Moreover, genes negatively correlated with let-7i-5p in TCGA-CESC were identified using LinkedOmics (http://www.linkedomics.org/login.php). The overlapping subset between the negatively correlated genes and predicted target genes was identified using Venn diagram analysis.

Cell culture

Human ccRCC cell lines 786-0 and 769-p were purchased from Cell Bank (Chinese Academy of Sciences, Shanghai, China). All cell lines were cultured in Dulbecco's Modified Eagle's Medium (DMEM) (HyClone, Thermo, USA) supplemented with 10% fetal bovine serum, 100 U/mL penicillin, and 100 mg/mL streptomycin and subsequently incubated at 37°C in a 5% CO_2 atmosphere.

Cell transfection

The mimics NC, inhibitor NC, siControl, let-7i-5p mimics, let-7i-5p inhibitor, siHABP4#1 and siHABP4#2 were designed and provided by Guangzhou RiboBio Co., Ltd., (Guangzhou, China). After reaching 70% confluence, cells were transfected or co-transfected with Lipofectamine 3000 (Invitrogen, Carlsbad, CA, USA) according to the manufacturer's instructions. Quantitative real-time polymerase chain reaction (qRT-PCR) and western blotting were then used to verify the transfection efficiency. After transfection for 48 h, ccRCC cells were collected for subsequent experiments. The sequences of miRNA mimics and miRNA inhibitor were as follows: hsa-let-7i-5p mimics, sense: 5′-UGAGGUAGUAGUUUGUGCUGUU-3′, antisense: 5′-CAGCACAAACUACUACCUCAUU-3′; miRNA mimics negative control (miRNA mimics NC), sense: 5′-UUCUCCGAACGUGUCACGUTT-3′, antisense: 5′-AGGUGACACGUUCGGAGAATT-3′; hsa-let-7i-5p inhibitor: 5′-AACAGCACAAACUACUAC CUCA-3′; miRNA inhibitor NC: 5′-CAGUACUUUUGU GUAGUACAA-3′. The siRNA sequences were as follows: siHABP4 #1, sense: 5′-AUCCCAGCUGGAGAUUAA UUUTT-3′ and antisense 5′-AAAUUAAUCUCCAGC UGGGAUTT-3′; siHABP4 #2, sense: 5′-CAAGUUCAA GAGAUGACUUUATT-3′ and antisense 5′-UAAAGU CAUCUCUUGAACUUGTT-3′.

RNA extraction and qRT-PCR analysis

Total RNA was extracted from the ccRCC cell lines using Trizol Universal reagent according to the manufacturer's instructions. The cDNA template used in mRNA qPCR was synthesized using reverse transcriptase and oligo (dT) primer (Promega). qRT-PCR was conducted on an ABI 7500 Sequence Detection System (Life Technologies, USA) using the corresponding PCR reagent according to the manufacturer's instructions. The primers used were as follows: HABP4, 5′-AAGAGCTGAGCGGAG ATCCTAC-3′ (forward) and 5′-TCCTCTCAACGGTCT GTCTCGA-3′ (reverse); GAPDH, 5′-GAAGGTGAA GGTCGGAGTC-3′ (forward) and 5′-GAAGATGGT GATGGGATTTC-3′ (reverse). cDNA template used in miRNA qPCR was synthesized using the miScript II Reverse Transcription Kit (Qiagen, Germany) according to the manufacturer's protocol. Quantification of let-7i-5p was carried out by miScript Primer Assay (Hs_let-7i_1 miScript Primer Assay MS00003157 Qiagen, Germany), normalizing over RNU6B control (Hs_RNU6-2_11 miScript Primer Assay MS00033740 Qiagen, Germany) and using the miScript SYBR Green PCR kit (Qiagen, Germany) on ABI 7500 Sequence Detection System (Life Technologies, USA). RNU6B and GAPDH served as internal controls. Relative expression was determined using the $2^{-\Delta\Delta CT}$ method.

Protein extraction and western blot analysis

After cells were trypsinized (0.05% Trypsin EDTA, Invitrogen), cell pellets were lysed with RIPA buffer (Beyotime, Shanghai, China) and kept in ice for 30 min with intermittent vortexing. The lysate was obtained through centrifugation at 12,000 rpm for 20 min at 4℃, after which its protein concentration was determined using BCA protein assay reagents (Beyotime, Shanghai, China). Protein samples were fractionated in a 10% sodium dodecyl sulfate–polyacrylamide gel and transferred to a polyvinylidene difluoride (PVDF) membrane (Immobilon-P transfer membrane, Millipore, Saint-Quentin-en-Yvelines, France). Membranes were blocked with 5% non-fat milk and washed with Tris-Buffered Saline and Tween 20 (TBST) and then incubated with primary antibody (anti-HABP4, Abnova, Taipei, Taiwan; anti-GAPDH, Proteintech, Wuhan, China) at 4℃ for 24 h. The PVDF membranes were extensively washed three times and then incubated with horseradish peroxidase-conjugated secondary antibody. After three washes with TBST, the membranes were detected using the ECL detection kit (Beyotime, Shanghai, China). GAPDH was used as an internal control. The integrated optical density (IOD) of the individual bands on blots was measured by ImageJ and the ratio of HABP4 protein to the housekeeping protein GAPDH was calculated.

Dual-luciferase reporter assay

The 3′-untranslated region (UTR) of HABP4 was synthesized, annealed, and inserted into the pmirGLO luciferase reporter vector (Promega Corporation, Madison, WI, USA). The 3′-UTR wild-type (WT) HABP4 sequence (ACTACCTC) complementary to the binding site of let-7i-5p was replaced with a mutated (MUT) HABP4 sequence (ACATGGTC). Let-7i-5p mimics were co-transfected with pmirGLO-WT-HABP4 or pmirGLO-MUT-HABP4 using Lipofectamine 3000 (Invitrogen, Carlsbad, CA, USA). After the cells were incubated for 48 h, luciferase activity was measured using the dual-luciferase reporter assay kit (Beyotime, Shanghai, China).

MTT assay

Transfected cells were seeded at 2.0×10^3 cells/well in 96-well plates. Subsequently, 10 μL of 5 mg/ml MTT (Beyotime, Shanghai, China) was added into each of the 96 wells for 4 h at 37℃, after which 100 μL DMSO was added to dissolve the purple crystals. Absorbance was determined using a spectrophotometer at 570 nm.

Wound healing assay

Transfected cells were seeded on 6-well plates with a fresh medium containing 10% FBS.

After forming a monolayer culture, cells were scratched using a sterile 200 μL pipette. The cells were washed twice with PBS, after which the medium was replaced with a serum-free medium. Images of the wound were taken on day 0 and after 24 h. The wound healing rate was calculated using the formula wound healing rate (%) = [(width at 0 h − width at 24 h)/(width at 0 h)] × 100.

Transwell invasion assay

Cells were seeded in the upper compartment of transwell chambers (Corning, NY, USA) that were pre-coated with Matrigel (BD Biosciences, CA, USA). DMEM containing 20% FBS was added to the bottom compartments as a chemoattractant. After 24 h, the non-invading cells were wiped out, whereas the invading cells on the lower surface were fixed with 4% paraformaldehyde and stained with crystal violet. Images were obtained using an Olympus microscope.

Statistical analysis

Statistical analysis was conducted using GraphPad Prism 6.0 (GraphPad Inc., La Jolla, CA, USA) or SPSS 23.0 software package (SPSS Inc., Chicago, IL, USA). Values were expressed as mean ± SD, with P values < 0.05 indicating statistical significance.

Results

High let-7i-5p expression was correlated with poor patient prognosis

To determine whether let-7i-5p expression was a prognostic factor for poor survival, expression data from the TCGA dataset were analyzed. Accordingly, ccRCC tissues had a higher let-7i-5p expression level than normal kidney tissues (Fig. 1a). Furthermore, we explored

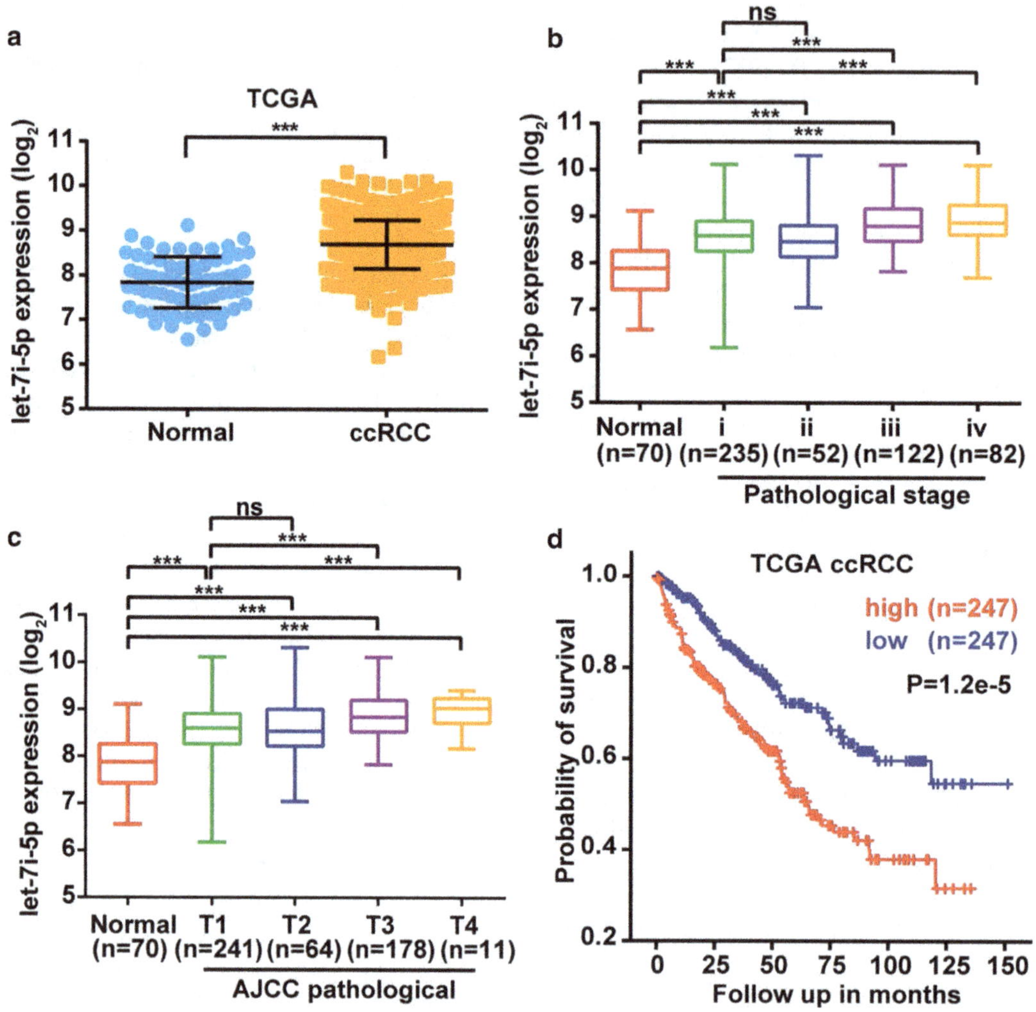

Fig. 1 Correlation between let-7i-5p expression and ccRCC pathological information. **a** The relative expression of let-7i-5p in TCGA dataset. **b, c** The relative expression of let-7i-5p across different pathological stages and AJCC pathological T stage. **d** Kaplan–Meier analysis of overall survival according to high or low let-7i-5p expression in the TCGA database. Data are presented as mean ± SD. ns > 0.05, $^{*}P < 0.05$; $^{**}P < 0.01$; $^{***}P < 0.001$

the relationship between let-7i-5p expression level and clinicopathological characteristics, with the results summarized in Table 1. Our results showed a significant difference between pathological stage, American Joint Committee on Cancer (AJCC) T, N, M stages, and tumor status. Meanwhile, the level of let-7i-5p expression increased significantly in the pathological stage (III and IV) and AJCC stages (T3 and T4) (Fig. 1b, 1c, Additional file 1: Table S1). Given that the patients with different survival outcomes had different levels of expression, we decided to explore whether let-7i-5p was a prognostic marker in ccRCC. Accordingly, Kaplan–Meier analysis showed that high let-7i-5p expression was associated with poor prognosis (Fig. 1d). These data indicated that let-7i-5p might play an oncogenic role in ccRCC.

Let-7i-5p enhanced cell proliferation, migration and invasion of ccRCC

Two kidney cancer cell lines (786-0 and 769-P) were used to examine the function of let-7i-5p in ccRCC. Accordingly, transfecting a let-7i-5p mimic into 786-0 and 769-P cells upregulated the expression of let-7i-5p, whereas transfecting a let-7i-5p inhibitor downregulated the same (Fig. 2a). MTT assay results showed that let-7i-5p overexpression could promote cell proliferation, whereas let-7i-5p downregulation could inhibit cell proliferation (Fig. 2b). Furthermore, a wound healing assay and transwell invasion were used to analyze the effects of

Table 1 Correlation between let-7i-5p expression and clinicopathological variables of ccRCC using The Cancer Genome Atlas datasets

Clinicopathological features	Cases	Let-7i-5p expression		*t*	*p*
		Low	High		
Group					
ccRCC	494	247	247	− 12.313	0.000
Normal	70	66	4		
Age					
≥ 60	265	125	140	− 1.502	0.134
< 60	229	122	107		
Gender					
Male	320	155	165	− 0.986	0.325
Female	174	92	82		
Race					
White	426	210	216	− 1.348	0.178
Black or African American	53	30	23		
Pathological stage					
III–IV	204	76	128	− 6.306	0.000
I–II	287	171	116		
AJCC pathological T					
T3–T4	189	69	120	− 5.892	0.000
T1–T2	305	178	127		
AJCC pathological N					
N1	17	3	14	− 2.843	0.005
N0	220	109	111		
AJCC pathological M					
M1	78	23	55	− 4.048	0.000
M0	387	209	178		
Tumor status					
With tumor	144	51	93	− 4.807	0.000
Tumor-free	308	178	130		
Hemoglobin					
Low	244	109	135	− 1.898	0.058
Normal	175	98	77		

let-7i-5p on ccRCC cell migration and invasion, respectively. Accordingly, we found that let-7i-5p overexpression could promote cell migration and invasion, whereas let-7i-5p downregulation could inhibit cell migration and invasion (Fig. 3a, b). Collectively, our results suggested that let-7i-5p played a facilitative role in ccRCC cell proliferation, migration, and invasion.

Predicted target genes of let-7i-5p

To explore the potential molecular mechanisms through which let-7i-5p promotes ccRCC cell proliferation, migration, and invasion, we used four different miRNA-target prediction programs (DIANA, miRanda, TargetScan, and miRmap) to predict the putative target genes of let-7i-5p. A total of 385 putative miRNA-target genes were predicted by DIANA, miRanda, TargetScan, and miRmap programs (Fig. 4a). Using LinkedOmics to analyze mRNA/miRNA expression data, we identified 234 genes that negatively correlated with let-7i-5p expression (Fig. 4a, Additional file 2: Table S2). Furthermore, five genes were obtained after comparing these two groups of genes. Statistical analysis of the binding score and the association between the five genes and let-7i-5p found that HABP4 had a high binding score in four different miRNA-target prediction programs (Table 2). To determine the function of HABP4 in ccRCC, the expression and prognosis of HABP4 were analyzed using the TCGA database. Accordingly, TCGA data showed that ccRCC tissues had lower HABP4 expression than normal kidney tissues (Fig. 4b). Moreover, Kaplan–Meier analysis showed that low HABP4 expression was associated with poor prognosis (Fig. 4c). Overall, our results suggested that HABP4 may be a novel target gene of let-7i-5p.

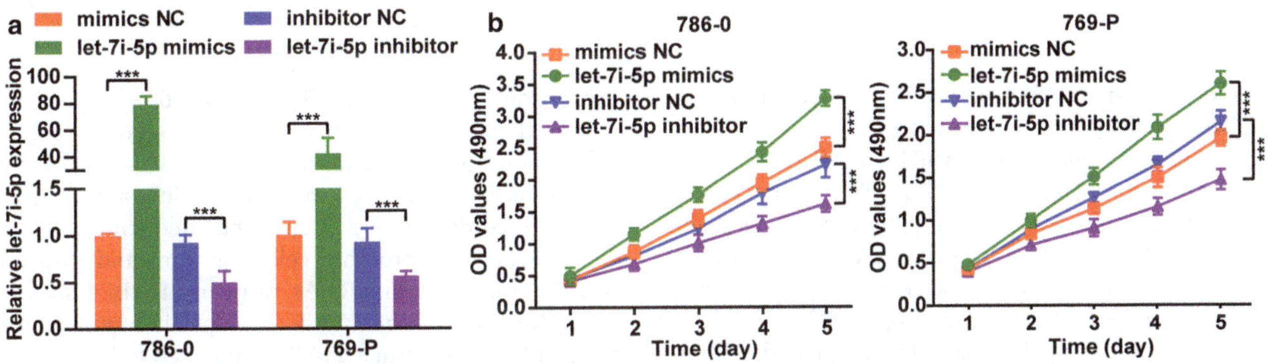

Fig. 2 The regulatory effect of let-7i-5p on ccRCC cell proliferation. **a** After transfecting 786-0 and 769-P cells with the let-7i-5p mimic or inhibitor, the expression of let-7i-5p was detected using qRT-PCR. **b** MTT assays were used to elucidate the effects of let-7i-5p on cell proliferation. Data are presented as mean ± SD. ***$P < 0.001$

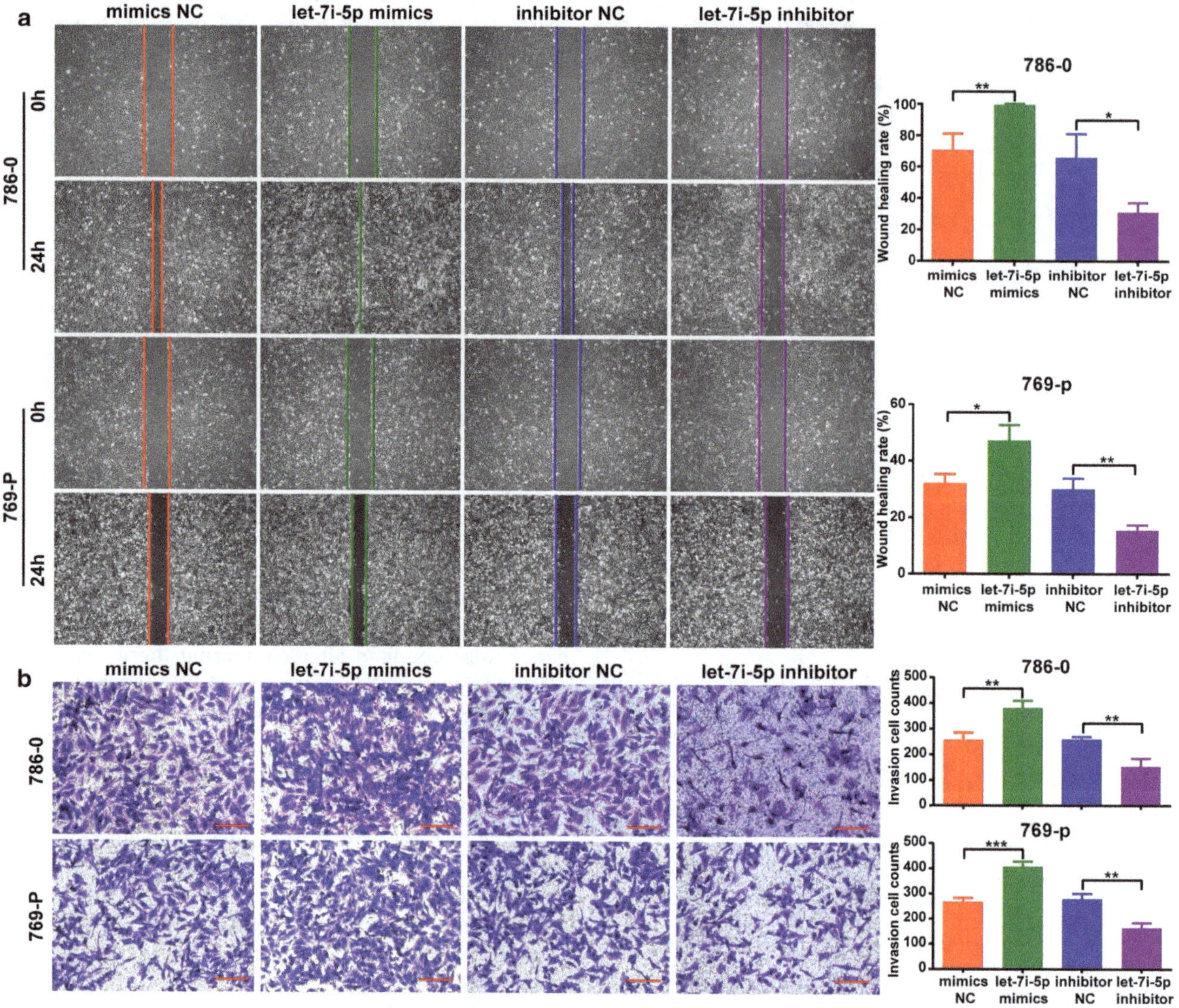

Fig. 3 The regulatory effect of let-7i-5p on ccRCC cell migration and invasion. **a** Wound healing assays were used to elucidate the effects of let-7i-5p on cell migration. **b** Transwell invasion assays were used to analyze the role of let-7i-5p on cell invasion. Scale bar = 100 μm. Data are presented as mean ± SD. *$P<0.05$; **$P<0.01$; ***$P<0.001$

Downregulation of HABP4 expression promoted cell proliferation, migration and invasion

To examine the effects of HABP4 on cell proliferation, migration, and invasion in ccRCC cells in vitro, HABP4 expression in cultured 796-0 and 769-P cells was downregulated using siRNA, an efficient approach used to extensively knock down specific gene expression in cells. Transfecting two siRNAs targeting HABP4 into 786-0 and 769-P cells significantly downregulated HABP4 protein expression. The two siRNAs targeting HABP4 showed nearly the same RNAi effects (Fig. 5a). MTT cell proliferation assays showed that decreased HABP4 expression could promote 786-0 and 769-P cell proliferation (Fig. 5b). Furthermore, we analyzed the effects of HABP4 on migration and invasion of ccRCC cells using wound healing analysis and transwell invasion, respectively. Accordingly, we found that reducing HABP4 expression could promote cell migration and invasion (Fig. 6a, b). The two siRNAs targeting HABP4 showed nearly the same inhibitory effects on proliferation, migration, and invasion. Thus, HABP4 appeared to have a negative regulatory effect on proliferation, migration, and invasion of ccRCC cells in vitro.

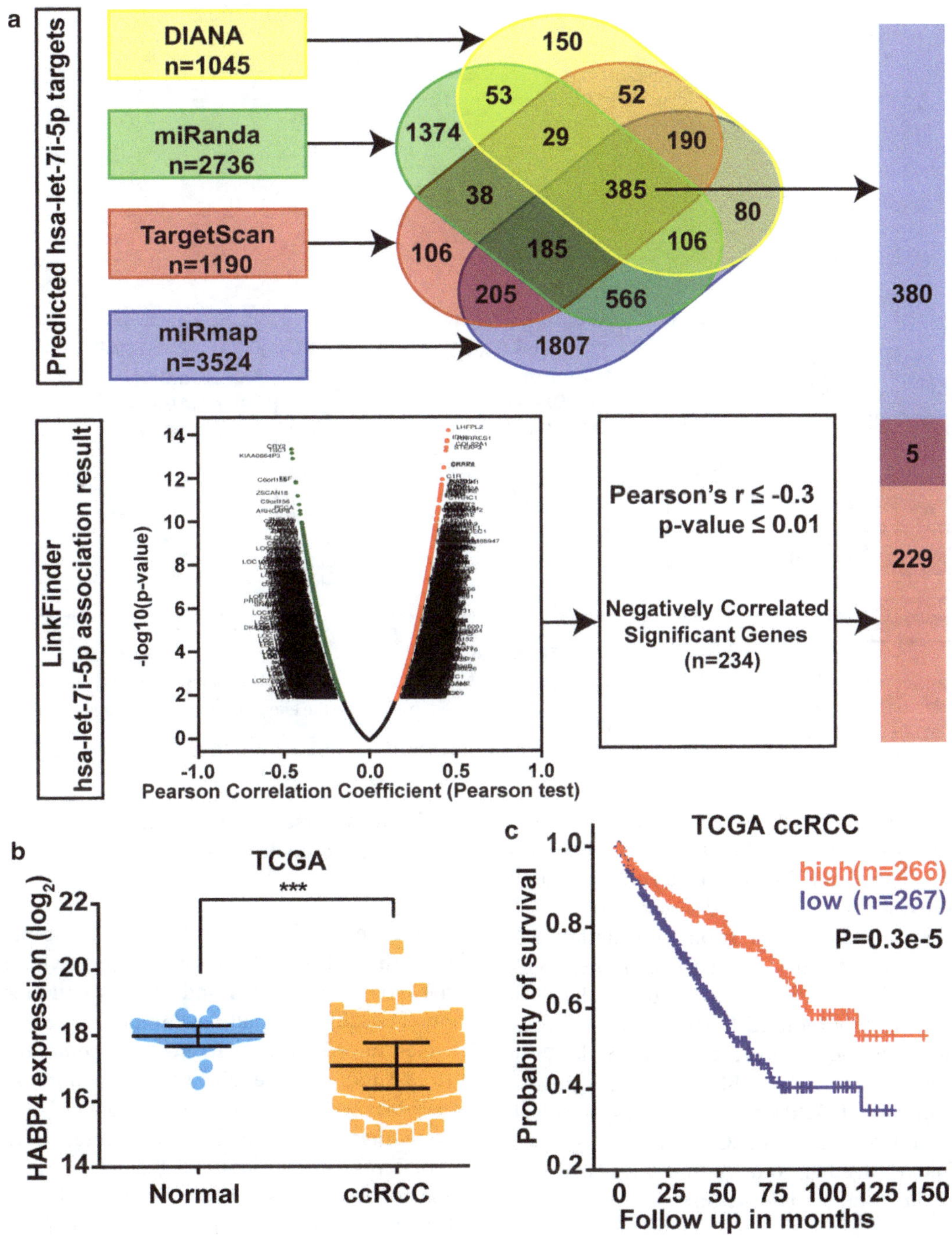

Fig. 4 Predicted target genes of let-7i-5p. **a** Four different miRNA-target prediction programs (DIANA, miRanda, TargetScan, and miRmap) were used to predict putative target genes of let-7i-5p. LinkedOmics database was used to analyze the negative correlation between let-7i-5p and mRNA expression. **b** The relative expression of HABP4 in the TCGA dataset. **c** Kaplan–Meier analysis of overall survival according to high or low HABP4 expression in the TCGA database. Data are presented as mean ± SD. ns > 0.05, $^{**}P < 0.01$; $^{***}P < 0.001$

HABP4 was a direct target of let-7i-5p

To determine the mechanism by which let-7i-5p regulated HABP4 expression through the HABP4 3′-UTR binding site using bioinformatics analysis, pmirGLO-WT-HABP4 and pmirGLO-MUT-HABP4 plasmids were synthesized, after which a HABP4 3′-UTR luciferase reporter assay was conducted in ccRCC cells (Fig. 7a). Accordingly, 786-0 and 769-P cells transfected with the let-7i-5p mimic and WT-HABP4 had significantly

Table 2 Statistical analysis of the binding score and association between the five genes and let-7i-5p

Target	Binding score				Association	
	miRmap	TargetScan	miRanda	DIANA	Pearson's r	p-value
HABP4	84.7	−0.35	−0.75	0.83	−0.33	5.82E−08
CPEB3	83.7	−0.19	−0.21	0.83	−0.30	9.47E−07
TSC1	79.6	−0.30	−0.35	0.82	−0.45	5.52E−14
SLC25A4	62.0	−0.33	−0.11	0.71	−0.38	6.06E−10
PPARGC1A	18.6	−0.18	−0.11	0.96	−0.30	9.18E−07

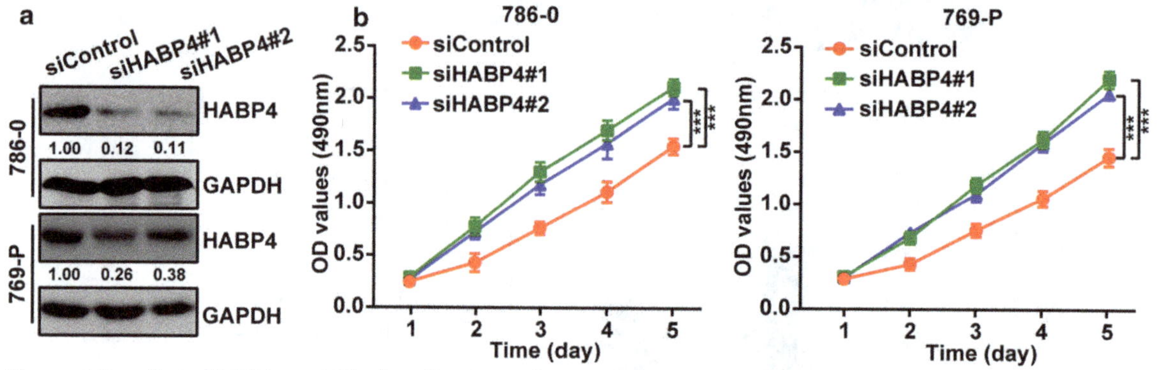

Fig. 5 The regulatory effect of HABP4 on ccRCC cell proliferation. **a** After transfecting 786-0 and 769-P cells with two siRNAs targeting HABP4, HABP4 expression was detected using western blotting. **b** MTT assays were used to elucidate the effects of HABP4 downregulation on cell proliferation. Data are presented as mean ± SD. ***$P<0.001$

reduced luciferase activity, whereas cells transfected with MUT-HABP4 showed no reduction (Fig. 7b). To confirm the relationship between HABP4 and let-7i-5p, qRT-PCR was used to investigate the expression levels of HABP4 in ccRCC cells 72 h after transfection with the let-7i-5p mimic, miR-3175 inhibitor, or corresponding NCs. Accordingly, ccRCC cells transfected with the let-7i-5p mimic had significantly reduced HABP4 mRNA expression levels, whereas those transfected with the let-7i-5p inhibitor showed increased HABP4 mRNA expression (Fig. 7c). Meanwhile, HABP4 expression was negatively correlated with let-7i-5p in ccRCC cells ($r=-0.335$) (Fig. 7d). Taken together, our results suggested that HABP4 was a direct target of let-7i-5p.

Discussion

The present study investigated the potential role and mechanism of let-7i-5p in ccRCC. Analysis of the TCGA database revealed that let-7i-5p expression was upregulated in ccRCC cells and that high let-7i-5p expression levels were positively correlated with poor survival. Moreover, our results showed that downregulating the expression of let-7i-5p might inhibit ccRCC cell proliferation, migration, and invasion by directly upregulating the expression of HABP4. Meanwhile, the present study has been the first to confirm that HABP4, a target gene of let-7i-5p, could be considered a tumor suppressor gene in ccRCC.

Evidence has shown that let-7i-5p, an important member of the miRNA let-7 family, played a vital role in both physiological processes and various pathological conditions [16–22], especially in tumor progression. Previous studies have shown that let-7i-5p could function as a tumor suppressor gene in various tumors, such as glioblastomas, colon cancer, gastric cancer, and esophageal carcinomas. Let-7i-5p directly targeted UDP-galactose-4-epimerase and Inhibitor of Nuclear Factor Kappa-B Kinase Subunit Epsilon to reduce glioblastoma cell proliferation and migration [11, 23]. Moreover, let-7i-5p had been found to inhibit the proliferation and metastasis of colon cancer cells by targeting kallikrein-related peptidase 6 [13] and significantly inhibit gastric cancer proliferation, invasion, and metastasis by targeting collagen type I alpha 1 chain [24]. Another study showed that let-7i-5p significantly inhibited esophageal carcinoma cell proliferation and promoted cisplatin-induced apoptosis by targeting the drug transporter ATP binding cassette subfamily C member 10 [25]. However, let-7i-5p exhibited both inhibitory and promotive functions (dual role) in the tumorigenesis of hepatocellular carcinoma. For

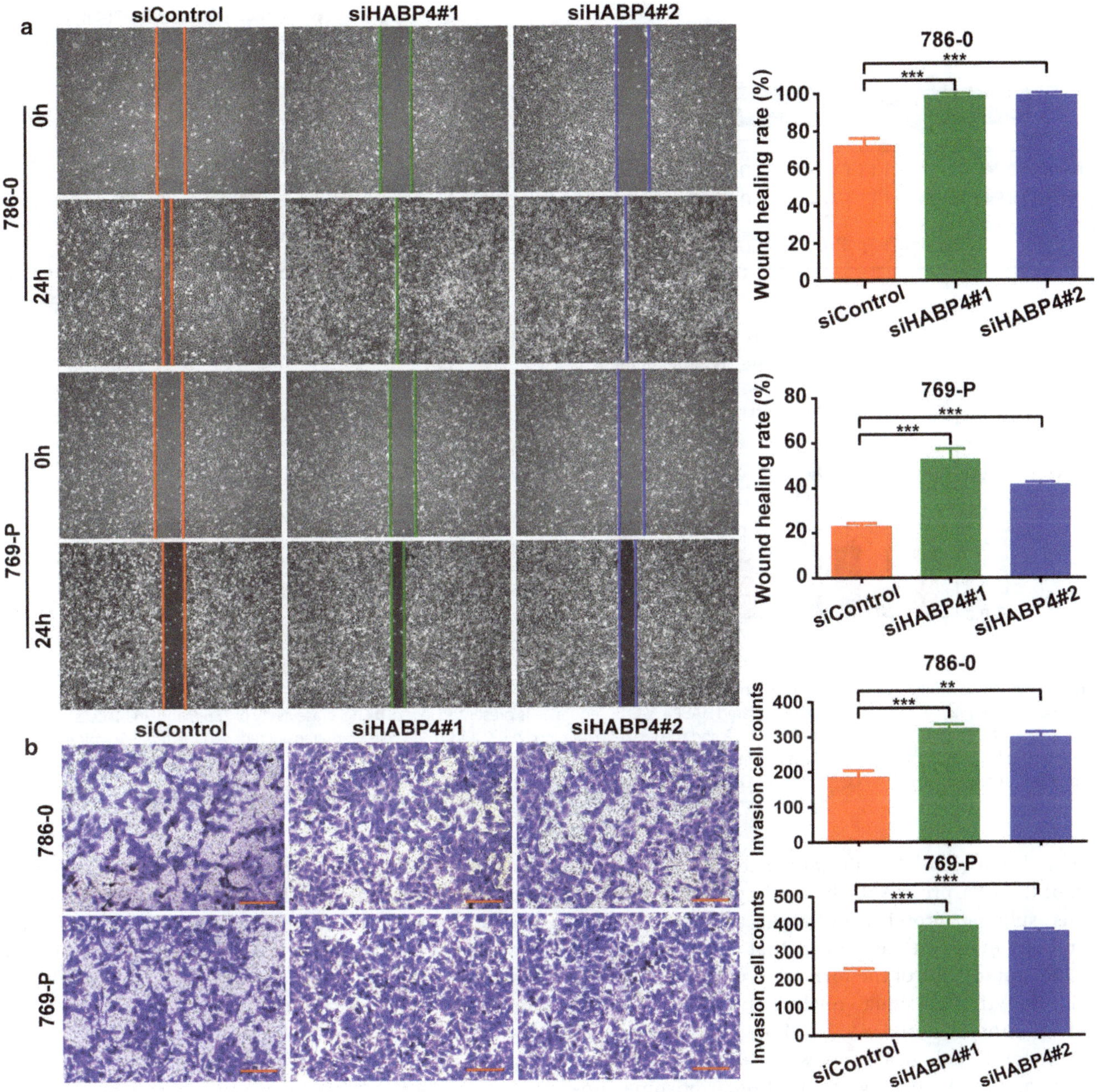

Fig. 6 The regulatory effect of HABP4 on ccRCC cell migration and invasion. **a** Wound healing assays were used to elucidate the effects of HABP4 downregulation on cell migration. **b** Transwell invasion assays were used to analyze the role of HABP4 downregulation on cell invasion. Data are presented as mean ± SD. $^{**}P < 0.01$; $^{***}P < 0.001$

instance, let-7i-5p had been found to not only inhibit hepatocellular carcinoma growth by targeting insulin-like growth factor 2-mRNA-binding proteins 1, 2, and 3 and the anti-apoptotic protein BCL2 like 1 [26, 27] but also rescue the tumor-suppressing effects of HDAC6 by targeting thrombospondin-1 in hepatocellular carcinoma cells [12]. Our results proved that let-7i-5p could serve to promote tumorigenesis of ccRCC.

HABP4, a nuclear and cytoplasmic regulatory protein first identified in malignant cells from Hodgkin's lymphoma [28, 29], had been found to participate in different physiological functions, including cell proliferation, tumorigenesis, RNA transcription and splicing, and telomere maintenance. Studies have shown that HABP4 overexpression resulted in reduced cancer cell proliferation, mainly because of a G1 phase arrest

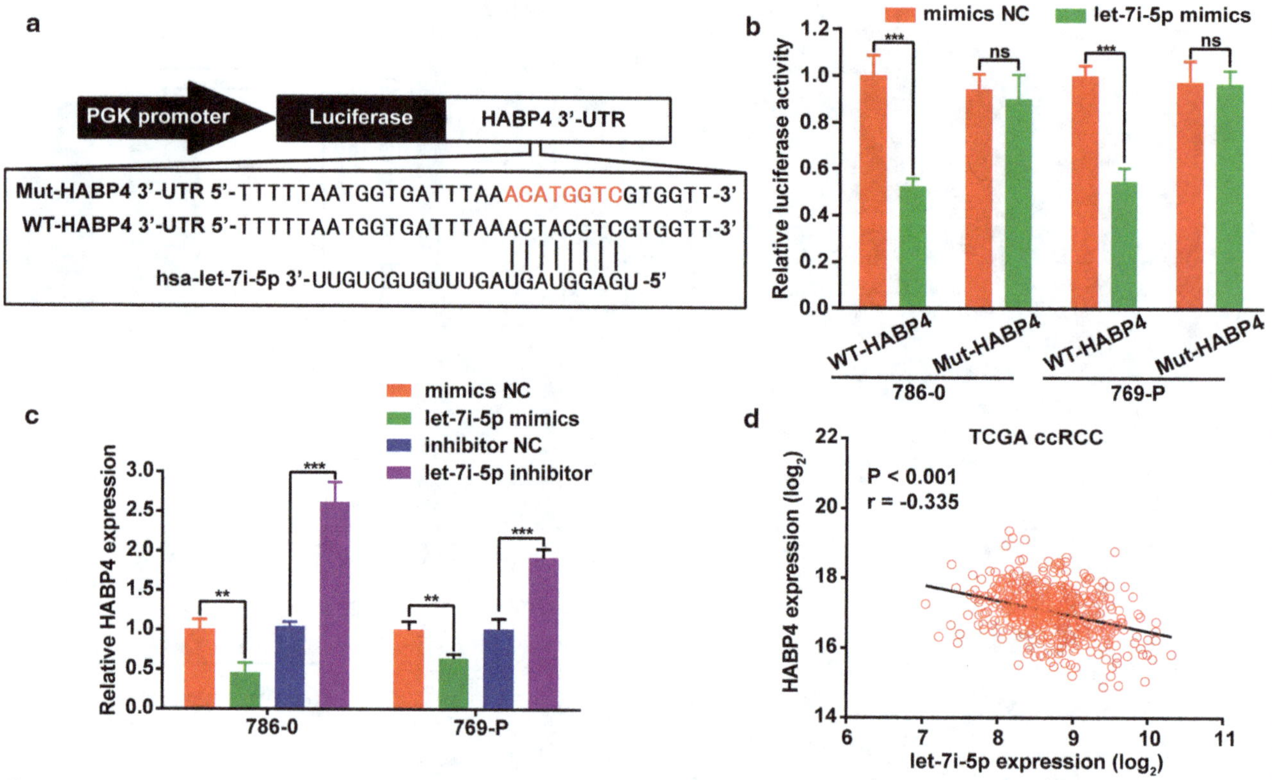

Fig. 7 HABP4 was modulated by let-7i-5p. **a** Schematic diagram of the let-7i-5p binding sites within the 3′-UTR of HABP4 mRNA (WT-HABP4) and mutated sequences (Mut-HABP4). The mutated HABP4 3′-UTR sequence is presented in red. **b** Luciferase assay of 786-0 and 769-P cells after co-transfection with WT or Mut HABP4 3′-UTR and the let-7i-5p mimic. **c** 786-0 and 769-P cells were transfected with the let-7i-5p mimic, let-7i-5p inhibitor, and corresponding NCs and incubated for 72 h. Cells were harvested and assayed using qRT-PCR. **d** Correlation between HABP4 expression and let-7i-5p in the TCGA database. Data are presented as mean ± SD. ns > 0.05; $^{**}P < 0.01$; $^{***}P < 0.001$

[15], and that HABP4 could influence the splicing pattern of the E1A pre-mRNA by binding with the endogenous splicing proteins hnRNPQ and SFRS9 [30]. Moreover, evidence has shown that SUMOylation of HANP4 could control the formation of As_2O_3-induced promyelocytic leukemia nuclear bodies. Although HABP4 modification via SUMO-1 was associated with several biological processes (i.e., transcription regulation, RNA splicing, translation, ribosome biogenesis, mitotic cell cycle, and apoptotic process), SUMO-2-modified HABP4 was strongly associated with biological processes related to the control of gene expression (transcription, splicing, and translation) and telomere maintenance [31]. The present study has been the first to report that HABP4, a target gene of let-7i-5p, functioned as a tumor suppressor gene in ccRCC.

Conclusion

The findings of the present study suggested that let-7i-5p could promote the proliferation, migration, and invasion of ccRCC cells by downregulating its target HABP4. Although we have preliminarily explored the molecular mechanism of let-7i-5p regulating the proliferation, migration, and invasion of ccRCC cells in vitro, further in vivo experiments are needed to verify the feasibility of let-7i-5p as a potential therapeutic target for ccRCC in future studies.

Abbreviations

ccRCC: Clear cell renal cell carcinoma; RCC: Renal cell carcinoma; nccRCC: Non-clear cell renal cell carcinoma; miRNAs: MicroRNAs; mRNA: Messenger RNA; HABP4: Hyaluronan-binding protein 4; qRT-PCR: Quantitative real-time PCR; DMEM: Dulbecco's Modified Eagle's Medium.

Supplementary Information

Additional file 1: Supplementary Table S1: The let-7i-5p expression data and clinical information of ccRCC patients.

Additional file 2: Supplementary Table S2: 234 genes that negatively correlated with let-7i-5p expression.

Acknowledgements

None.

Authors' contributions

All authors had full access to all data in the current study. YL and XH take responsibility for the integrity of the data and the accuracy of the data analysis. XL critically revised the manuscript for important intellectual content. All authors have read and approved the final manuscript.

Author details

[1] Department of Geriatric Medicine, The Affiliated Hospital of Southwest Medical University, Luzhou 646000, China. [2] Department of General Practice, The Affiliated Hospital of Southwest Medical University, Luzhou 646000, China. [3] Department of Cardiovascular Surgery, The General Hospital of Western Theater Command, Chengdu 610083, China. [4] Department of Pharmacy, The Affiliated Hospital of Southwest Medical University, Luzhou 646000, China.

References

1. Hsieh JJ, Purdue MP, Signoretti S, Swanton C, Albiges L, Schmidinger M, et al. Renal cell carcinoma. Nat Rev Dis Primers. 2017;3:17009.
2. Kovacs G, Akhtar M, Beckwith BJ, Bugert P, Cooper CS, Delahunt B, et al. The Heidelberg classification of renal cell tumours. J Pathol. 1997;183:131–3.
3. Wang ZG, Wei M, Ren Y, Liu H, Wang M, Shi KH, et al. miR149 rs71428439 polymorphism and risk of clear cell renal cell carcinoma: a case-control study. Tumor Biol. 2014;35:12127–30.
4. Ran LJ, Liang J, Deng X, Wu JY. miRNAs in prediction of prognosis in clear cell renal cell carcinoma. Biomed Res Int. 2017. https://doi.org/10.1155/2017/4832931.
5. Barth DA, Slaby O, Klec C, Juracek J, Drula R, Calin GA, et al. Current concepts of non-coding RNAs in the pathogenesis of non-clear cell renal cell carcinoma. Cancers (Basel). 2019;11:1580.
6. Yang GH, Ren ZX, Yang X, Zhang YG. KIF4A promotes clear cell renal cell carcinoma (ccRCC) proliferation in vitro and in vivo. Onco Targets Ther. 2020;13:2667–76.
7. Medina PP, Slack FJ. MicroRNAs and cancer: an overview. Cell Cycle. 2008;7:2485–92.
8. Wang RH, He LY, Zhou SH. The role of gene sculptor microRNAs in human precancerous lesions. Onco Targets Ther. 2018;11:5667–75.
9. Roush S, Slack FJ. The let-7 family of microRNAs. Trends Cell Biol. 2008;18:505–16.
10. Lee H, Han S, Kwon CS, Lee D. Biogenesis and regulation of the let-7 miRNAs and their functional implications. Protein Cell. 2016;7:100–13.
11. Sun XP, Xue H, Xiong Y, Yu R, Gao X, Qian MY, et al. GALE promotes the proliferation and migration of glioblastoma cells and is regulated by miR-let-7i-5p. Cancer Manag Res. 2019;11:10539–54.
12. Yang HD, Kim HS, Kim SY, Na MJ, Yang G, Eun JW, et al. HDAC6 suppresses Let-7i-5p to elicit TSP1/CD47-mediated anti-tumorigenesis and phagocytosis of hepatocellular carcinoma. Hepatology. 2019;70:1262–79.
13. Song J, Wang L, Ma Q, Yang Y, Yang Z, Wang B, et al. Let7i5p inhibits the proliferation and metastasis of colon cancer cells by targeting kallikreinrelated peptidase 6. Oncol Rep. 2018;40:1459–66.
14. Goncalves Kde A, Bressan GC, Saito A, Morello LG, Zanchin NI, Kobarg J. Evidence for the association of the human regulatory protein Ki-1/57 with the translational machinery. FEBS Lett. 2011;585:2556–60.
15. Costa FC, Saito A, Goncalves KA, Vidigal PM, Meirelles GV, Bressan GC, et al. Ki-1/57 and CGI-55 ectopic expression impact cellular pathways involved in proliferation and stress response regulation. Biochim Biophys Acta. 2014;1843:2944–56.
16. Chen D, Li L, Wang Y, Xu R, Peng S, Zhou L, et al. Ischemia-reperfusion injury of brain induces endothelial-mesenchymal transition and vascular fibrosis via activating let-7i/TGF-betaR1 double-negative feedback loop. FASEB J. 2020;34:7178–91.
17. Ge P, Guo Y, Shen J. IcarisideII facilitates the differentiation of ADSCs to SCs via let-7i/STAT3 axis to preserve erectile function. Biol Res. 2019;52:54.
18. Nguyen T, Su C, Singh M. Let-7i inhibition enhances progesterone-induced functional recovery in a mouse model of ischemia. Proc Natl Acad Sci U S A. 2018;115:E9668–77.
19. Qi M, Yin L, Xu L, Tao X, Qi Y, Han X, et al. Dioscin alleviates lipopolysaccharide-induced inflammatory kidney injury via the microRNA let-7i/TLR4/MyD88 signaling pathway. Pharmacol Res. 2016;111:509–22.
20. Syed M, Ball JP, Romero DG. Let-7i: lethal weapon against angiotensin II-induced cardiac injury. Hypertension. 2015;66:739–41.
21. Wang X, Wang HX, Li YL, Zhang CC, Zhou CY, Wang L, et al. MicroRNA Let-7i negatively regulates cardiac inflammation and fibrosis. Hypertension. 2015;66:776–85.
22. Giroud M, Karbiener M, Pisani DF, Ghandour RA, Beranger GE, Niemi T, et al. Let-7i-5p represses brite adipocyte function in mice and humans. Sci Rep. 2016;6:1–11.
23. Tian Y, Hao S, Ye M, Zhang A, Nan Y, Wang G, et al. MicroRNAs let-7b/i suppress human glioma cell invasion and migration by targeting IKBKE directly. Biochem Biophys Res Commun. 2015;458:307–12.
24. Shi Y, Duan Z, Zhang X, Zhang X, Wang G, Li F. Down-regulation of the let-7i facilitates gastric cancer invasion and metastasis by targeting COL1A1. Protein Cell. 2019;10:143–8.
25. Wu K, Yang Y, Zhao J, Zhao S. BAG3-mediated miRNA let-7g and let-7i inhibit proliferation and enhance apoptosis of human esophageal carcinoma cells by targeting the drug transporter ABCC10. Cancer Lett. 2016;371:125–33.
26. Fawzy IO, Hamza MT, Hosny KA, Esmat G, Abdelaziz AI. Abrogating the interplay between IGF2BP1, 2 and 3 and IGF1R by let-7i arrests hepatocellular carcinoma growth. Growth Factors. 2016;34:42–50.
27. Wu LJ, Wang QF, Yao J, Jiang H, Xiao C, Wu FS. MicroRNA let-7g and let-7i inhibit hepatoma cell growth concurrently via downregulation of the anti-apoptotic protein B-cell lymphoma-extra large. Oncol Lett. 2015;9:213–8.
28. Colleti C, Melo-Hanchuk TD, da Silva FRM, Saito A, Kobarg J. Complex interactomes and post-translational modifications of the regulatory proteins HABP4 and SERBP1 suggest pleiotropic cellular functions. World J Biol Chem. 2019;10:44–64.
29. Goncalves KD, Bressan GC, Saito A, Morello LG, Zanchin NIT, Kobarg J. Evidence for the association of the human regulatory protein Ki-1/57 with the translational machinery. Febs Lett. 2011;585:2556–60.
30. Bressan GC, Quaresma AJ, Moraes EC, Manfiolli AO, Passos DO, Gomes MD, et al. Functional association of human Ki-1/57 with pre-mRNA splicing events. FEBS J. 2009;276:3770–83.
31. Saito A, Souza EE, Costa FC, Meirelles GV, Goncalves KA, Santos MT, et al. Human regulatory protein Ki-1/57 is a target of SUMOylation and affects PML nuclear body formation. J Proteome Res. 2017;16:3147–57.

25

Computer-aided diagnosis with a convolutional neural network algorithm for automated detection of urinary tract stones on plain X-ray

Masaki Kobayashi[1], Junichiro Ishioka[2], Yoh Matsuoka[2*], Yuichi Fukuda[1], Yusuke Kohno[1], Keizo Kawano[1], Shinji Morimoto[1], Rie Muta[3], Motohiro Fujiwara[3], Naoko Kawamura[3], Tetsuo Okuno[3], Soichiro Yoshida[2], Minato Yokoyama[2], Rumi Suda[4], Ryota Saiki[4], Kenji Suzuki[5], Itsuo Kumazawa[5] and Yasuhisa Fujii[2]

Abstract

Background: Recent increased use of medical images induces further burden of their interpretation for physicians. A plain X-ray is a low-cost examination that has low-dose radiation exposure and high availability, although diagnosing urolithiasis using this method is not always easy. Since the advent of a convolutional neural network via deep learning in the 2000s, computer-aided diagnosis (CAD) has had a great impact on automatic image analysis in the urological field. The objective of our study was to develop a CAD system with deep learning architecture to detect urinary tract stones on a plain X-ray and to evaluate the model's accuracy.

Methods: We collected plain X-ray images of 1017 patients with a radio-opaque upper urinary tract stone. X-ray images ($n=827$ and 190) were used as the training and test data, respectively. We used a 17-layer Residual Network as a convolutional neural network architecture for patch-wise training. The training data were repeatedly used until the best model accuracy was achieved within 300 runs. The F score, which is a harmonic mean of the sensitivity and positive predictive value (PPV) and represents the balance of the accuracy, was measured to evaluate the model's accuracy.

Results: Using deep learning, we developed a CAD model that needed 110 ms to provide an answer for each X-ray image. The best F score was 0.752, and the sensitivity and PPV were 0.872 and 0.662, respectively. When limited to a proximal ureter stone, the sensitivity and PPV were 0.925 and 0.876, respectively, and they were the lowest at mid-ureter.

Conclusion: CAD of a plain X-ray may be a promising method to detect radio-opaque urinary tract stones with satisfactory sensitivity although the PPV could still be improved. The CAD model detects urinary tract stones quickly and automatically and has the potential to become a helpful screening modality especially for primary care physicians for diagnosing urolithiasis. Further study using a higher volume of data would improve the diagnostic performance of CAD models to detect urinary tract stones on a plain X-ray.

*Correspondence: yoh-m.uro@tmd.ac.jp
[2] Department of Urology, Tokyo Medical and Dental University, Tokyo, Japan
Full list of author information is available at the end of the article

Keywords: Artificial intelligence, Convolutional neural network, Deep learning, X-ray, Urinary tract stone, Urolithiasis

Background

Urolithiasis is a common disease. Non-contrast computed tomography (CT) has become the gold standard modality as an imaging examination for diagnosing urolithiasis because of its high accuracy, which is reportedly 92–100%, and its excellent ability to detect other acute flank pain conditions [1–3]. However, some problems have emerged. CT is generally an expensive examination compared with others such as intravenous urography [4], and it is not preferred for pregnant women or children [5, 6]. Therefore, the repetitive use of CT is unsuitable for follow-up based on cost-effectiveness and radiation exposure. To reduce radiation exposure, low-dose CT is a promising option [7]. However, CT is not necessarily available in small-sized medical institutions such as in a medical office [8] because a CT scanner is expensive and requires a high level of interpretation capability. Conversely, a plain X-ray is a low-cost examination that has low-dose radiation exposure and high availability, although its accuracy, which is reportedly 44–77%, is inferior to that of CT [9].

An increased use of medical images induces further burden of their interpretation for physicians. Recently, a considerable amount of evidence has demonstrated the utility of artificial intelligence for diagnostic imaging. A computer-aided diagnosis (CAD) has been especially receiving attention in recent years. A neural network is a machine learning model that was designed to mimic human neural systems. Since the advent of a convolutional neural network (CNN) via deep learning in the 2000s, which is an advanced form of a neural network, CAD accuracy has increased and CAD has had a great impact on automatic image analysis in the urological field, leading to some successful reports about the detection of prostate cancer on magnetic resonance imaging (MRI) or the differentiation of distal ureteral stones and pelvic phleboliths [10, 11]. A combination of X-ray and CAD has also become successful in improving the diagnostic ability for various diseases, although its efficacy for identifying urinary tract stones has not been studied [12, 13]. In this study, we developed a CAD algorithm with deep learning architecture to automatically detect urinary tract stones on a plain X-ray image and evaluated the efficacy of this new model.

Methods

Study design and datasets

Ethics board approval was obtained from the Tokyo Medical and Dental University Ethics Review Committee (approval number M2018-176). This was a multicenter retrospective study. We collected plain X-ray images of 1123 patients who were diagnosed with upper urinary tract urolithiasis from 2013 to 2018 at three institutions. The diagnosis of urolithiasis was confirmed by urologists based on the CT images in all cases. We excluded 106 cases that had only radiolucent urinary tract stones. X-ray images of 1017 patients with a radio-opaque urinary tract stone were used for this study. We enrolled 616 patients from Tsuchiura Kyodo General Hospital, 211 from Tokyo Medical and Dental University, and 190 from JA Toride Medical Center. We included only one image per patient. If the X-ray was repeated, only the image that was performed at diagnosis was included. Images with a visible artificial foreign body on the X-ray were included. We divided all X-ray images into two datasets, as follows: a training dataset consisting of 827 X-ray images from Tsuchiura Kyodo General Hospital and Tokyo Medical and Dental University, which were used to develop the CAD algorithm; and a test dataset consisting of 190 X-ray images from the JA Toride Medical Center, which were used to evaluate the model that we created. Figure 1 shows the inclusion and exclusion criteria and the outline of the present study.

Labeling stone lesions

Among all of the X-ray images, all visible stone lesions were labeled as the correct information by urologists who manually traced the stone outline (Fig. 2a, b), with reference to the CT scan images. Invisible stone lesions on the X-ray were ignored in this study.

Image pre-processing

All X-ray images were resized to 1328 × 1328 pixels to accommodate the different image size in each hospital. Histogram equalization was used to enhance contrast. In the training data, patches that were 166 × 166 pixels were cropped from resized X-ray images to randomly reduce the amount of calculations based on the following rules: (1) patches were forced to include a urinary tract stone or not at the same rate; (2) a urinary tract stone was forced to be centered in the patch if it was included; and (3) patches without any part of a urinary tract stone were forced to be created if the stone was not included (Fig. 2c). These patches were then divided into the follow

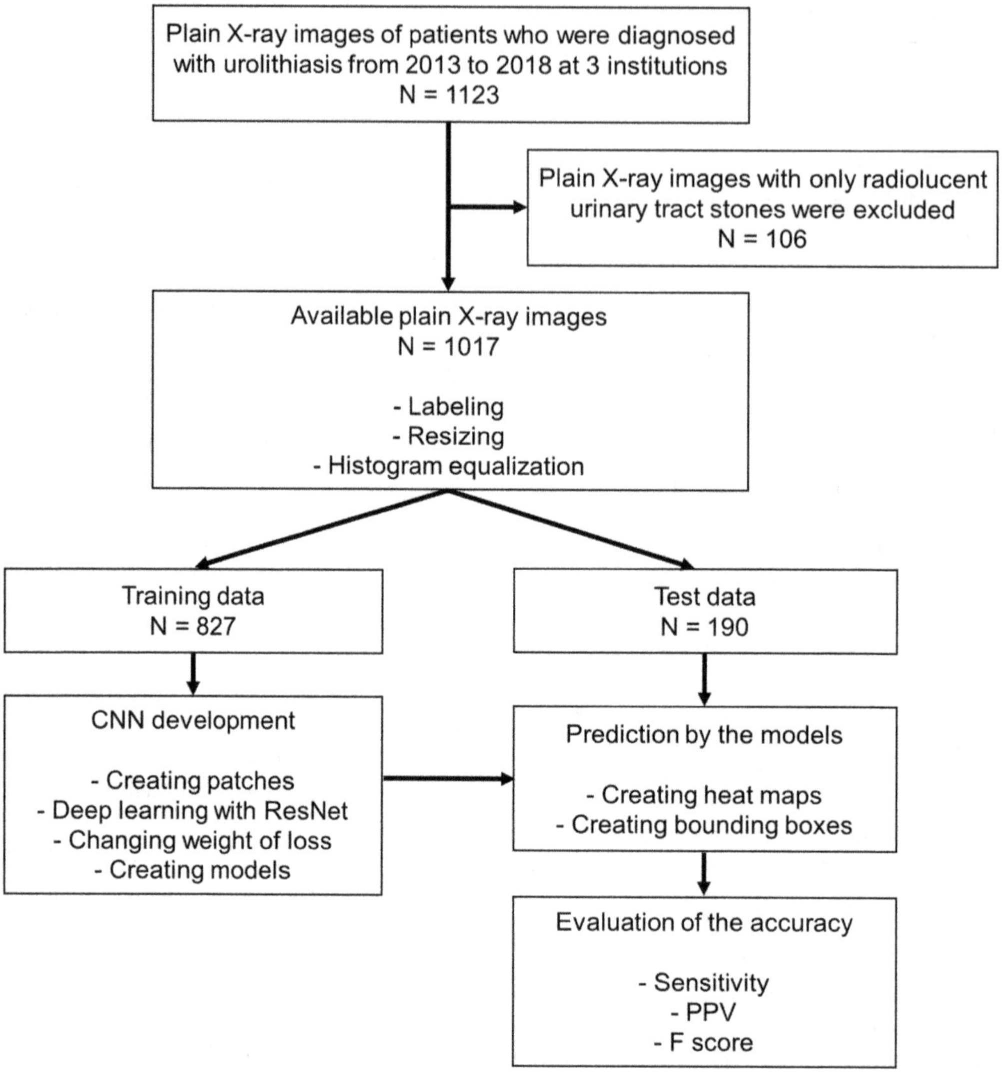

CNN: convolutional neural network, ResNet: residual network, PPV: positive predictive value

Fig. 1 Flowchart of the inclusion and exclusion criteria and study outline. Eight hundred and twenty-seven X-ray images were used for training and 190 X-ray images were used for evaluating the model's accuracy

ing two groups based on whether or not the urinary tract stone lesion was contained in the patch: patches including or not including a stone lesion.

Deep learning for training

To develop the CAD algorithm, deep learning with graphics processing unit (GPU) computing using a computer equipped with GeForce GTX 1080 graphics card (Nvidia, Santa Clara, CA, USA) was performed. As a CNN architecture for a patch-wise training, we used a 17-layer Residual Network (ResNet) in this study [14]. Figure 3 shows the ResNet architecture. The patches including or not including a stone lesion were used as input data and the computer determined whether or not a stone lesion was contained in the patch. The outputs were normalized to show a probability of stone's existence with the softmax function. There were two types of errors: overlooking and misdetection. An overlooking was an error that the patch included a stone lesion but the computer could not identify the stone, while a misdetection was an error that the patch included no stone lesion but the computer determined that a stone was present. Each error was calculated as a loss according to the probability of stone's existence which the computer

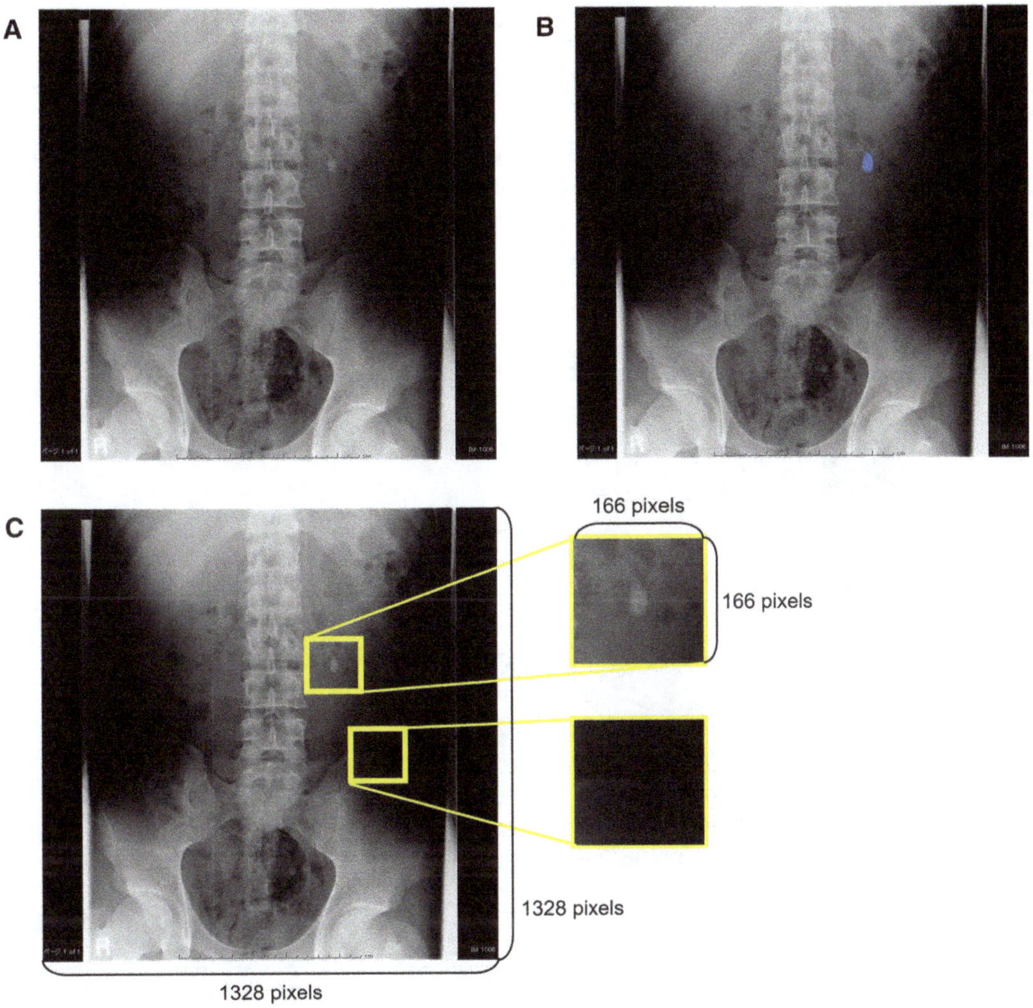

Fig. 2 Labeling stone lesions and image division into patches. **a** Resized plain X-ray image of a patient with a left ureteral stone. **b** Labeling of stone lesions by urologists. A blue area in the image is a label showing the correct location of the stone lesion. **c** Random cropping and creating patches. Patches of 166 × 166 pixels were randomly cropped from a plain X-ray image and divided into two groups: patches including or not including a stone lesion

output as a result of prediction. Using the back propagation method, the CNN's parameters were optimized to minimize each loss, which resulted in a model with fewer errors. In addition, several different weights of loss were tried for overlooking against misdetection to find a model with the most balanced diagnostic performance. The weight of loss for overlooking was a coefficient that we set up to adjust for the influence of overlooking when the weight of loss for misdetection was set to 1. For example, when the weight of loss for overlooking was set to 1, the loss was equally calculated among overlooking and misdetection. When the weight of loss for overlooking was set to 10, the loss for overlooking was calculated as 10 times more than that of misdetection. The weight of loss for overlooking affected how easily the model would overlook a stone lesion, and we could create models with different accuracies by changing this value. The training dataset was repeatedly used for the training, which was stopped when the model's best accuracy was determined within 300 runs.

Evaluation of the model's accuracy

The test data were used to evaluate the accuracy of the model that we created using deep learning. The computer was forced to identify urinary tract stones in each whole X-ray image of the test data, not in the patches. As the result of prediction by the computer, the probability of stone's existence was calculated in each pixel and demonstrated in each input image as heat maps that represented the probability of stone's existence by the color

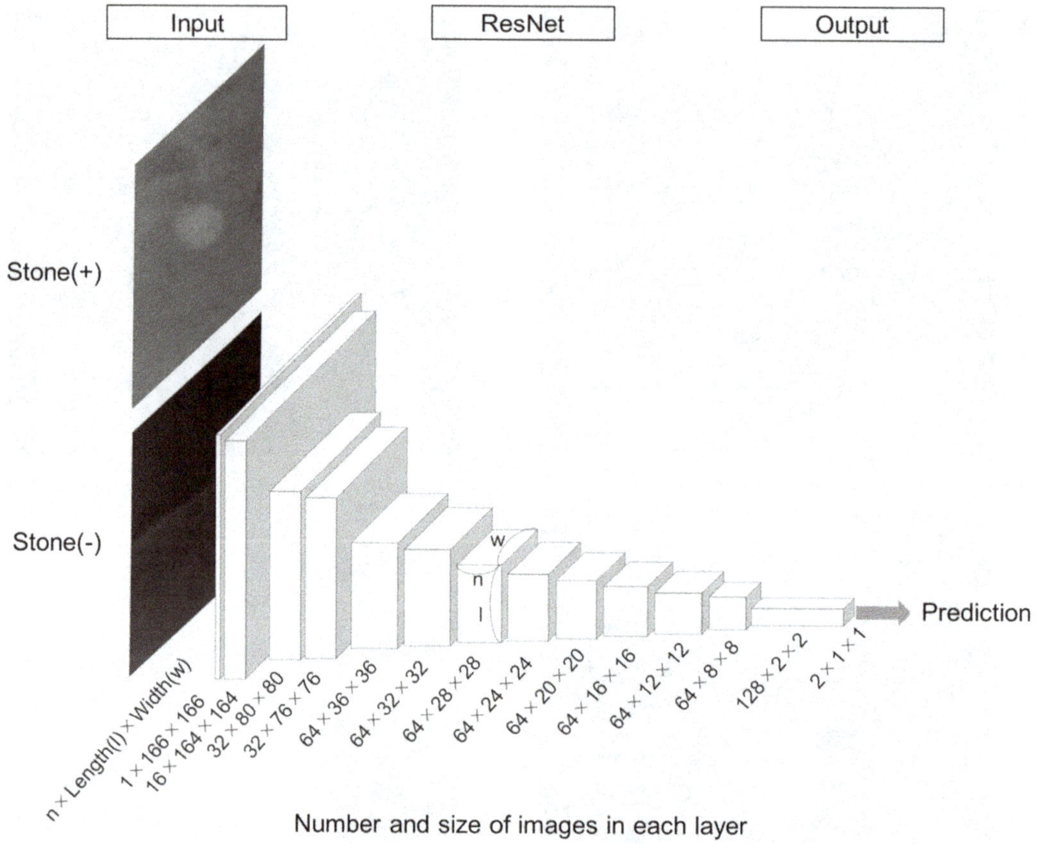

Fig. 3 ResNet architecture. The patches were input and convoluted as they passed through each layer. Each box indicates the number (n) and size (length (l) × width (w) = pixels) of images in each layer. The computer's prediction of whether an input patch was included was output and each loss was calculated if the output was not concordant with the input. The parameters were optimized using the back propagation method, in which each loss was supposed to be minimized

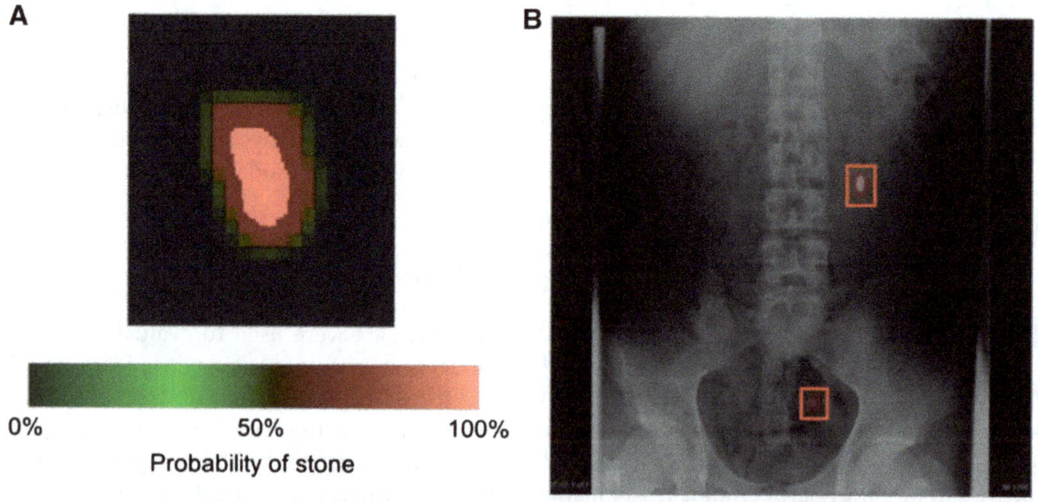

Fig. 4 Preparation to evaluate the model's accuracy. **a** Heat map representing the possibility of a stone lesion by color between light red at 100% and dark green at 0%. **b** Bounding boxes were automatically created to enclose three pixels outside of the heat maps

between light red at 100% and dark green at 0% (Fig. 4a). In addition, bounding boxes were automatically created to enclose three pixels outside of the heat maps (Fig. 4b). If the bounding box completely contained the stone label, it was considered to be a true positive (TP), and if not, it was considered to be a false positive (FP). Additionally, if a stone lesion was ignored, it was considered to be a false negative (FN). TP or FP were assigned to each bounding box and FN to each ignored stone lesion, and they were then counted. We measured the sensitivity, positive predictive value (PPV), and F score of the models that we created, with three different weights of loss for overlooking, as follows: 1, 10, and 20. The F score, which is usually used to compare the models' accuracies, is the harmonic mean of the sensitivity and PPV, and it reaches its maximum value at one and its worst value at zero. The closer the F score is to one, the more balanced is the diagnostic performance. Sensitivity, PPV, and the F score were calculated using the formulas that are described below.

$$Sensitivity = \frac{TP}{TP + FN}$$

$$Positive\ predictive\ value\ (PPV) = \frac{TP}{TP + FP}$$

$$F\ score = \frac{2 \times Sensitivity \times PPV}{Sensitivity + PPV}$$

Statistical analyses

Statistical analyses were performed using the JMP software program, version 10.0 (SAS, Cary, NC, USA). Data were compared between each group using Pearson's chi-square test or Fisher's exact test for categorical variables and Student's t-test or Mann–Whitney U test for continuous variables. Chi-square test was also used for comparing sensitivity or PPV. $P < 0.05$ was considered statistically significant.

Results

Patients and images characteristics

The characteristics of patients and images that are assigned to the training and test datasets are summarized in Table 1. There were no significant differences between both datasets for gender and the number of labeled lesions per image ($P = 0.132$ and 0.486, respectively). Patients in the training dataset were significantly older than those in the test dataset (58 vs. 56 years old, $P = 0.038$). The proportion of images with a urinary tract stone located at mid-ureter was significantly lower in the training dataset than in the test dataset (9.1% vs. 14.2%, $P = 0.046$). However, the proportion of images with a urinary tract stone that was located in the distal ureter was significantly higher in the training dataset than in the test dataset (22.2% vs. 9.5%, $P < 0.001$). In the present study, images with an artificial foreign body such as a ureteral stent, a nephrostomy tube, an artificial joint, and a screw

Table 1 Characteristics of patients and X-ray images assigned to the training and test datasets

	Training dataset	Test dataset	*P* value
Number of patients	827	190	
Gender, n (%)			0.132
Male	537 (64.9)	143 (75.3)	
Female	290 (35.1)	47 (24.7)	
Age, median (range), years	58 (17–89)	56 (14–87)	0.038
Number of labeled lesions per image, n (%)			0.486
One	656 (79.4)	144 (75.8)	
Two	112 (13.5)	32 (16.8)	
More than two	59 (7.1)	14 (7.4)	
Location of urinary tract stone, n (%)			
Kidney	428 (51.8)	106 (55.8)	0.895
Proximal ureter	334 (40.4)	72 (37.9)	0.582
Mid-ureter	75 (9.1)	27 (14.2)	0.046
Distal ureter	184 (22.2)	18 (9.5)	<0.001
Staghorn calculus, n (%)			0.553
Yes	17 (2.1)	2 (1.1)	
No	810 (97.9)	188 (98.9)	
Artificial foreign body in image, n (%)			0.672
Yes	53 (6.4)	10 (5.3)	
No	774 (93.6)	180 (94.7)	

for spinal surgery were included, resulting in no significant differences between the training and test datasets (6.4% vs. 5.3%, $P=0.672$).

Deep learning results and the model's accuracy

The GPU needed 9 h to finish learning the training data. The model that we created needed 110 ms to provide an answer for each image. Figure 5 shows four representative cases in which the computer's predictions were visualized. The sensitivity when the weights of loss for overlooking were 1, 10, and 20 was 0.872, 0.916, and 0.960, respectively. For each weight of loss, the PPV was 0.662, 0.488, and 0.418, and the F score was 0.752, 0.637, and 0.582, respectively. Figure 6 demonstrates a line graph showing the models' diagnostic performances that was created for each weight of loss for overlooking, indicating that the sensitivity was increased and the PPV and F score were decreased as the weight of loss for overlooking increased. Based on the F score, the diagnostic performance of the model that was created when weight of loss for overlooking was set to 1 was considered to be the most balanced.

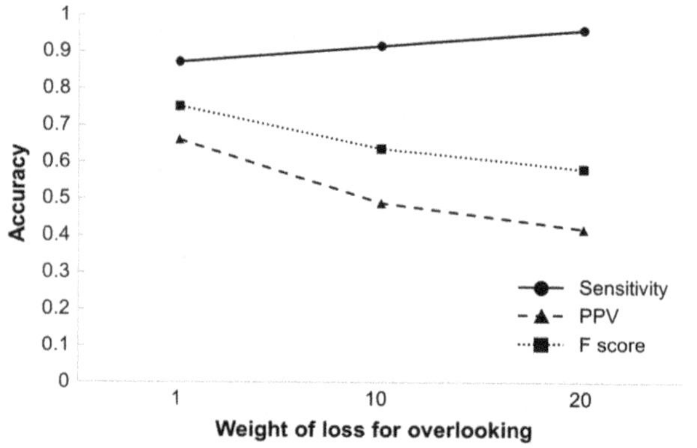

Fig. 6 The models' diagnostic performance that was created for each weight of loss for overlooking. This line graph indicates that the sensitivity was increased and that the PPV and F score were decreased as the weight of loss for overlooking was increased

The model accuracy for each urinary tract stone location

In our test dataset of 190 patients, 106 kidney stones, 107 proximal ureteral stones, 22 mid-ureteral stones, and 30 distal ureteral stones were identified by urologists. We studied the differences in the model's diagnostic performance based on the location of a urinary tract stone, using the model that was created when the weight of loss for overlooking was set to 1. In this case, the CAD model was able to detect 95 stones in the kidney, 99 stones in the proximal ureter, 13 at mid-ureter, and 24 in the distal ureter. Conversely, there were 72 FPs in the kidney, 14 in the proximal ureter, 13 in the mid-ureter, and 19 in the distal ureter. The diagnostic performance was as follows: the sensitivity was 0.896 in the kidney, 0.925 in

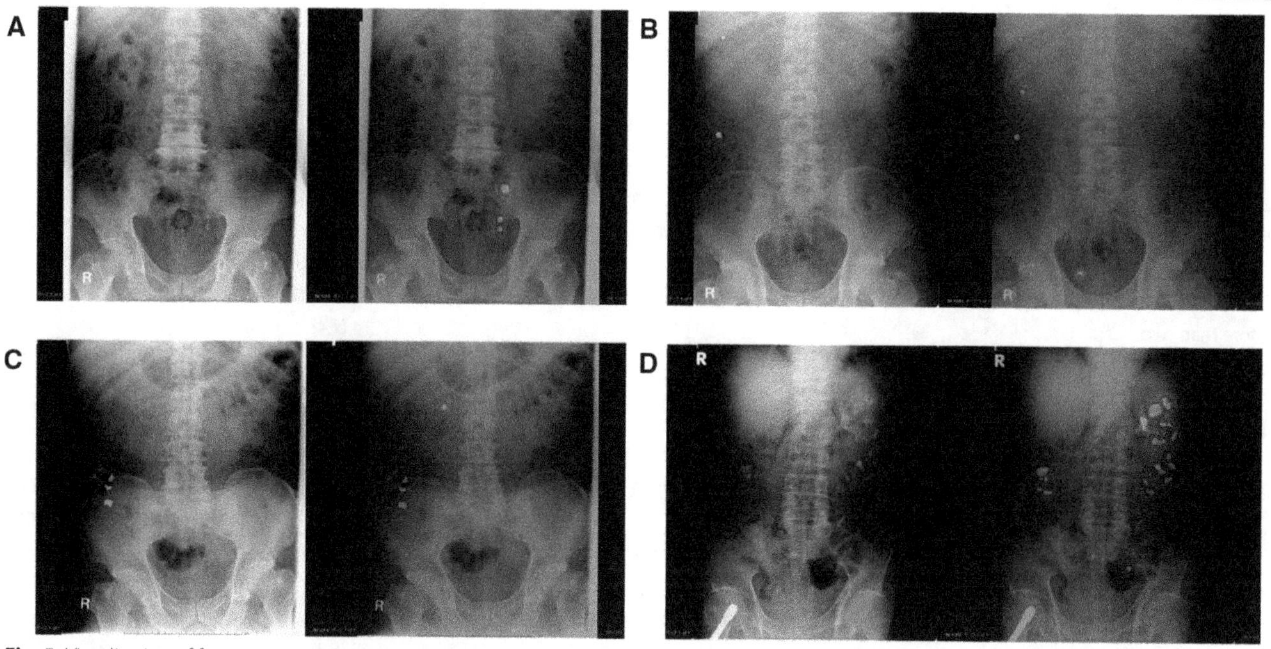

Fig. 5 Visualization of four representative cases. **a** A case with multiple calculi including a mid-ureteral stone. **b** A case in which a calculus was able to be distinguished from pelvic phleboliths. **c** A case with residual barium in the colon. **d** A case with multiple calculi and an artificial joint

the proximal ureter, 0.591 at mid-ureter, and 0.800 in the distal ureter. The sensitivity for mid-ureter stone was significantly lower than that for kidney and proximal ureter stone ($P = 0.001$ and < 0.001, respectively). The PPV was 0.569 in the kidney, 0.876 in the proximal ureter, 0.500 at mid-ureter, and 0.558 in the distal ureter (Table 2). The PPV for proximal ureter was significantly higher than that for kidney, mid-ureter and distal ureter stone ($P < 0.001$, < 0.001, and < 0.001, respectively). There were no significant differences except for the above-mentioned comparisons.

Discussion

In this study, we used deep learning to develop a CAD system to detect radio-opaque urinary tract stones on a plain X-ray. To our knowledge, there has been no report about automatic detection of urinary tract stones on plain X-ray. Our model was able to detect urinary tract stones quickly with a high sensitivity. This might become a new screening modality for diagnosing urolithiasis.

Automatic detection of urinary tract stones using a CAD system has several advantages. First, a CAD system is always able to provide quick and consistent interpretation without fatigue or fickleness. This capability is helpful in emergency medicine. Second, a CAD system is economical and easy to access because it can function as an application on a computer. There is no need to purchase any special machine and all we need to do is to install the application. Third, a CAD system with deep learning can have a self-learning system. Learning the mistakes that were made using a CAD system allows improvement of its diagnostic performance. Given these advantages, a plain X-ray with a CAD system may become a reliable modality in clinical practice as a screening tool, although the main problem is its accuracy.

We studied the diagnostic performance of a CAD system with a focus on a balance by changing the weight of loss for overlooking. In this study, we measured the F score, which represented a balance of the CAD system's diagnostic performance between overlooking and misdetection. The F score was best when the weight of loss for overlooking was set to 1, and the sensitivity and PPV were 0.872 and 0.662. According to the previous report about automatic detection of abnormality on chest X-ray, the sensitivity and specificity were 0.887 and 0.696, which are similar to our results [13]. The sensitivity seemed to be so satisfactory that the CAD system could help primary care physicians to find a urinary tract stone. In fact, this CAD model was able to detect a kidney stone of 2 mm in diameter (Fig. 5b). However, PPV was low, particularly in the kidney, at mid-ureter, and in the distal ureter. It was probably because the computer was likely to misdiagnose calcifications or bones as urinary tract stones. The computer did not have knowledge about the structure of the human body, resulting in mistakes that would not be made by physicians. On the other hand, another study reported that the combination of CAD system and CT had high accuracy in automatic differentiation of distal ureteral stones and pelvic phleboliths with the sensitivity of 0.94 and the specificity of 0.9 [11]. Another possible reason is the small amount of training data that we used in this study. We prepared only 1017 images for deep learning. This amount was low for training data for adequate deep learning. For example, in a previous report about deep learning for chest X-ray, over 100,000 images were used [15]. In the future, if we are able to prepare an adequate amount of training data and combine it with another algorithm to identify the human body's structure, the accuracy may be further enhanced. The CAD system that we created in this study seems to be useful as a screening tool, because X-ray has the several advantages such as low-cost, low-dose radiation and high availability.

Data augmentation is a method that is used to amplify training data by adding a change to an original image. We did not perform data augmentation in this study. In our pilot analysis, data augmentation did not improve accuracy (i.e. the best F score was 0.636), which was probably because the computer identified urinary tract stones based on their shape or orientation. Data augmentation by transformation or rotation might not be helpful for developing the CAD system to detect urinary tract stones. However, data augmentation without transformation or rotation may improve the accuracy. One such

Table 2 The accuracy of the model for each urinary tract stone location

Urinary tract stone location	Number of TP	Number of FP	Number of FN	Sensitivity	PPV
Kidney	95	72	11	0.896	0.569
Proximal ureter	99	14	8	0.925	0.876
Mid-ureter	13	13	9	0.591	0.500
Distal ureter	24	19	6	0.800	0.558
All locations	231	118	34	0.872	0.662

TP true positive, *FP* false positive, *FN* false negative, *PPV* positive predictive value

method is embedding augmentation, which means making a fake image that is similar to a real image [16]. Using stone embedding, we can create a large amount of fake images of urolithiasis and increase the training data for deep learning, leading to an improvement in the CAD system's diagnostic performance.

The present study has several limitations. First, we excluded cases with only radiolucent urinary tract stones, which is reportedly observed in 10% of patients with urolithiasis, because the diagnostic ability of the algorithm depends on the contrast information in the image [17]. This model can identify only lesions visible on plain X-ray. A radiolucent urinary tract stone will not be detected by models using a plain X-ray trained with CNN algorithm, although the combination with ultrasonography or intravenous pyelogram may be effective. Although the diagnostic performance of a CAD system would currently be inferior to CT for diagnosing radiolucent stones, a CAD system could be improved in the future, and it is expected to be used in various situations such as follow-up until stone expulsion or objective evaluation of stone treatment. In addition, if trained based on CT or MRI, the CAD system seems to gain the ability to accommodate various types of lesions, as we reported about automatic detection of prostate cancer in the previous study [10]. The efficacy of a CAD system combined with CT or MRI images for the urological field including not only urolithiasis but also neoplastic disease is under investigation. Second, the proportion of X-ray images with a distal ureteral stone was lower in the test dataset than in the training dataset. Distal ureteral stones were difficult to distinguish from pelvic phleboliths, which might tend to increase the number of FP results. Therefore, the test dataset in the present study might contribute to reducing the number of FPs. Third, we did not include negative images without a stone lesion. Therefore, the specificity and negative predictive value could not be calculated in this study. Prospective investigations of the CAD system's usefulness are required for urinary stone clinical practice.

Conclusions

We developed a CAD system using deep learning to detect radio-opaque urinary tract stones on a plain X-ray. The sensitivity was high enough to use the CAD model in clinical practice, although there was still room to improve the PPV. The CAD model can detect urinary tract stones quickly and automatically, and has the potential to help primary care physicians to diagnose urolithiasis as a screening modality. Further study using higher-volume data would improve the CAD models' diagnostic performance for detecting urinary tract stones on a plain X-ray.

Abbreviations

CAD: Computer-aided diagnosis; CNN: Convolutional neural network; CT: Computed tomography; FN: False negative; FP: False positive; GPU: Graphics processing unit; MRI: Magnetic resonance imaging; PPV: Positive predictive value; ResNet: Residual network; TP: True positive.

Acknowledgements

Not applicable.

Authors' contributions

MK, JI, YM contributed to study conception and design. MK, JI, RM, MF contributed to data acquisition. Suda R, Saiki R, KS, IK contributed to analysis and interpretation. MK and YM contributed to drafting the manuscript. YF, YK, KK, SM, NK, TO, SY, MY, YF contributed to editing the manuscript. YM and YF were the supervisors of this study. All authors read and approved the final manuscript.

Author details

[1]Department of Urology, Tsuchiura Kyodo General Hospital, Tsuchiura, Japan. [2]Department of Urology, Tokyo Medical and Dental University, Tokyo, Japan. [3]Department of Urology, JA Toride Medical Center, Toride, Japan. [4]Department of Information and Communications Engineering, Tokyo Institute of Technology, Tokyo, Japan. [5]Laboratory for Future, Interdisciplinary Research of Science and Technology, Institute of Innovative Research, Tokyo Institute of Technology, Tokyo, Japan.

References

1. Niall O, Russell J, Macgregor R, Duncan H, Mullins J. A comparison of noncontrast computerized tomography with excretory urography in the assessment of acute flank pain. J Urol. 1999;161:534–7.
2. Pfister SA, Deckart A, Laschke S, Dellas S, Otto U, Buitrago C, et al. Unenhanced helical computed tomography vs intravenous urography in patients with acute flank pain: accuracy and economic impact in a randomized prospective trial. Eur Radiol. 2003;13:2513–20.
3. Wang JH, Shen SH, Huang SS, Chang CY. Prospective comparison of unenhanced spiral computed tomography and intravenous urography in the evaluation of acute renal colic. J Chin Med Assoc. 2008;71:30–6.
4. Li J, Kennedy D, Levine M, Kumar A, Mullen J. Absent hematuria and expensive computerized tomography: case characteristics of emergency urolithiasis. J Urol. 2001;165:782–4.
5. Brenner DJ, Hall EJ. Computed tomography—an increasing source of radiation exposure. N Engl J Med. 2007;357:2277–84.
6. Goodman TR, Mustafa A, Rowe E. Pediatric CT radiation exposure: where we were, and where we are now. Pediatr Radiol. 2019;49:469–78.
7. Rodger F, Roditi G, Aboumarzouk OM. Diagnostic accuracy of low and ultra-low dose CT for identification of urinary tract stones: a systematic review. Urol Int. 2018;100:375–85.
8. Bellolio MF, Bellew SD, Sangaralingham LR, Campbell RL, Cabrera D, Jeffery MM, et al. Access to primary care and computed tomography use in the emergency department. BMC Health Serv Res. 2018;18:154.
9. Heidenreich A, Desgrandschamps F, Terrier F. Modern approach of diagnosis and management of acute flank pain: review of all imaging modalities. Eur Urol. 2002;41:351–62.
10. Ishioka J, Matsuoka Y, Uehara S, Yasuda Y, Kijima T, Yoshida S, et al. Computer-aided diagnosis of prostate cancer on magnetic resonance imaging using a convolutional neural network algorithm. BJU Int. 2018;122:411–7.
11. Jendeberg J, Thunberg P, Lidén M. Differentiation of distal ureteral stones and pelvic phleboliths using a convolutional neural network. Urolithiasis. 2020. https://doi.org/10.1007/s00240-020-01180-z.
12. Singh R, Kalra MK, Nitiwarangkul C, Patti JA, Homayounieh F, Padole A, et al. Deep learning in chest radiography: detection of findings and presence of change. PLoS ONE. 2018;13:e0204155.

13. Hwang EJ, Nam JG, Lim WH, Park SJ, Jeong YS, Kang JH, et al. Deep learning for chest radiograph diagnosis in the emergency department. Radiology. 2019;293:573–80.
14. He K, Zhang X, Ren S, Sun J. Deep residual learning for image recognition. Comput Vis Pattern Recognit. 2016. https://doi.org/10.1109/CVPR.2016.90.
15. Rajpurkar P, Irvin J, Ball RL, Zhu K, Yang B, Mehta H, et al. Deep learning for chest radiograph diagnosis: a retrospective comparison of the CheXNeXt algorithm to practicing radiologists. PLoS Med. 2018;15:e1002686.
16. Pezeshk A, Petrick N, Chen W, Sahiner B. Seamless lesion insertion for data augmentation in CAD training. IEEE Trans Med Imaging. 2017;36:1005–15.
17. Sakhaee K. Epidemiology and clinical pathophysiology of uric acid kidney stones. J Nephrol. 2014;27:241–5.

Development and validation of a preoperative nomogram for predicting patients with impacted ureteral stone

Chenglu Wang[1], Lu Jin[2], Xinyang Zhao[2], Boxin Xue[2] and Min Zheng[1*]

Abstract

Background: To develop and validate a practical nomogram for predicting the probability of patients with impacted ureteral stone.

Methods: Between June 2020 to March 2021, 214 single ureteral stones received ureteroscopy lithotripsy (URSL) were selected in development group. While 82 single ureteral stones received URSL between April 2021 to May 2021 were included in validation group. Independent factors for predicting impacted ureteral stone were screened by univariate and multivariate logistic regression analysis. The relationship between preoperative factors and stone impaction was modeled according to the regression coefficients. Discrimination and calibration were estimated by area under the receiver operating characteristic (AUROC) curve and calibration curve respectively. Clinical usefulness of the nomogram was evaluated by decision curve analysis.

Results: Age, ipsilateral stone treatment history, hydronephrosis and maximum ureteral wall thickness (UWT_{max}) at the portion of stone were identified as independent predictors for impacted stone. The AUROC curve of development and validation group were 0.915 and 0.882 respectively. Calibration curve of two groups showed strong concordance between the predicted and actual probabilities. Decision curve analysis showed that the predictive nomogram had a superior net benefit than UWT_{max} for all examined probabilities.

Conclusions: We developed and validated an individualized model to predict impacted ureteral stone prior to surgery. Through this prediction model, urologists can select an optimal treatment method and decrease intraoperative and postoperative complications for patients with impacted ureteral calculus.

Keywords: Impacted stone, Nomograms, Ureteroscopy, Urolithiasis, Computed tomography (CT)

Background

Urinary lithiasis has plagued more than 12% of the worldwide population during last several decades [1]. Impacted ureteral stones are defined as the stones staying in the same location for a prolonged time and causing ureteral obstruction [2]. Stone impaction is common in clinical practice and often lead to obstructive hydronephrosis, which may cause urosepsis even renal failure. It was reported that a patient with impacted stone caused

*Correspondence: reprodw@foxmail.com
[1] Reproductive Medicine Center, Department of Reproductive Endocrinology, Affiliated People's Hospital, Zhejiang Provincial People's Hospital, Hangzhou Medical College, No.158 Shangtang Road, Hangzhou 310014, Zhejiang, People's Republic of China
Full list of author information is available at the end of the article

urosepsis and required amputation of all 4 extremities [3]. Impacted stones are more common with intra-operative and postoperative complications because of the longer operation time and more complicated surgical procedures compared with non-impacted ones [4, 5]. Therefore, there is an urgent need for developing a tool to predict stone impaction prior to surgery. In previous research, ureteral wall thickness at the portion of impacted stone was identified as a critical predictor for SWL outcome [6]. Sarica et al. [7] indicated that the serum acute phase reactants CRP (C-reactive protein) and ESR (erythrocyte sedimentation rate) values as well as the UWT were helpful to estimate the presence of stone impaction. In recent, it was found that several preoperative factors, such as age, stone location and UWT, were strongly associated with the impacted ureteral stone [8]. Based on a review of previous studies, the present study aimed to evaluate the ability of preoperative factors for screening and identifying the stone impaction prior to surgery. In addition, established models for predicting ureteral calculi associated with urosepsis exist but the model for predicting the ureteric stone impaction is still in development [9]. Therefore, we subsequently developed and validated a preoperative model for predicting these stones.

Methods

Patients

After getting approval from institutional review board, we retrospectively analyzed 376 URSL for single ureteral stone removal at The Second Affiliated Hospital of Soochow University hospital between June 2020 to May 2021. Of these 376 procedures, 80 were excluded because of the lack of preoperative NCCT. Between June 2020 to March 2021, 214 single ureteral stones received URSL were selected in development group. While 82 single ureteral stones received URSL between April 2021 to May 2021 were included in validation group.

Data collection

Preoperative factors including patients baseline characteristics, laboratory values and radiological investigations were reviewed from medical records. Baseline characteristics recorded included age in years, gender, physical examination, medical history and ipsilateral stone treatment history. Stone impaction was defined intra-operatively, as failure to pass a guidewire or the smallest ureteric catheter pass the stone at 1st attempt. Patients were divided into 2 groups : Group1: impacted and Group2: Non impacted stones. Ipsilateral stone treatment history including the previous medical treatment or surgery for the same side ureteral stone. For radiologic evaluation, the preoperative NCCT was performed in all patients. Based on NCCT images, stone characteristics such as stone location, stone side, degree of hydronephrosis, maximum stone diameter, maximum cross-sectional area of the stone, stone volume, stone density (Hounsfield Unit) and UWT_{max} were reviewed by a blinded expert urologist. UWT_{max} was measured at an 8 times magnification in the axial view with an abdominal window (Fig. 1). Stone volume was estimated by scalene ellipsoid volume formula ($L \times W \times H \times \pi \times 0.167$) after measuring stone length, width and height. The degree of hydronephrosis was assigned as 0–2 values based upon follows: 0 = no or mild hydronephrosis (no calyces or renal pelvis dilation or renal pelvis dilation alone); 1 = moderate hydronephrosis (mild calyces dilation); 2 = severe hydronephrosis (severe calyces dilation).

Surgical procedures

After spinal or general anesthesia, all URSL procedures was performed in the lithotomy position using an 8/9.5 F semi-rigid ureteroscope (Karl Storz,

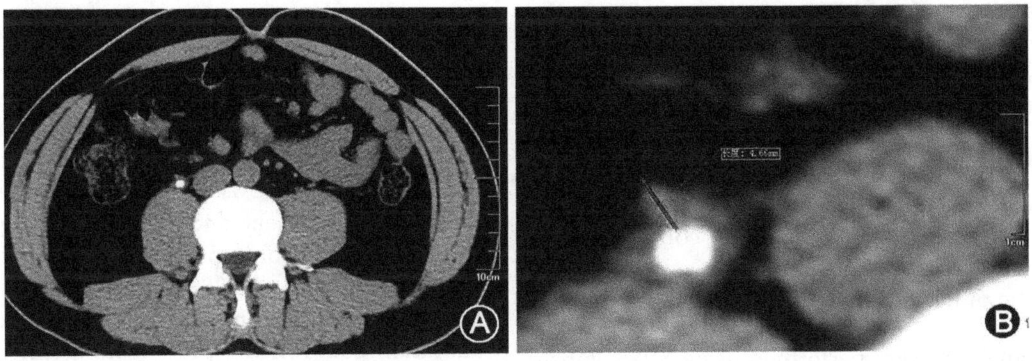

Fig. 1 **A** The ureteral calculus is demonstrated in axial section. **B** UWT max is calculated by the imaging software. Maximal (8 ×) magnification is used to facilitate

Tuttlingen, Germany), a holmium laser lithotripsy system (Lumenis, Santa Clara, Amercia) and a pressure-controlled irrigation pump (JingRui, Zhejiang, China). Before lithotripsy, a 0.035-inch guidewire (Terumo, Shizuoka, Japan) was employed to attempt to pass through the stone by a semi-rigid ureteroscope. If guidewire failed to pass the stone, URSL was firstly conducted for space creation between the stone and the ureteral wall. The stones were fragmented using holmium laser lithotripsy after guidewire placed in the ureter. If patients were diagnosed as proximal impacted ureteral stone, after space creating, a ureteral occlusion device was utilized for the prevention of stone migration before continuing stone fragmentation. A double J stent (size 4.7 F of 6 F) was inserted in ureter at the end of procedure. Four weeks after surgery, the stent was removed and abdominal x-ray film was taken to detect the stone-free status in the follow up evaluation. All procedures were finished by the same experienced endourologist.

Statistical analysis

All clinical factors were compared by Mann-Whitney *U* and chi-square tests. Continuous variables are presented as mean and categorical variables are presented as percentage. The factors showing statistical significance in univariate analysis were further included in the multivariate logistic regression analysis. A variable selection method of $P < 0.1$ was selected for variable elimination in the model. Before variable selection, nomogram variables were coded by a blinded investigator. Based on regression coefficients of selected variables, an individualized nomogram prediction model for ureteral stone impaction was established. The predictive ability of nomogram was evaluated according to discrimination and calibration. The discrimination refers to the ability to correctly distinguish between patients with impacted stones from those without impaction. Area under the ROC curve was calculated for the assessment of model discrimination. The calibration refers to the ability of concordance between the average predicted probability and the out prevalence in patients with impacted stones. Calibration curve was used to investigate the goodness of fit for prediction model. Additionally, the clinical usefulness of the nomogram was investigated by decision curve analysis. The net benefit of decision curve analysis, combined the number of true positives and false positives, was used to evaluate the practical value of risk model.

Statistical analyses were performed using SPSS statistical software (ver 24.0, USA) and R statistical software (ver 3.5.3, USA). Two-tailed analysis with $P < 0.05$ was considered as statistically significant.

Results

Patient data

A total of 296 patients were included in the present study. The stone-free rate in development group were 97.7% (non-impacted patients) and 89.0% (impacted patients) respectively, whereas stone-free rate in validation group were 98.0% (non-impacted patients) and 87.5% (impacted patients) respectively ($P < 0.05$). All clinical characteristics were presented in Table 1. Comparison of factors in development and validation groups indicated that no significant differences were found between patients in two groups. Significant differences between the impacted and non-impacted patients in the development group were viewed for the following parameters: age ($P < 0.001$), ipsilateral stone treatment history ($P < 0.001$), stone density ($P = 0.008$), hydronephrosis ($P < 0.001$), maximum stone diameter ($P = 0.002$), maximum cross-sectional area of the stone ($P = 0.002$), stone volume ($P = 0.002$), percussion tenderness over kidney region ($P < 0.001$) and UWT_{max} ($P < 0.001$).

Nomogram development

Statistically significant factors screened from the univariate analysis were further compared by multivariate logistic regression analysis. The four variables including age ($P = 0.046$), degree of hydronephrosis ($P = 0.026$), ipsilateral stone treatment history ($P < 0.001$) and UWT_{max} ($P = 0.001$) were identified as independent risk predictors of impacted stones (Table 2). Based on multivariate logistic regression analysis, the prediction model was established using the abovementioned four preoperative characteristics. An individualized nomogram was then developed (Fig. 2). According to the nomogram, the total score was obtained from the individual score of each prediction indicator, and the predicted risk corresponding to the sum of points is viewed as the probability of stone impaction.

Nomogram validation

The predictive ability of the model was evaluated according to discrimination and calibration. ROC curves along with AUC values were used to access the accuracy of the model in development and validation group. The estimated AUC values for impaction risk of these two groups were 0.915 (Fig. 3) and 0.882 (Fig. 4) respectively, demonstrating excellent discrimination for the predictive model. Calibration curve of the present model in both groups showed strong concordance between the predicted and actual probabilities (Figs. 5 and 6). Moreover, decision curve analysis reviewed that the practical nomogram

Table 1 Comparison of patients and stone characteristics according to the impacted stones and non-impacted stones

Variable	Development group (n = 214)		Validation group (n = 82)		*P* value
	Impacted (n = 82)	Non-impacted (n = 132)	Impacted (n = 32)	Non-impacted (n = 50)	
Gender (%)					0.203
Male	49 (59.8)	73 (55.3)	19 (59.3)	21 (42.0)	
Female	33 (40.2)	59 (44.7)	13 (40.6)	29 (58.0)	
Mean (SD) age, year	58.85 (12.34)	45.12 (12.78)	57.72 (12.19)	46.39 (12.92)	0.655
Hypertension (%)					0.267
Yes	29 (35.3)	40 (30.3)	8 (25.0)	13 (26.0)	
No	53 (64.6)	92 (69.7)	24 (75.0)	37 (74.0)	
Diabetes (%)					0.803
Yes	8 (9.8)	15 (11.3)	3 (9.4)	5 (10.0)	
No	74 (90.2)	117 (88.6)	29 (90.6)	45 (90.0)	
Ipsilateral stone treatment history (%)					0.885
Yes	50 (61.0)	20 (15.2)	18 (56.3)	8 (16.0)	
No	32 (39.0)	112 (84.8)	14 (43.8)	42 (84.0)	
Stone side (%)					0.543
Right	37 (45.1)	68 (51.5)	19 (59.4)	18 (36.0)	
Left	45 (54.9)	64 (48.5)	13 (40.6)	32 (64.0)	
Stone location (%)					0.707
Proximal ureter	40 (48.8)	69 (52.3)	14 (43.8)	24 (48.0)	
Middle ureter	18 (22.0)	21 (15.9)	8 (25.0)	10 (20.0)	
Distal ureter	24 (29.3)	42 (31.8)	10 (31.3)	16 (32.0)	
Hydronephrosis (%)					
NO or mild	4 (4.9)	89 (67.4)	1 (3.1)	29 (58.0)	0.252
Moderate	41 (50.0)	39 (29.5)	13 (40.6)	19 (38.0)	
Severe	37 (45.1)	4 (3.0)	18 (56.3)	2 (4.0)	
Mean (SD)					
Maximum diameter of stone, mm	8.67(2.28)	7.17(2.75)	8.52(2.54)	7.32(2.69)	0.872
Maximum cross-sectional area of the stone, mm^2	43.83(23.65)	31.14(23.64)	41.53(25.12)	32.97(25.06)	0.619
Stone volume, mm^3	386.20(296.60)	253.04(296.29)	373.57(292.37)	265.13(292.71)	0.335
Stone density, HU	847.66(282.39)	698.65(325.50)	858.92(281.87)	688.27(326.29)	0.329
UWT_{max}, mm	4.15(0.94)	2.58(0.76)	4.08(0.82)	2.53(0.78)	0.913
Percussion tenderness over kidney region (%)					
Positive	18 (22.0)	8 (6.1)	12 (37.5)	3 (6.0)	0.356
Weak positive	54 (65.9)	75 (56.8)	15 (46.9)	29 (58.0)	
Negative	10 (12.2)	49 (37.1)	5 (15.6)	18 (36.0)	
Stone-free rate	89.0% (73)	97.7% (129)	87.5% (28)	98.0% (49)	0.871

had a superior net benefit than that risk predicting with UWT_{max} for all of the examined probabilities (Fig. 7).

Discussion

Ureteral calculous disease is highly prevalent and affects both males and females in all age groups. Impacted ureteral stone is defined as the calculi staying at the same place in ureter for at least 2 months, causing inflammatory changes in the ureteral mucosa and resulting in epithelial hypertrophy as well as extensive ureteral edema [2]. For a prolonged period of obstruction, impacted stone may cause pyonephrosis, urosepsis, and even severe renal failure. Such stone is not uncommon in clinical practice. Thus, early diagnosis and treatment of impacted ureteral stone to avoid serious complications and consequences is essential for urologists. However, the development of new diagnostic methods had seen little progress during the last three decades. Previously, stone impaction has been defined as the calculi that has not progressed

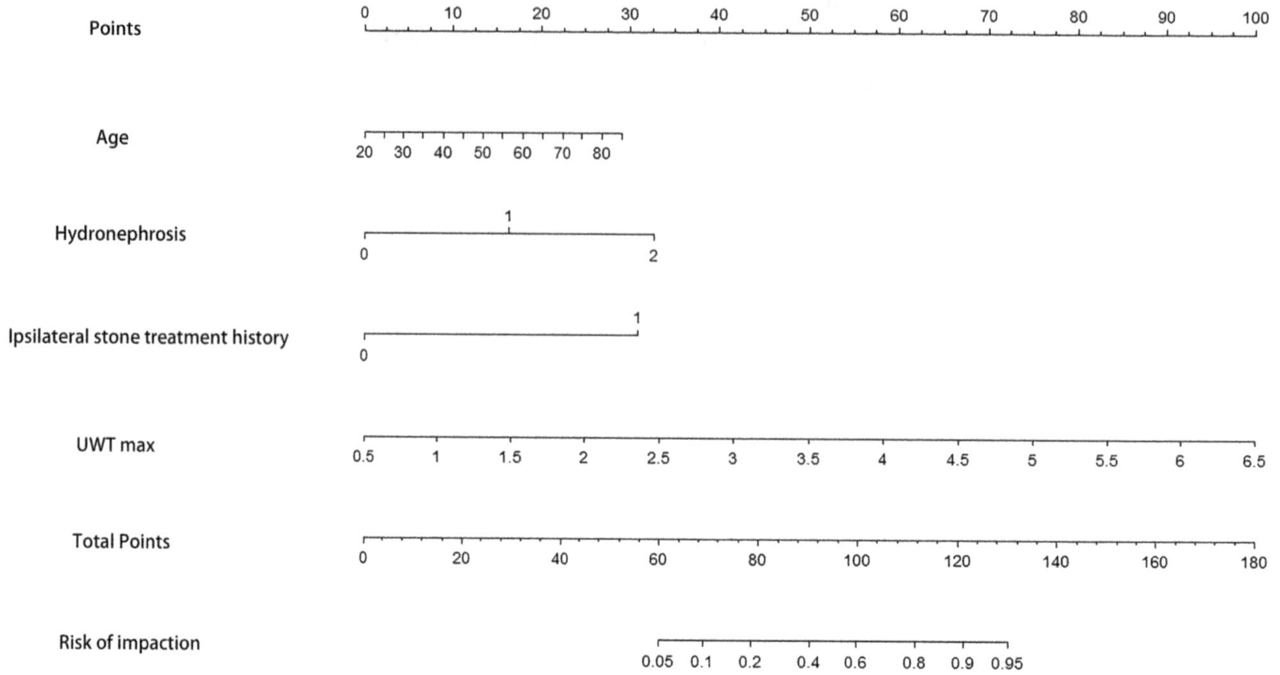

Fig. 2 Preoperative nomogram for predicting patients with impacted stone

Table 2 Univariate and multivariate logistic regression analysis of impacted prediction

Variable	Univariate analysis		Multivariate analysis	
	OR (95 %CI)	*P* value	OR (95 %CI)	*P* value
Gender	1.20 (0.69–2.10)	0.253	NA	
Age	1.12 (1.07–1.16)	< 0.001	1.06 (1.00–1.13)	0.046
Hypertension	1.26 (0.70–2.26)	0.441	NA	
Diabetes	0.84 (0.34–2.09)	0.712	NA	
Ipsilateral stone treatment history	8.75 (4.57–16.77)	< 0.001	5.20 (2.17–12.79)	< 0.001
Stone side	0.77 (0.45–1.35)	0.363	NA	
Stone location	1.48 (0.71–3.10)	0.300	NA	
Hydronephrosis	15.31 (7.41–31.62)	< 0.001	6.14 (1.22–11.29)	0.026
Maximum diameter of stone	1.24 (1.06–1.46)	0.002	NA	
Maximum cross-sectional area of the stone	1.02 (1.01–1.04)	0.002	NA	
Stone volume	1.00 (1.00–1.00)	0.002	NA	
Stone density	1.00 (1.00–1.00)	0.008	NA	
UWT max	10.17 (4.20–24.60)	< 0.001	6.23 (2.02–19.22)	0.001
Percussion tenderness over kidney region	0.91 (0.03–0.27)	< 0.001	NA	

proximally or distally for more than 2 months. Nevertheless, it is challenge for urologists to determine precisely the duration of calculi in the ureter. In addition, some researchers have defined an impacted stone as the antegrade or retrograde contrast cannot readily pass through it [10]. Nonetheless, using this method may precludes the opportunity for the selection of suitable surgical procedures because urologists cannot discover the impaction until the time of surgery.

Reviewing several studies published in the last few decades, UWT has aroused much attention since it was initially reported. After analyzing the clinical factors of 80 patients with single proximal ureteral stone, Kemal and colleagues found that the value of CRP, ESR and

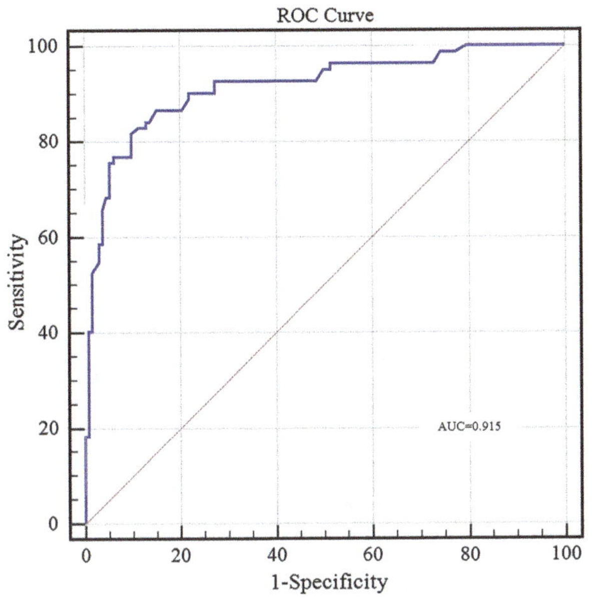

Fig. 3 The ROC AUCs of the development group

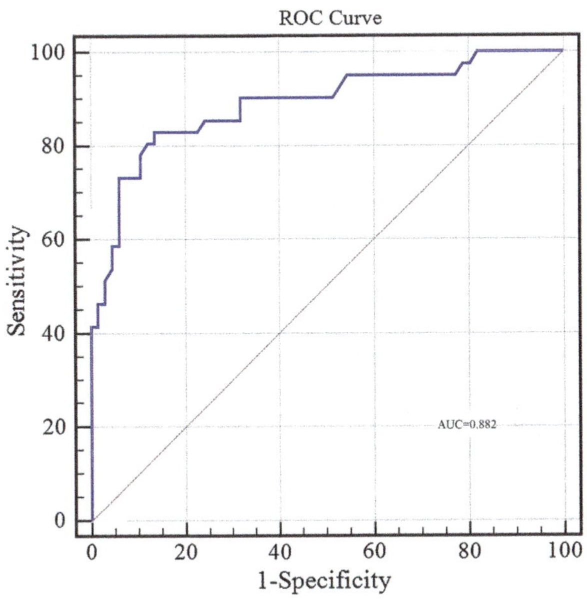

Fig. 4 The ROC AUCs of the validation group

UWT are associated with the presence of ureteric stone impaction [7]. They also noted that UWT can serve as a predictor for the final SWL outcome in patients with impacted proximal ureteral stones [6]. The recently-introduced study indicated that applying a cut-off of 3.49 mm, high UWT is closely related with a higher risk of stone impaction as well as more adverse outcomes of URSL [8].

Consistent with previous study, UWT_{max} was found as one of the independent pretreatment predictors for stone impaction in the present study. Apart from UWT_{max}, multivariate logistic regression analysis suggested that age in years, ipsilateral stone treatment history and degree of hydronephrosis were also as the preoperative independent predictors. Previous research found that ureteral hypertrophy, interstitial fibrosis as well as secretion of fibrinous exudate were basic pathologic changes of impacted ureteral stone [11, 12]. Endoscopic features including inflammatory ureteral polyps and ureteral stricture have been described by Mugiya et al. [12] Because of large stone burden and long period of obstruction, server inflammatory and immune response at the ureteral mucosa were recognized as the pathological causes of impaction [13]. The above-mentioned chronic and repeat episodes can further cause fibroepithelial ureteral polyps and ureteral stricture. Bolton et al. [13] retrospectively evaluated the records of 140 patients who were diagnosed as fibroepithelial ureteral polyps and discovered concomitant urolithiasis in 10 cases. Roberts et al. [2] found that 24% patients was associated with ureteral stricture during 5 to 17 months of stone impaction.

Except urinary calculi, there were several important risk factors including urinary crystals, stents, infection and residual fragments were identified as reasons for inflammatory response of ureteral tissues. Among four preoperative independent predictors, ipsilateral stone treatment history especially URSL was one of the most important factors which has strong correlation with the ureteral polyps and stricture. During URSL, ureteroscope was introduced into ureter by a guide wire and varying degrees of injury can be obtained by this invasive manipulation. Other operative risk events such as residual fragments after surgery, thermal tissue injury by the holmium and double J stent placement after stone extraction can happen during URSL. In view of the importance of stone treatment history, therefore, we hypothesized that the stone impaction can be avoided by minimizing intraoperative injury and reducing the residue rate of stone.

Extracorporeal shock wave lithotripsy (SWL), ureteroscopy lithotripsy (URSL), and percutaneous nephrolithotomy (PCNL) are the available noninvasive management strategies for ureteral stones [14]. Nonetheless, treatment of impacted ureteral stone remained a controversial issue for the urologists and the optimal treatment method for such stone still needs to be established. Compared with non-impacted stone, disintegration of impacted stone is more difficult because of the tissue changes at the surrounding ureteral wall and the lack of natural expansion space. Therefore, impacted ureteral calculi are considered as a high-risk factor for treatment failure, stone residue as well as the

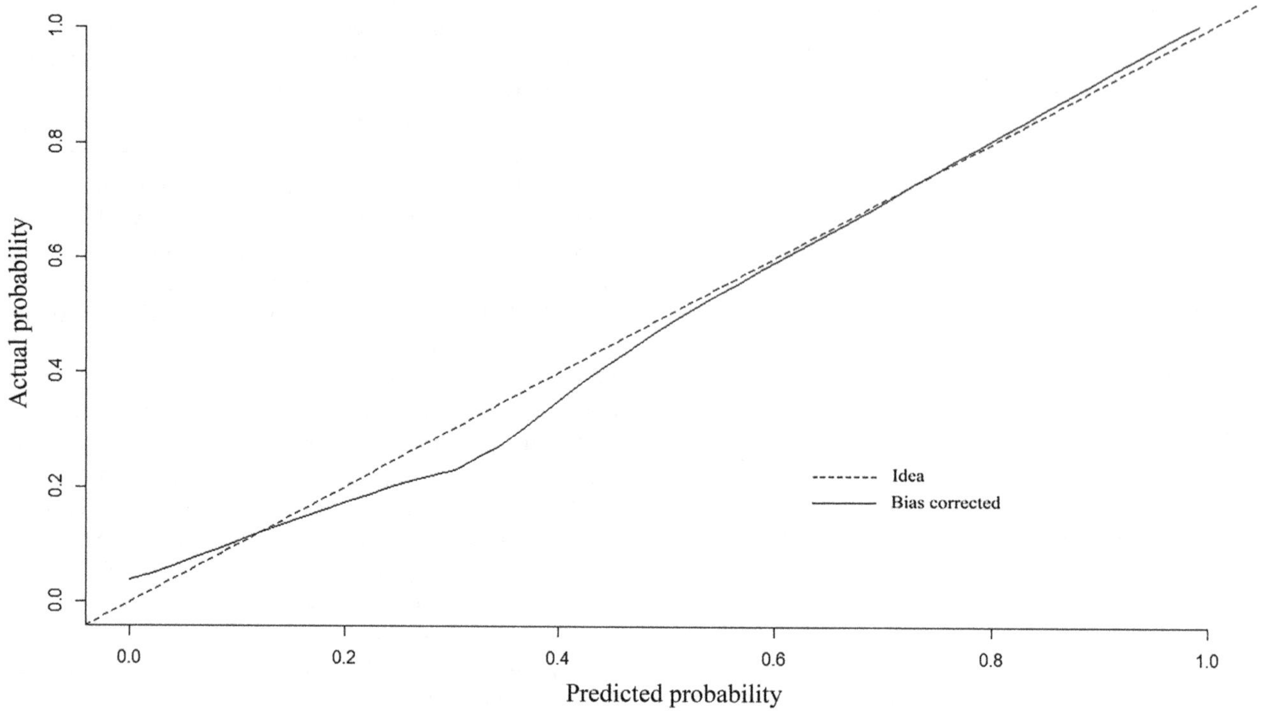

Fig. 5 The calibration curve of the actual vs. predicted probability of the preoperative nomogram for predicting impacted ureteral stone in the development group

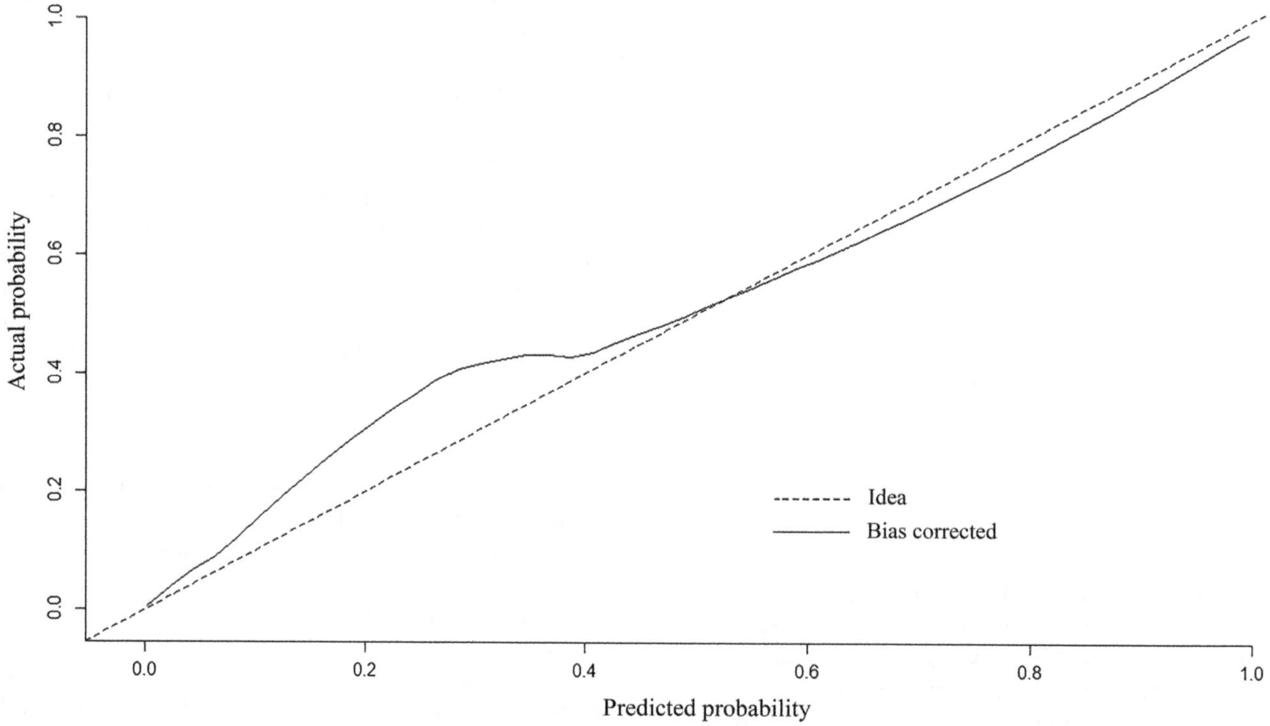

Fig. 6 The calibration curve of the actual vs. predicted probability of the preoperative nomogram for predicting impacted ureteral stone in the validation group

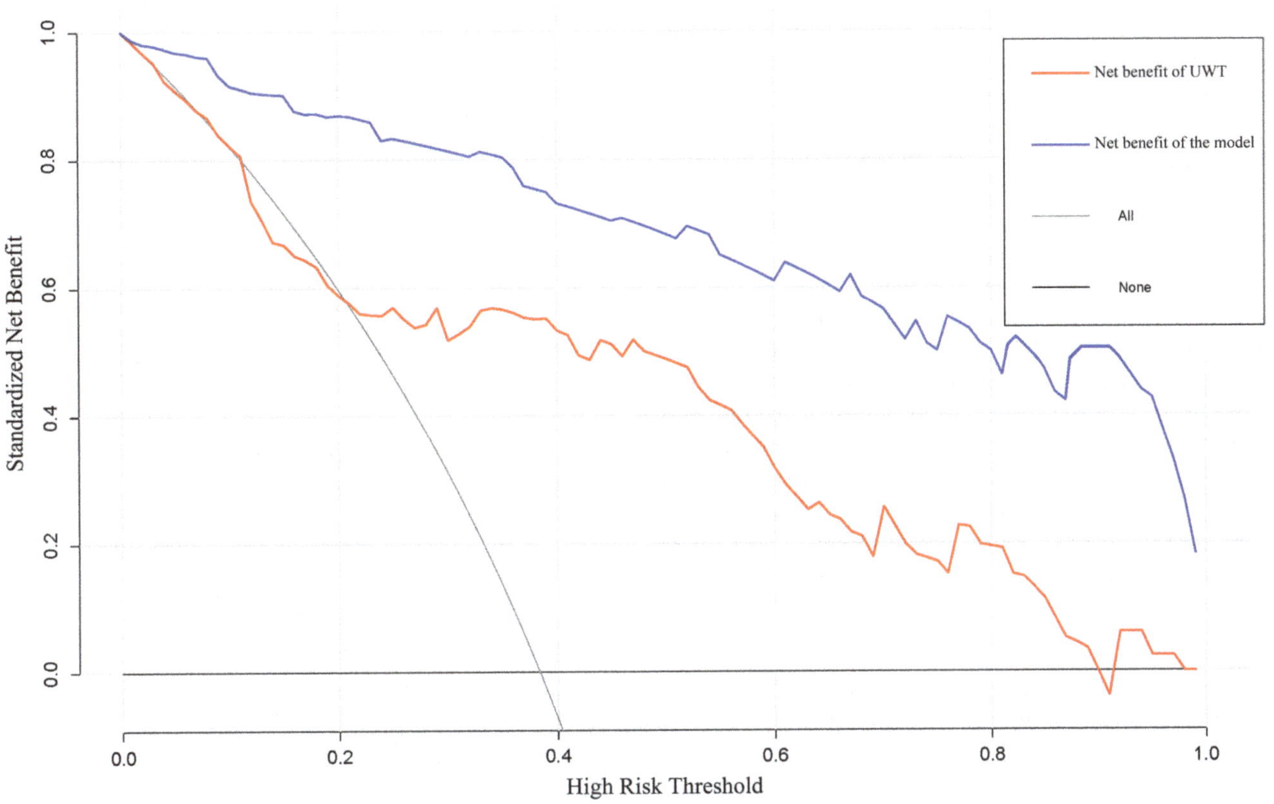

Fig. 7 The DCA of the nomogram

occurrence of intraoperative and postoperative complications [5]. Published studies so far have clearly demonstrated that SWL is a first line choice with acceptable and effective results for proximal ureteral stones [15, 16]. However, stone-free rates are greatly decreased as stone impaction with reported success rate of 45–60% [17–19]. With the predictive model for identifying proximal impacted ureteral stone before management, urologist could choose the antegrade approach strategies for these stones. Moufid et al. [20] reported that antegrade approach had significantly higher stone-free rate (95.5% v 66.7%) and lower failure rate (0% *v* 33%) for impacted upper ureteral stone > 15 mm. Long et al. [21] retrospectively reviewed 163 patients after treatment of mini-PCNL (MPCNL) and found 95.7% stone-free rate without any complications such as ureteral perforations or postoperative strictures in 6 months follow-up. In addition, a comparative study carried out by Wang et al. [22] showed that outcomes of MPCNL and retroperitoneal ureterolithotomy (RPUL) were more favorable than URSL in patients with impacted upper ureteral stone. Consequently, instead of URSL, MPCNL and RPUL are more recommended as suitable procedures if the patients' impaction risk predicted from the nomogram is high. Nephrostomy tube placement before URSL allows for decompression of the obstructed renal collecting system with minimal complications. This treatment procedure also could be considered as an option in case of impacted stones. Additionally, in a recently published study, tip-flexible semirigid ureterorenoscope was introduced as a novel management strategy for safely and effectively treating impacted stones with a low rate of complications [23].

Moreover, a report in recent research indicated that adjunctive tamsulosin therapy plays a critical role in relaxing ureteral smooth muscles, which allows a successful retrograde access for stone extraction and ureteral access sheath placement [24]. Consequently, if a urologist notes the predictive model suggesting stone impaction, alpha-blockers therapy prior to surgery were advocated for these patients.

Present study also has some limitations. Firstly, as a retrospective study, the selection bias cannot be avoided. Secondly, the data from clinical samples were derived from only one center. The validation of the nomogram needs more procedures from other centers. Therefore, in the following research, we will conduct a multicenter external validation with a large number of patients. Thirdly, the slice thickness of NCCT in our hospital is 1.25 mm. The UWT_{max} could be evaluated more accurate by the NCCT with optimal slice thickness.

Conclusions

This is the 1st attempt at developing a Nomogram to predict using preoperative parameters the possibility of impacted stones. From our study age/past history of stone treatment/degree of hun (will be ideal to say which grade) and UWT max are the 4 key criteria. This will help urologists to plan and counsel patients for a better ureteroscopic intervention outcome. To our best of our knowledge, this is the first study of a nomogram for predicting impacted ureteral stone prior to treatment. Through this prediction model, urologists can accurately identify impacted ureteral stone and select optimal treatment for patients.

Abbreviations

URSL: Ureteroscopy lithotripsy; AUROC: Area under the receiver operating characteristic curve; UWT_{max}: Maximum ureteral wall thickness; CT: Computed tomography; CRP: C-reactive protein; ESR: Erythrocyte sedimentation rate; NCCT: Non-contrast computed tomography; SWL: Extracorporeal shock wave lithotripsy; PCNL: Percutaneous nephrolithotomy; MPCNL: Mini-percutaneous nephrolithotomy; RPUL: Retroperitoneal ureterolithotomy.

Acknowledgements

There was no acknowledgements for this manuscript.

Author's contribution

CLW: Project development, data collection and management, data analysis, manuscript writing and editing. LJ: Data collection and management, manuscript editing. XYZ: Data collection, manuscript editing. BXX: Data collection, manuscript editing. MZ: Project development, data collection and manage ment, data analysis, manuscript writing and editing. All authors read and approved the final manuscript.

Author details

[1]Reproductive Medicine Center, Department of Reproductive Endocrinology, Affiliated People's Hospital, Zhejiang Provincial People's Hospital, Hangzhou Medical College, No.158 Shangtang Road, Hangzhou 310014, Zhejiang, People's Republic of China. [2]Department of Urology, Second Affiliated Hospital of Soochow University, Suzhou, Jiangsu, People's Republic of China.

References

1. Brener ZZ, Winchester JF, Salman H, Bergman M. Nephrolithiasis: evaluation and management. South Med J. 2011;104(2):133–9. https://doi.org/10.1097/SMJ.0b013e318206f6bd.
2. Roberts WW, Cadeddu JA, Micali S, Kavoussi LR, Moore RG. Ureteral stricture formation after removal of impacted calculi. J Urol. 1998;159(3):723–6.
3. Bender LC, Dubinsky TJ. The impacted ureteral stone. Ultrasound Q. 2012;28(3):235–7. https://doi.org/10.1097/RUQ.0b013e3182673795.
4. Degirmenci T, Gunlusoy B, Kozacioglu Z, Arslan M, Kara C, Koras O, et al. Outcomes of ureteroscopy for the management of impacted ureteral calculi with different localizations. Urology. 2012;80(4):811–5. https://doi.org/10.1016/j.urology.2012.05.007
5. Seitz C, Tanovic E, Kikic Z, Fajkovic H. Impact of stone size, location, composition, impaction, and hydronephrosis on the efficacy of holmium:YAG-laser ureterolithotripsy. Eur Urol. 2007;52(6):1751–7. https://doi.org/10.1016/j.eururo.2007.04.029.
6. Sarica K, Kafkasli A, Yazici O, Cetinel AC, Demirkol MK, Tuncer M, et al. Ureteral wall thickness at the impacted ureteral stone site: a critical predictor for success rates after SWL. Urolithiasis. 2015;43(1):83–8. https://doi.org/10.1007/s00240-014-0724-6.
7. Sarica K, Eryildirim B, Sahin C, Sabuncu K, Cetinel C, Narter F. Impaction of ureteral stones into the ureteral wall: Is it possible to predict? Urolithiasis. 2016;44(4):371–6. https://doi.org/10.1007/s00240-015-0850-9.
8. Yoshida T, Inoue T, Omura N, Okada S, Hamamoto S, Kinoshita H, et al. Ureteral wall thickness as a preoperative indicator of impacted stones in patients with ureteral stones undergoing ureteroscopic lithotripsy. Urology. 2017;106:45–9. https://doi.org/10.1016/j.urology.2017.04.047.
9. Hu M, Zhong X, Cui X, Xu X, Zhang Z, Guan L, et al. Development and validation of a risk-prediction nomogram for patients with ureteral calculi associated with urosepsis: a retrospective analysis. PLoS One. 2018;13(8):e0201515. https://doi.org/10.1371/journal.pone.0201515.
10. Deliveliotis C, Chrisofos M, Albanis S, Serafetinides E, Varkarakis J, Protogerou V. Management and follow-up of impacted ureteral stones. Urol Int. 2003;70(4):269–72. https://doi.org/10.1159/000070133.
11. Yamaguchi K, Minei S, Yamazaki T, Kaya H, Okada K. Characterization of ureteral lesions associated with impacted stones. Int J Urol. 1999;6(6):281–5.
12. Mugiya S, Ito T, Maruyama S, Hadano S, Nagae H. Endoscopic features of impacted ureteral stones. J Urol. 2004;171(1):89–91. https://doi.org/10.1097/01.ju.0000100960.08768.81.
13. Bolton D, Stoller ML, Irby P, 3rd. Fibroepithelial ureteral polyps and urolithiasis. Urology. 1994;44(4):582–7.
14. Preminger GM, Tiselius HG, Assimos DG, Alken P, Buck AC, Gallucci M, et al. 2007 Guideline for the management of ureteral calculi. Eur Urol. 2007;52(6):1610–31.
15. Lopes Neto AC, Korkes F, Silva JL, Amarante RD, Mattos MH, Tobias-Machado M, et al. Prospective randomized study of treatment of large proximal ureteral stones: extracorporeal shock wave lithotripsy versus ureterolithotripsy versus laparoscopy. J Urol. 2012;187(1):164–8. https://doi.org/10.1016/j.juro.2011.09.054.
16. Tiselius HG, Ackermann D, Alken P, Buck C, Conort P, Gallucci M, et al. Guidelines on urolithiasis. Eur Urol. 2001;40(4):362–71.
17. Chaussy CG, Fuchs GJ. Current state and future developments of noninvasive treatment of human urinary stones with extracorporeal shock wave lithotripsy. J Urol. 1989;141(3 Pt 2):782–9.
18. Mueller SC, Wilbert D, Thueroff JW, Alken P. Extracorporeal shock wave lithotripsy of ureteral stones: clinical experience and experimental findings. J Urol. 1986;135(4):831–4.
19. Dretler SP, Keating MA, Riley J. An algorithm for the management of ureteral calculi. J Urol. 1986;136(6):1190–3.
20. Moufid K, Abbaka N, Touiti D, Adermouch L, Amine M, Lezrek M. Large impacted upper ureteral calculi: A comparative study between retrograde ureterolithotripsy and percutaneous antegrade ureterolithotripsy in the modified lateral position. Urol Ann. 2013;5(3):140–6. https://doi.org/10.4103/0974-7796.115729.
21. Long Q, Guo J, Xu Z, Yang Y, Wang H, Zhu Y, et al. Experience of mini-percutaneous nephrolithotomy in the treatment of large impacted proximal ureteral stones. Urol Int. 2013;90(4):384–8. https://doi.org/10.1159/000343668.
22. Wang Y, Zhong B, Yang X, Wang G, Hou P, Meng J. Comparison of the efficacy and safety of URSL, RPLU, and MPCNL for treatment of large upper impacted ureteral stones: a randomized controlled trial. BMC Urol. 2017;17(1):50. https://doi.org/10.1186/s12894-017-0236-0.
23. Gao X, Zeng G, Chen H, Cheng Y, Wang K, Li J, et al. A novel ureterorenoscope for the management of upper urinary tract stones: initial experience from a prospective multicenter study. J Endourol. 2015;29(6):718–24. https://doi.org/10.1089/end.2015.0046.
24. Ahmed AF, Maarouf A, Shalaby E, Alshahrani S, El-Feky M, Khaled S, et al. Semi-rigid ureteroscopy for proximal ureteral stones: does adjunctive tamsulosin therapy increase the chance of success? Urol Int. 2017;98(4):411–7. https://doi.org/10.1159/000452926.

Low bone mineral density is a potential risk factor for symptom onset and related with hypocitraturia in urolithiasis patients: A single-center retrospective cohort study

Kazumi Taguchi, Shuzo Hamamoto*, Atsushi Okada, Yutaro Tanaka, Teruaki Sugino, Rei Unno, Taiki Kato, Ryosuke Ando, Keiichi Tozawa and Takahiro Yasui

Abstract

Background: Patients with urolithiasis have a lower bone mineral density (BMD) than those without stones, suggesting a potential correlation between calcium stone formation and bone resorption disorders, including osteopenia and osteoporosis.

Methods: To investigate the influence of BMD on clinical outcomes in urolithiasis, we performed a single-center retrospective cohort study to analyze patients with urolithiasis who underwent both BMD examination and 24-h urine collection between 2006 and 2015. Data from the national cross-sectional surveillance of the Japanese Society on Urolithiasis Research in 2015 were utilized, and additional data related to urinary tract stones were obtained from medical records. The primary outcome was the development of stone-related symptoms and recurrences during follow-up. A total of 370 patients were included in this 10-year study period.

Results: Half of the patients had recurrent stones, and the two-thirds were symptomatic stone formers. While only 9% of patients had hypercalciuria, 27% and 55% had hyperoxaluria and hypocitraturia, respectively. There was a positive correlation between T-scores and urinary citrate excretion. Both univariate and multivariate analyses demonstrated that female sex was associated with recurrences (odds ratio $= 0.44$, $p = 0.007$), whereas a T-score < -2.5 and hyperoxaluria were associated with symptoms (odds ratio $= 2.59$, $p = 0.037$; odds ratio $= 0.45$, $p = 0.01$; respectively).

Conclusion: These results revealed that low T-scores might cause symptoms in patients with urolithiasis, suggesting the importance of BMD examination for high-risk Japanese patients with urolithiasis having hypocitraturia.

Keywords: Urolithiasis, 24-h urine, Bone mineral density, T-score, Hypocitraturia

Background

The prevalence of urolithiasis is increasing worldwide [1], with a reported recurrence rate of 15 per 100 person-years [2]. With the recognized relationship between urolithiasis and metabolic syndrome, the increasing prevalence of metabolic syndrome, such as obesity and diabetes mellitus, is also speculated to increase the prevalence of urolithiasis [3]. Urolithiasis is not a direct life-threatening disease, but a recent study indicated that it could indirectly cause death with its slightly increasing trend [4]. Therefore, prevention is essential in reducing its economic and medical burden; however, there are few useful biomarkers for monitoring and predicting disease severity and recurrence except for 24-h urine parameters.

*Correspondence: hamamo10@med.nagoya-cu.ac.jp
Department of Nephro-urology, Nagoya City University Graduate School of Medical Sciences, Kawasumi 1, Mizuho-cho, Mizuho-ku, Nagoya 4678601, Japan

Calcium-containing stones are the most prevalent, and this disease pathology is clearly based on the mineralization process [5]. Patients with urolithiasis, especially those whose stones are composed of calcium oxalate and phosphate, are reported to have abnormal mineral laboratory findings, such as hypercalcemia and hypercalciuria, as well as bone metabolic symptoms including fractures [6]. The bone mineral density (BMD) of patients with urolithiasis is lower than that of those without stones [7]; even the male adolescent population demonstrates similar findings [8]. In particular, osteoporotic states often cause hypercalciuria in patients with urolithiasis due to deterioration in bone resorption [9]. This evidence indicates that the pathogenesis of urolithiasis is linked to osteogenesis via mineral metabolism.

Worldwide guidelines [10–12] recommend 24-h urine collection for patients considered high-risk stone formers, such as those with staghorn stones, recurrences, and comorbidities like metabolic syndromes. However, the examination of osteogenesis parameters, including BMD, is usually not recommended by experts despite the overlap between urolithiasis and osteogenesis. In contrast, with 24-h urine collection, few urologists examine BMD in patients with urolithiasis; hence, the clinical importance of monitoring BMD in patients with urolithiasis has not been fully understood.

We previously investigated the potential therapeutic influence of bisphosphonates on postmenopausal women with urolithiasis, who showed improved BMD and reduced risk of calcium phosphate stone formation [13]. Since then, we have been monitoring BMD in patients with urolithiasis to better understand its role in the pathogenesis of urolithiasis. This study aimed to evaluate the association between BMD and clinical outcomes in urolithiasis, including not only mineral parameters such as 24-h urine collection but also symptoms and incidence of recurrences.

Methods

Study design and patient selection

This retrospective cohort study was conducted at Nagoya City University (NCU) Hospital, a high-volume center. The institutional review board (IRB) approval was obtained from the medical research review board at NCU Graduate School of Medical Sciences (#60-19-0044), as well as Chiba University Graduate School of Medicine (#1962), Kanazawa Medical University (#226), and Osaka City University (#970) as national cross-sectional surveillance. The patients provided written informed consent. At the time of the national cross-sectional survey by the Japanese Society on Urolithiasis Research in 2015, all our patients with urinary stone disease diagnosed by radiographic evidence were included, as previously reported [14]. We utilized this surveillance data at NCU Hospital and selected patients with both 24-h urine collection and BMD examination at least once between 2006 and 2015 (Fig. 1). Patients younger than 18 years and those who had severe conditions due to other diseases were excluded from the study.

The primary outcome was the presence of symptoms during the follow-up and any recurrence, and the secondary outcome was the association between BMD data and 24-h urine parameters. The stone-related symptoms were confirmed by patients' self-reports of pain, discomfort, hematuria, and/or stone passage, which seemed to be related to urolithiasis; recurrence was confirmed by past medical history with either patients' self-reports or image findings.

Data collection

Patient characteristics, stone-related symptoms, treatment history of urolithiasis, comorbidities, and BMD examination results, blood tests, and 24-h urine collection were obtained from the survey data and institutional electronic medical records. We also captured doctor's lifestyle recommendations for fluid (> 2.5 L/day) and nutrition (increasing calcium-rich food and vegetables/fruits and reducing sodium and animal protein intake), which were obtained from the electronic medical records.

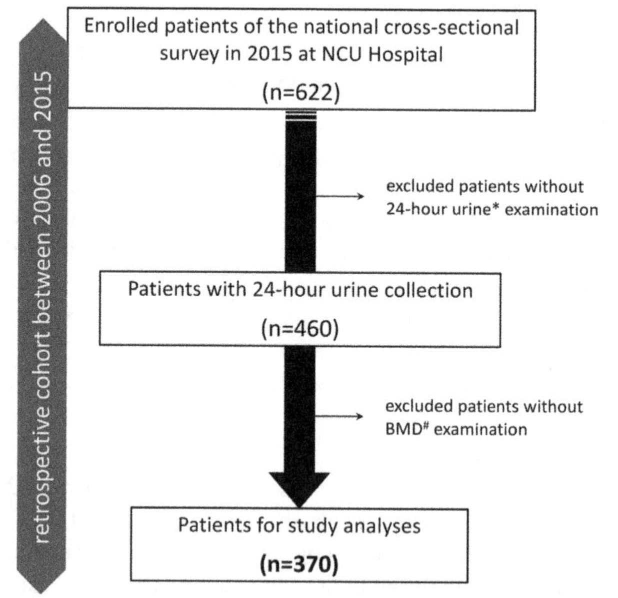

Fig. 1 Study design chart. *Examined for high-risk stone formers using at least one collection after surgical intervention and/or during clinic follow-up. #Examined for high-risk stone formers with suspicion of bone mineral abnormalities within 6 months of 24-h urine collection. NCU, Nagoya City University Hospital; BMD, bone mineral density

BMD was measured from the lumbar vertebra (L2-4) using dual-energy X-ray absorptiometry (DEXA) DELPHI A™; Hologic, Inc., Marlborough, MA, USA). With standard deviation (SD) based on the average BMD of young adults, the T-score was utilized for standard evaluation. The T-scores were categorized as normal (> -1.0), osteopenia (between -1.0 and -2.5), and osteoporosis (< -2.5), according to the World Health Organization guidelines.

Statistical analysis

We utilized means ± SD and medians (25% and 75% interquartile range) for normally and non-normally distributed variables, respectively. Differences were identified using either Two-sample t test, Mann–Whitney U tests, or Fisher's exact test. Differences were considered statistically significant at $\alpha < 0.05$ with analyses using EZR (R Project, Vienna, Austria) [15].

Results

Among 622 patients with urolithiasis at our institution from the national cross-sectional survey year in 2015, 370 were included in this 10-year study period. The background and sex comparison of the enrolled patients are summarized in Table 1. The sex comparison revealed that female patients were significantly younger at both disease onset and clinic visits and had lower BMI, lower recurrence rates, lower BMD and T-score/Z-scores, higher serum phosphate and urinary pH, and lower urinary phosphate, sodium, and oxalate excretion than male patients.

Among female patients, 77% were postmenopausal women, were significantly older, had a larger population with hypocitraturia and hypertension as comorbidities, and had much lower BMD and T-scores than premenopausal women (Table 2). The other background characteristics affecting bone and/or calcium metabolism, including nutrition recommendation, bisphosphonate/sodium potassium citrate/thiazide usage, and vitamin D supplementation, did not differ between premenopausal and postmenopausal women.

Additional univariate analysis comparing T-score ranges demonstrated that among patients with urolithiasis, those who had low T-scores were older and had lower BMI, higher prevalence of pseudohypoparathyroidism and renal tubular acidosis, higher bisphosphonate and thiazide use, and a lower and higher probability of having hyperphosphaturia and hypocitraturia, respectively (Table 3).

Figure 2 shows the scatterplots of the correlation analyses between T-scores and urinary parameters from the 24-h urine collection. There were positive correlations between T-scores and urinary phosphate excretion in male and postmenopausal female patients and urinary citrate excretion in male and premenopausal female patients. No association was found between T-scores and urinary calcium and oxalate excretion.

We further performed logistic regression analyses to determine the potential risks associated with patients' clinical outcomes with urolithiasis, such as the presence of symptoms during the follow-up period and the existence of stone recurrence before and during the follow-up period. Although the univariate analysis did not show any association between stone recurrence and BMD as well as urinary parameters, both univariate and multivariate analyses demonstrated that female sex was negatively associated with recurrences (odds ratio = 0.44, $p = 0.007$ in the multivariate analysis) (Table 4). In addition to recurrence, both univariate and multivariate analyses showed that hyperoxaluria was associated with a lower chance of developing symptoms during follow-up (odds ratio = 0.45, $p = 0.01$); however, a T-score < -2.5 was associated with a higher possibility of developing symptoms (odds ratio = 2.59, $p = 0.037$) (Table 5).

Discussion

Urolithiasis is known for its high prevalence and recurrence rate; therefore, close follow-up is important for preventing stone relapse and symptomatic events for better patient care [1, 2] In this study, we tried to investigate the relationship between the BMD and follow-up outcomes of patients with urolithiasis in clinical practice. Patients at high risk of urolithiasis, such as those with metabolic syndrome and metabolic abnormalities [16] should be carefully evaluated and followed-up; we speculate that the screening of BMD could be useful for reduce urinary risk factors including hypocitraturia and future symptom onset.

The relationship between urolithiasis and BMD was first reported in 1976 by Alhava et al. [17]. In their cohort of 21 male and 54 female participants, they found that the BMD was statistically lower in patients with urolithiasis than in healthy controls of both sexes. Since then, the association of urolithiasis with hypercalciuria and low BMD, particularly in postmenopausal women, has been recognized [18]. The main concern regarding bone metabolism in patients with urolithiasis is not only about having a higher chance of recurrence but also having a potential risk for fractures. A retrospective cohort study in the United Kingdom demonstrated that urolithiasis was associated with higher fracture risk, especially in adolescent boys and older women [19]. Similarly, two large cohort studies in the United States revealed that nephrolithiasis was associated with a markedly high risk of wrist fractures in both men and women (relative risk: 1.20) [20]. Interestingly,

Table 1 Patients' background and sex comparison of study population

	Total (n = 370)	Male (n = 233)	Female (n = 137)	*p* value
Age (years)	57.5 ± 14.6	55.5 ± 14.7	60.9 ± 13.9	0.001
BMI (kg/m^2)	24.4 ± 4.9	25.2 ± 4.7	23.2 ± 4.8	0.002
Age of onset (years)	46.5 ± 16.7	44.5 ± 16.1	50.1 ± 17.5	0.01
Previous history of urolithiasis	174 (53.7)	122 (58.9)	52 (44.4)	0.02
Presence of symptoms at clinic visits	216 (62.1)	142 (64.3)	74 (58.3)	0.30
Family history of stone	26 (22.2)	16 (19.3)	10 (29.4)	0.23
DM	50 (14.1)	32 (14.3)	18 (13.8)	1.00
HLP	94 (26.6)	63 (28.3)	31 (23.8)	0.39
HTN	109 (30.7)	65 (29.0)	44 (33.6)	0.40
PHP	11 (3.3)	4 (1.9)	7 (5.6)	0.11
RTA	3 (0.9)	1 (0.5)	2 (1.6)	0.56
Fluid recommendation	295 (82.9)	193 (85.8)	102 (77.9)	0.12
Nutrition recommendation	332 (93.3)	211 (93.8)	121 (92.4)	0.84
Thiazide use	1 (0.3)	0 (0.0)	1 (0.8)	0.37
VitD supplementation	4 (1.2)	0 (0.0)	4 (3.1)	0.02
BMD (g/cm^2)	0.91 ± 0.18	0.95 ± 0.17	0.84 ± 0.18	< 0.001
T-score	− 1.00 ± 1.48	− 0.58 ± 1.13	− 1.71 ± 1.72	< 0.001
Z-score	0.40 ± 1.48	0.12 ± 1.23	0.86 ± 1.73	< 0.001
Serum Ca (mg/dL)	9.3 ± 0.4	9.3 ± 0.4	9.3 ± 0.5	0.44
Serum P (mg/dL)	3.2 ± 0.5	3.1 ± 0.5	3.5 ± 0.4	< 0.001
Serum PTH (mg/dL)	46.7 ± 22.9	44.5 ± 21.8	49.6 ± 24.2	0.16
Urinary pH	6.50 [6.00, 7.00]	6.50 [6.00, 7.00]	6.75 [6.25, 7.25]	0.01
Urinary volume (L/day)	1.45 [1.05, 2.00]	1.50 [1.10, 2.05]	1.35 [1.00, 1.95]	0.05
Hypercalciuria	32 (8.6)	23 (9.9)	9 (6.6)	0.34
Hyperphosphaturia	35 (9.5)	30 (12.9)	5 (3.6)	0.003
Hypernatriuria	1 (0.3)	0 (0.0)	1 (0.7)	0.37
Hyperoxaluria	98 (26.5)	71 (30.5)	27 (19.7)	0.03
Hypocitraturia	203 (54.9)	124 (53.2)	79 (57.7)	0.45
Urinary Ca (g/day)	0.14 [0.09, 0.20]	0.14 [0.09, 0.21]	0.15 [0.09, 0.20]	0.97
Urinary P (g/day)	0.66 [0.50, 0.83]	0.71 [0.54, 0.87]	0.58 [0.41, 0.73]	< 0.001
Urinary Na (g/day)	2.54 [1.84, 3.31]	2.85 [1.98, 3.51]	2.13 [1.65, 2.96]	< 0.001
Urinary Ox (mg/day)	27.7 [20.6, 37.2]	29.7 [22.8, 40.8]	23.5 [16.9, 32.4]	< 0.001
Urinary Cit (mg/day)	347 [209, 508]	362 [216, 512]	329 [204, 508]	0.53

Values are presented as mean ± SD, n (%), or medians [interquartile range]

Definitions of urine abnormalities: hypercalciuria ≥ 300 mg/day; hyperphosphaturia ≥ 3 g/day; hypernatriuria ≥ 5.8 g/day; hyperoxaluria ≥ 40 mg/day; hypocitraturia ≤ 320 mg/day

BMI, body mass index; DM, diabetes mellitus, HLP, hyperlipidemia; HTN, hypertension, PHP, pseudohypoparathyroidism; RTA, renal tubular acidosis; VitD, vitamin D; BMD, bone mineral density, SD, standard deviation, Ca, calcium, P, phosphorus, PTH, parathyroid hormone; Na, sodium; Ox, oxalate; Cit, citrate

the Women's Health Initiative report indicated a significant association between urolithiasis and incidental total fractures in postmenopausal women by unadjusted analyses; however, covariate-adjusted analyses revealed no statistical association between them [21]. Although there is no absolute conclusion, a recent meta-analysis suggested that patients with nephrolithiasis had significantly lower T-scores, was four times more likely to have osteoporosis, and had a potentially increased risk of fractures [7].

The low BMD in patients with urolithiasis, especially calcium-containing stone formers, is caused by calcium metabolism disorders including hypercalciuria [6, 22]. In fact, patients with urolithiasis have a high occurrence rate of hypercalciuria, up to 50% reported in the literature [23]. Unlike the results of previous reports from Europe and the United States [9, 24], our cohort had only 8.6% hypercalciuria in both men and women but had a higher prevalence of hypocitraturia. Similar to our study cohort, a Japanese cohort also had a lower

Table 2 Background differences between premenopausal and postmenopausal women with urolithiasis

	Premenopausal female (n = 30)	Postmenopausal female (n = 103)	*p* value
Age (years)	41.1 ± 7.7	70.0 ± 9.2	< 0.001
BMI (kg/m^2)	23.1 ± 4.6	23.4 ± 4.9	0.77
Age of onset (years)	33.2 ± 9.0	56.4 ± 16.2	< 0.001
Previous history of urolithiasis	14 (46.7)	38 (44.7)	0.67
Presence of symptoms at clinic visits	15 (50.0)	55 (58.5)	0.53
Family history of stone	5 (16.7)	5 (21.7)	0.22
DM	2 (6.7)	16 (16.7)	0.24
HLP	3 (10.0)	28 (29.2)	0.05
HTN	4 (13.3)	40 (41.2)	0.01
PHP	2 (6.9)	5 (5.3)	0.67
RTA	0 (0.0)	2 (2.1)	1.00
Fluid recommendation	24 (80.0)	74 (76.3)	0.85
Nutrition recommendation	28 (93.3)	89 (91.8)	1.00
Bisphosphonate use	2 (6.7)	14 (13.6)	0.52
NaKCit use	10 (33.3)	27 (28.4)	0.65
Thiazide use	0 (0.0)	1 (1.1)	1.00
VitD supplementation	1 (3.3)	3 (3.2)	1.00
BMD (g/cm^2)	0.93 ± 0.15	0.81 ± 0.18	0.001
T-score	− 0.83 ± 1.47	− 2.01 ± 1.72	0.001
Serum Ca (mg/dL)	9.1 ± 0.5	9.3 ± 0.4	0.05
Serum P (mg/dL)	3.5 ± 0.5	3.5 ± 0.4	0.84
Serum PTH (mg/dL)	44.7 ± 16.5	51.8 ± 26.4	0.28
Urinary pH	7.00 [6.50, 7.25]	6.75 [6.38, 7.12]	0.56
Urinary volume (L/day)	1.25 [0.96, 1.64]	1.40 [1.05, 1.95]	0.36
Hypercalciuria	0 (0.0)	9 (8.7)	0.21
Hyperphosphaturia	2 (6.7)	3 (2.9)	0.32
Hypernatriuria	1 (3.4)	0 (0.0)	0.29
Hyperoxaluria	6 (20.0)	20 (19.4)	1.00
Hypocitraturia	11 (36.7)	66 (64.1)	0.01
Urinary Ca (g/day)	0.12 [0.08, 0.19]	0.15 [0.09, 0.22]	0.19
Urinary P (g/day)	0.60 [0.41, 0.76]	0.56 [0.40, 0.73]	0.44
Urinary Na (g/day)	2.05 [1.52, 3.01]	2.17 [1.66, 2.92]	0.96
Urinary Ox (mg/day)	24.9 [21.0, 34.3]	23.3 [16.2, 29.1]	0.21
Urinary Cit (mg/day)	395 [242, 548]	296 [178, 458]	0.07

Values are presented as mean ± SD, n (%), or medians [interquartile range]

BMI, body mass index; DM, diabetes mellitus, HLP, hyperlipidemia; HTN, hypertension, PHP, pseudohypoparathyroidism; RTA, renal tubular acidosis; NaKCit, sodium potassium citrate; VitD, vitamin D; BMD, bone mineral density, SD, standard deviation, Ca, calcium, P, phosphorus, PTH, parathyroid hormone; Na, sodium; Ox, oxalate; Cit, citrate

prevalence of hypercalciuria [18]. Low BMD is found to be associated with hypercalciuria; this could be an independent risk factor for developing urolithiasis [25–27]. Owing to our unique demography, a low prevalence of hypercalciuria was observed in those with low BMD and postmenopausal women; we hypothesize that a different mechanism from hypercalciuria may cause a lower BMD in Japanese patients with urolithiasis. This needs further essential investigation. Our study also demonstrated the demographic differences between premenopausal and postmenopausal women with urolithiasis. Despite the relatively low number of patients in our study, the finding that postmenopausal women had a higher prevalence of hypertension, lower BMD, and hypocitraturia was consistent with current evidence [28], implying that postmenopausal status was associated with a higher risk of urolithiasis.

The current study also demonstrated some correlation between BMD and urinary parameters, such as hyperphosphaturia and hypocitraturia. There was a positive

Table 3 Association between bone mineral density, disease severity, and osteogenesis parameters in patients with urolithiasis

	T-score			*p* value
	> − 1.0 (n = 186)	− 1 to − 2.5 (n = 135)	< − 2.5 (n = 49)	
Age (years)	55.3 ± 14.6	57.8 ± 14.6	64.9 ± 12.4	< 0.001
BMI (kg/m^2)	25.8 ± 5.1	23.5 ± 4.5	21.6 ± 2.5	< 0.001
Age of onset (years)	44.9 ± 16.0	46.1 ± 17.1	54.3 ± 17.3	0.01
Recurrence	89 (54.3)	65 (56.0)	20 (45.5)	0.48
Previous history of urolithiasis	113 (63.8)	69 (56.1)	34 (70.8)	0.16
Presence of symptoms during clinic visits	9.3 ± 0.4	9.3 ± 0.4	9.3 ± 0.5	0.39
Family history of stones	13 (19.4)	12 (32.4)	1 (7.7)	0.13
DM	24 (13.3)	19 (15.0)	7 (14.9)	0.91
HLP	51 (28.5)	32 (25.2)	11 (23.4)	0.70
HTN	56 (31.1)	36 (28.3)	17 (35.4)	0.66
PHP	2 (1.2)	4 (3.2)	5 (11.1)	0.004
RTA	1 (0.6)	0 (0.0)	2 (4.4)	0.02
Fluid recommendation	149 (82.3)	105 (82.7)	41 (85.4)	0.54
Nutrition recommendation	169 (93.4)	119 (93.7)	44 (91.7)	0.66
Bisphosphonate use	1 (0.5)	6 (4.4)	15 (30.6)	< 0.001
NaKCit use	37 (20.7)	31 (24.4)	12 (26.1)	0.63
Thiazide use	0 (0.0)	0 (0.0)	1 (2.2)	0.04
VitD supplementation	2 (1.2)	0 (0.0)	2 (4.3)	0.07
Serum Ca (mg/dL)	9.3 ± 0.4	9.3 ± 0.4	9.3 ± 0.5	0.39
Serum P (mg/dL)	3.2 ± 0.5	3.2 ± 0.6	3.4 ± 0.4	0.33
Serum PTH (mg/dL)	44.5 ± 21.4	47.2 ± 23.8	56.4 ± 26.3	0.21
Urinary pH	6.50 [6.00, 7.00]	6.58 [6.00, 7.00]	6.75 [6.12, 7.00]	0.47
Urinary volume (L/day)	1.50 [1.03, 2.15]	1.40 [1.10, 1.95]	1.40 [1.13, 1.88]	0.72
Hypercalciuria	13 (7.0)	17 (12.6)	2 (4.1)	0.10
Hyperphosphaturia	23 (12.4)	12 (8.9)	0 (0.0)	0.03
Hyperoxaluria	56 (30.1)	32 (23.7)	10 (20.4)	0.26
Hypocitraturia	92 (49.5)	76 (56.3)	35 (71.4)	0.02

Values are presented as means ± SD, n (%), or medians [interquartile range]

Definitions of urine abnormalities: hypercalciuria ≥ 300 mg/day; hyperphosphaturia ≥ 3 g/day; hypernatriuria ≥ 5.8 g/day; hyperoxaluria ≥ 40 mg/day; hypocitraturia ≤ 320 mg/day

BMI, body mass index; DM, diabetes mellitus, HLP, hyperlipidemia; HTN, hypertension, PHP, pseudohypoparathyroidism; RTA, renal tubular acidosis; VitD, vitamin D; SD, standard deviation, Ca, calcium, P, phosphorus, PTH, parathyroid hormone

association between T-scores and urinary phosphate excretion in men and postmenopausal women with urolithiasis. Although no prior research directly detected this relationship, a few papers indicated the relationship between low BMD and phosphaturia [29, 30]. Since the bone resorption mechanism involves phosphate metabolism, which is also regulated by the intestinal phosphate absorption, hyperphosphaturia in urolithiasis may be linked to lower BMD; this may explain the risk for stone development. Furthermore, we found that urinary citrate excretion was positively associated with T-scores in men and premenopausal women with urolithiasis. Citrate is considered to decrease with acidosis under circumstances of increasing bone resorption; therefore, patients with urolithiasis with osteopenia or osteoporosis tend to have hypocitraturia [24, 31]. In fact, some papers indicated that potassium citrate treatment reversed low BMD [32, 33]. Such evidence suggests that awareness of urinary citrate levels is essential for evaluating stone development risk factors, including BMD.

Most importantly, logistic regression analyses revealed that female sex was associated with a decreased odds ratio for stone recurrence, whereas osteoporosis status (T-score < − 2.5) was associated with an increased odds ratio for developing stone symptoms; however, hyperoxaluria was associated with a decreased odds ratio for developing stone symptoms. Interestingly, this result of association between T-scores < − 2.5 and symptomatic

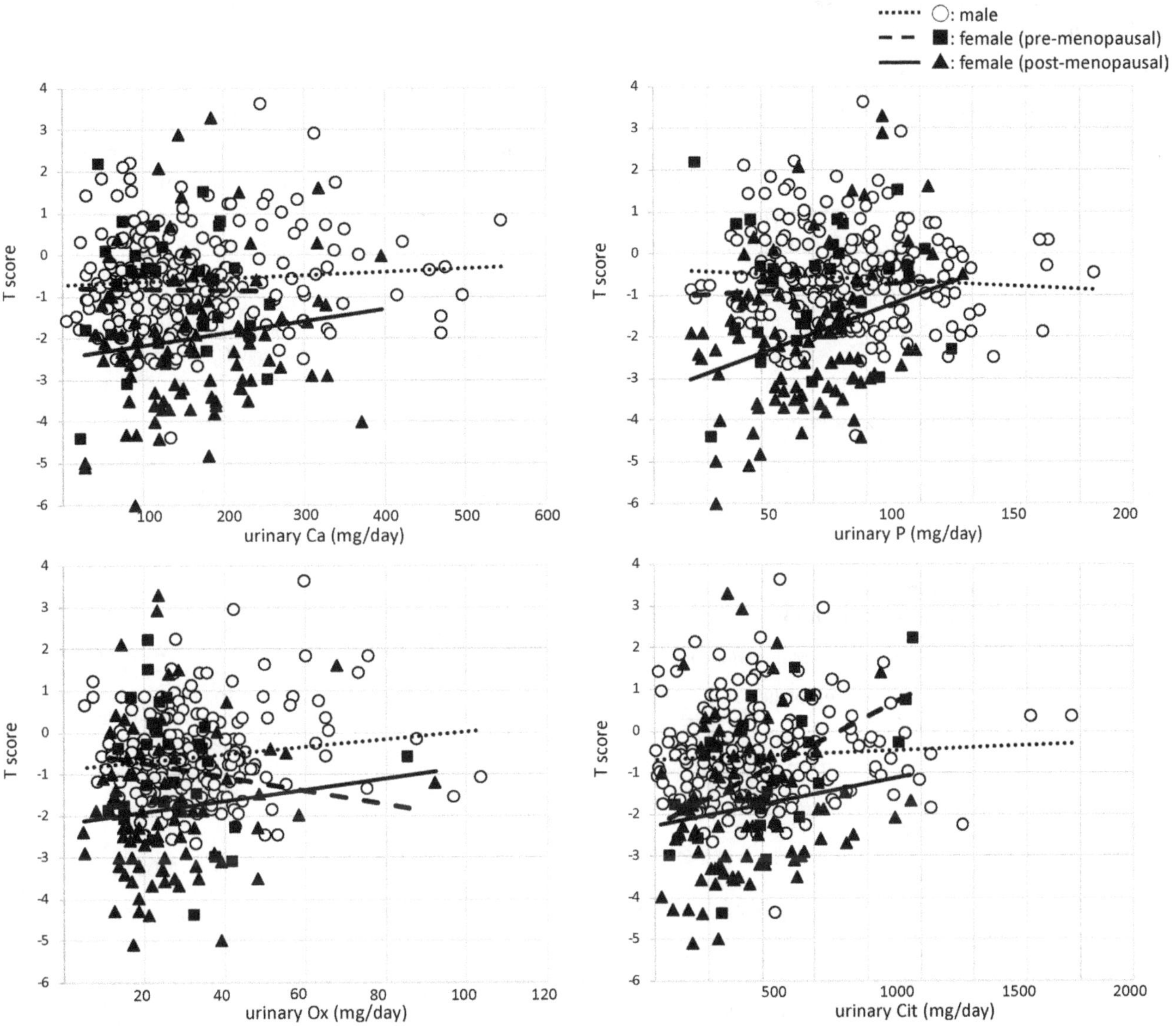

Fig. 2 Scatterplots of the results of Spearman's rank correlation tests between T-scores and urinary calcium (male: coefficient = 0.06, $p = 0.40$; premenopausal female: coefficient = − 0.03, $p = 0.89$; postmenopausal female: coefficient = 0.11, $p = 0.41$), phosphate (male: coefficient = 0.23, $p < 0.001$; premenopausal female: coefficient = 0.07, $p = 0.70$; postmenopausal female: coefficient = 0.32, $p = 0.01$), oxalate (male: coefficient = 0.14, $p = 0.05$; premenopausal female: coefficient = 0.21, $p = 0.31$; postmenopausal female: coefficient = 0.11, $p = 0.44$), and citrate excretion (male: coefficient = 0.18, $p = 0.01$; premenopausal female: coefficient = 0.57 $p = 0.003$; postmenopausal female: coefficient = 0.22, $p = 0.12$). Ca, calcium; P, phosphate; Ox, oxalate; Cit, citrate

stones was not observed on univariate analysis; this was probably due to the presence of confounders such as age, BMI, sex, and presence of urinary abnormalities. Examining BMD in patients with urolithiasis is important for effective follow-up; therefore, in real-world practice, this BMD evaluation may be performed in patients with a high-risk of urolithiasis at initial metabolic evaluation.

This study has several limitations, the primary being the study design. Although we could capture a large number of follow-up patients with urolithiasis who had both BMD and 24-h urine examinations, this single-center retrospective cohort study may not reflect daily practice data around the world. As described above, the prevalence of hypercalciuria was quite low, unlike previously reported rates among other ethnicities, suggesting a potential difference in calcium metabolism between the Asian population and others. Additionally, there is a lack of evidence regarding the stone composition and dietary/fluid records, which affect data interpretation. Preventive measures, such as bisphosphonates and NaKCit, may be

Table 4 Logistic regression analyses of bone mineral density and urinary parameters for stone recurrence

Factors	Univariate analysis		Multivariate analysis	
	OR (95% CI)	*p* value	OR (95% CI)	*p* value
T-score < − 2.5	0.68 (0.36–1.29)	0.24	0.86 (0.36–2.05)	0.73
Hypercalciuria	2.05 (0.86–4.86)	0.1	3.12 (0.92–10.60)	0.068
Hyperoxaluria	1.38 (0.83–2.28)	0.22	0.92 (0.48–1.75)	0.8
Hyperphosphaturia	1.29 (0.62–2.71)	0.5	0.79 (0.26–2.43)	0.68
Hypocitraturia	0.97 (0.63–1.51)	0.91	1.01 (0.56–1.81)	0.98
Female sex	0.56 (0.35–0.88)	0.012	0.44 (0.24–0.80)	0.007
age	1.01 (0.99–1.03)	0.47	1.00 (0.98–1.02)	0.83
body mass index	1.00 (0.95–1.06)	0.99	0.98 (0.92–1.04)	0.46

Data were adjusted by age, body mass index, T-score, hypercalciuria, hyperoxaluria, hyperphosphaturia, hypocitraturia, and female sex

Definitions of urine abnormalities: hypercalciuria ≥ 300 mg/day; hyperphosphaturia ≥ 3 g/day; hypernatriuria ≥ 5.8 g/day; hyperoxaluria ≥ 40 mg/day; hypocitraturia ≤ 320 mg/day

Table 5 Logistic regression analyses of bone mineral density and urinary parameters for symptomatic stones

Factors	Univariate analysis		Multivariate analysis	
	OR (95% CI)	*p* value	OR (95% CI)	*p* value
T-score < − 2.5	1.57 (0.81–3.06)	0.18	2.59 (1.06–6.36)	0.037
Hypercalciuria	1.18 (0.53–2.61)	0.69	1.35 (0.49–3.71)	0.56
Hyperoxaluria	0.60 (0.37–0.97)	0.038	0.45 (0.24–0.83)	0.01
Hyperphosphaturia	0.99 (0.48–2.04)	0.97	1.20 (0.43–3.36)	0.72
Hypocitraturia	0.88 (0.57–1.36)	0.57	1.24 (0.72–2.13)	0.44
Female sex	0.78 (0.50–1.21)	0.27	0.82 (0.46–1.45)	0.49
age	0.99 (0.98–1.01)	0.25	1.00 (0.98–1.01)	0.63
body mass index	1.00 (0.95–1.05)	0.88	1.01 (0.96–1.07)	0.66

Data were adjusted by age, body mass index, T-score, hypercalciuria, hyperoxaluria, hyperphosphaturia, hypocitraturia, and female gender

Definitions of urine abnormalities: hypercalciuria ≥ 300 mg/day; hyperphosphaturia ≥ 3 g/day; hypernatriuria ≥ 5.8 g/day; hyperoxaluria ≥ 40 mg/day; hypocitraturia ≤ 320 mg/day

biased by the preferences of physicians who diagnose and record the appropriate disease codes for connecting with the national insurance system. Lastly, our study did not include some bone turnover markers [6, 9] such as osteocalcin, β-cross-laps, and 25-hydroxy vitamin D, useful for evaluating bone metabolism; however, we believe that the current data set represents real-world data more accurately than currently available data.

Conclusion

Our cross-sectional study on 370 patients with urolithiasis undergoing BMD and 24-h urine examinations revealed that lower BMD represented as T-scores, was associated with hyperphosphaturia and hypocitraturia. Moreover, logistic regression analyses revealed that a lower T-score was associated with increased odds ratios for stone symptoms during follow-up. These novel findings suggest that examining BMD could be a useful tool for effective follow-up of urolithiasis; this may prevent future risks of stone development and may influence current practice strategy.

Abbreviations

BMD: Bone mineral density; BMI: Body mass index; DEXA: Dual-energy X-ray absorptiometry; NCU: Nagoya City University; SD: Standard deviation.

Acknowledgements

We thank the urology outpatient clinic staff and radiology staff of Nagoya City University Hospital, who provided the DEXA images. We also thank Momoko Noda, who helped analyze the BMD data from image files.

Authors' contributions

The study conception was performed by KTa, SH, and AO. The study design was performed by YT, TS, RU, and KTo. Data collection was performed by YT, TS, SH, AO, RU, RA, and KTo. Data analysis was performed by KTa, SH, TK, and RA. Interpretation of data was assessed by SH and TY. The first draft of the manuscript was written by KTa. AO, TK, and KTo substantively revised the manuscript. All authors commented on previous versions of the manuscript. All authors read and approved the final manuscript.

References

1. Sorokin I, Mamoulakis C, Miyazawa K, Rodgers A, Talati J, Lotan Y. Epidemiology of stone disease across the world. World J Urol. 2017;35:1301–20.
2. Ferraro PM, Curhan GC, D'Addessi A, Gambaro G. Risk of recurrence of idiopathic calcium kidney stones: analysis of data from the literature. J Nephrol. 2017;30:227–33.
3. Antonelli JA, Maalouf NM, Pearle MS, Lotan Y. Use of the National Health and Nutrition Examination Survey to calculate the impact of obesity and diabetes on cost and prevalence of urolithiasis in 2030. Eur Urol. 2014;66:724–9.
4. Kum F, Mahmalji W, Hale J, Thomas K, Bultitude M, Glass J. Do stones still kill? An analysis of death from stone disease 1999–2013 in England and Wales. BJU Int. 2016;118:140–4.
5. Yasui T, Okada A, Hamamoto S, Ando R, Taguchi K, Tozawa K, et al. Pathophysiology-based treatment of urolithiasis. Int J Urol. 2017;24:32–8.
6. Arrabal-Polo MA, Cano-García Mdel C, Canales BK, Arrabal-Martin M. Calcium nephrolithiasis and bone demineralization: pathophysiology, diagnosis, and medical management. Curr Opin Urol. 2014;24:633–8.
7. Lucato P, Trevisan C, Stubbs B, Zanforlini BM, Solmi M, Luchini C, et al. Nephrolithiasis, bone mineral density, osteoporosis, and fractures: a systematic review and comparative meta-analysis. Osteoporos Int. 2016;27:3155–64.
8. Kusumi K, Schwaderer AL, Clark C, Budge K, Hussein N, Raina R, et al. Bone mineral density in adolescent urinary stone formers: is sex important? Urolithiasis. 2020;48:329–35.
9. Arrabal-Polo MA, Girón-Prieto MS, Cano-García Mdel C, Poyatos-Andujar A, Quesada-Charneco M, Abad-Menor F, et al. Retrospective review of serum and urinary lithogenic risk factors in patients with osteoporosis and osteopenia. Urology. 2015;85:782–5.
10. Taguchi K, Cho SY, Ng AC, Usawachintachit M, Tan YK, Deng YL, et al. The Urological Association of Asia clinical guideline for urinary stone disease. Int J Urol. 2019;26:688–709.
11. Türk C, Petřík A, Sarica K, Seitz C, Skolarikos A, Straub M, et al. EAU guidelines on diagnosis and conservative management of urolithiasis. Eur Urol. 2016;69:468–74.

12. Pearle MS, Goldfarb DS, Assimos DG, Curhan G, Denu-Ciocca CJ, Matlaga BR, et al. Medical management of kidney stones: AUA guideline. J Urol. 2014;192:316–24.
13. Yasui T, Itoh Y, Okada A, Hamamoto S, Hirose M, Kobayashi T, et al. Alendronate reduces the excretion of risk factors for calcium phosphate stone formation in postmenopausal women with osteoporosis. Urol Int. 2009;83:226–9.
14. Sakamoto S, Miyazawa K, Yasui T, Iguchi T, Fujita M, Nishimatsu H, et al. Chronological changes in the epidemiological characteristics of upper urinary tract urolithiasis in Japan. Int J Urol. 2018;25:373–8.
15. Kanda Y. Investigation of the freely available easy-to-use software 'EZR' for medical statistics. Bone Marrow Transplant. 2013;48:452–8.
16. Kohjimoto Y, Sasaki Y, Iguchi M, Matsumura N, Inagaki T, Hara I. Association of metabolic syndrome traits and severity of kidney stones: results from a nationwide survey on urolithiasis in Japan. Am J Kidney Dis. 2013;61:923–9.
17. Alhava EM, Juuti M, Karjalainen P. Bone mineral density in patients with urolithiasis. A preliminary report. Scand J Urol Nephrol. 1976;10:154–6.
18. Tsuji H, Umekawa T, Kurita T, Uemura H, Iguchi M, Kin K, et al. Analysis of bone mineral density in urolithiasis patients. Int J Urol. 2005;12:335–9.
19. Denburg MR, Leonard MB, Haynes K, Tuchman S, Tasian G, Shults J, et al. Risk of fracture in urolithiasis: a population-based cohort study using the health improvement network. Clin J Am Soc Nephrol. 2014;9:2133–40.
20. Taylor EN, Feskanich D, Paik JM, Curhan GC. Nephrolithiasis and risk of incident bone fracture. J Urol. 2016;195:1482–6.
21. Carbone LD, Hovey KM, Andrews CA, Thomas F, Sorensen MD, Crandall CJ, et al. Urinary tract stones and osteoporosis: findings from the women's health initiative. J Bone Miner Res. 2015;30:2096–102.
22. Arrabal-Polo MÁ, Sierra Girón-Prieto M, Orgaz-Molina J, Zuluaga-Gómez A, Arias-Santiago S, Arrabal-Martín M. Calcium renal lithiasis and bone mineral density. Importance of bone metabolism in urinary lithiasis. Actas Urol Esp. 2013;37:362–7.
23. Coe FL, Worcester EM, Evan AP. Idiopathic hypercalciuria and formation of calcium renal stones. Nat Rev Nephrol. 2016;12:519–33.
24. Patel ND, Ward RD, Calle J, Remer EM, Monga M. CT-based diagnosis of low vertebral bone mineral density is associated with hypercalciuria and hypocitraturia on opportunistic imaging. J Endourol. 2018;32:878–83.
25. Prochaska M, Taylor E, Vaidya A, Curhan G. Low bone density and bisphosphonate use and the risk of kidney stones. Clin J Am Soc Nephrol. 2017;12:1284–90.
26. Sakhaee K, Maalouf NM, Poindexter J, Adams-Huet B, Moe OW. Relationship between urinary calcium and bone mineral density in patients with calcium nephrolithiasis. J Urol. 2017;197:1472–7.
27. Tugcu V, Ozbek E, Aras B, Ozbay B, Islim F, Tasci AI. Bone mineral density measurement in patients with recurrent normocalciuric calcium stone disease. Urol Res. 2007;35:29–34.
28. Prochaska M, Taylor EN, Curhan G. Menopause and risk of kidney stones. J Urol. 2018;200:823–8.
29. Pointillart A. Enhancement of phosphorus utilization in growing pigs fed phytate-rich diets by using rye bran. J Anim Sci. 1991;69:1109–15.
30. Casado JL, Santiuste C, Vazquez M, Bañón S, Rosillo S, Gomez A, et al. Bone mineral density decline according to renal tubular dysfunction and phosphaturia in tenofovir-exposed HIV-infected patients. AIDS. 2016;30:1423–31.
31. Arrabal-Polo MA, Arrabal-Martin M, Arias-Santiago S, Garrido-Gomez J, Poyatos-Andujar A, Zuluaga-Gomez A. Importance of citrate and the calcium:citrate ratio in patients with calcium renal lithiasis and severe lithogenesis. BJU Int. 2013;111:622–7.
32. Alshara L, Batagello CA, Armanyous S, Gao T, Patel N, Remer EM, et al. The impact of thiazides and potassium citrate on bone mineral density evaluated by CT scan in stone formers. J Endourol. 2018;32:559–64.
33. Granchi D, Torreggiani E, Massa A, Caudarella R, Di Pompo G, Baldini N. Potassium citrate prevents increased osteoclastogenesis resulting from acidic conditions: implication for the treatment of postmenopausal bone loss. PLoS ONE. 2017;12:e0181230.

28

CTCs detection from intraoperative salvaged blood in RCC–IVC thrombus patients by negative enrichment and iFISH identification

Xiaoqing Zhang[1], Xiangyang Guo[1], Yanan Zong[1], Chuanya Xu[1], Jilian Wang[1], Bin Zhang[1], Chang Liu[1], Yueqing Gong[2], Lixiang Xue[2], Lulin Ma[3], Shudong Zhang[3], Yi Li[1*] and Hong Zeng[1*]

Abstract

Background: Intra-operative cell salvage (IOCS) and leukocyte-depleted filter (LDF) are widely used and effective in saving blood. However, the safety issue concerning reinfusion of IOCS–LDF processed blood to renal cell carcinoma (RCC) patients with inferior vena cava (IVC) thrombus were inconclusive for fear of increased risk of cancer metastases. This study intends to analyze the circulating tumor cell (CTC) eliminating effect of IOCS–LDF in 5 RCC–IVC thrombus patients.

Methods: A novel strategy integrating negative enrichment by immunomagnetic beads and immunostaining-fluorescence in situ hybridization with probes identifying aneuploid of 8 and/or 7 were used to detect CTCs from salvages blood. Blood samples were collected from 4 stages in each patient.

Results: Of the 5 RCC patients, the number of CTCs decreased (from 3, 4, 10, 7, 3, respectively, to all zero) after IOCS–LDF treatment. The triploid of chromosome 7 and/or chromosome 8 were most common karyotype for RCC patients with IVC thrombus. Tetraploid of chromosome 8 occurred in only one sample and no polypoid (number of chromosome > 4) were found.

Conclusion: IOCS–LDF might be a promising way of reducing of allogeneic product transfusion based on current preliminary outcome. More convincing conclusions are to be drawn with enlarged sample size and long-term follow-up for patients prognosis.

Keywords: Renal cell carcinoma, Inferior vena cava thrombus, Intra-operative cell salvage, Leukocyte depletion filter, Aneuploidy

Background

Renal cell carcinoma (RCC) ranks the sixth most frequently diagnosed cancer in men and the 10th in women worldwide. It is the 13th most common cause of cancer death worldwide according to data provided by the World Health Organization, as more than 140,000 RCC-related deaths yearly. The incidence rates of RCC is still rising, and this is partially because the increase in the imaging examination. Although most detected lesions are small tumors, locally advanced disease continues to be diagnosed in a notable proportion of patients, with up to 17% of patients harboring distant metastases at the time of diagnosis [1].

*Correspondence: liyicomeon@yahoo.com; dr_zeng@sina.com
[1] Department of Anesthesia, Peking University Third Hospital, Huayuan 49# Rd, Haidian Dist., Beijing, China
Full list of author information is available at the end of the article

It is observed in 4–10% RCC patients who have a unique propensity for vascular invasion (into the renal vein and inferior vena cava) in the advanced stage [2]. Current guidelines recommend surgical excision of non-metastatic RCC with inferior vena cava (IVC) thrombosis in patients with acceptable performance status [3]. Patients with RCC–IVC tumor thrombus had a significant blood loss during operation despite improvements in surgical technique. The median estimated blood loss was 1900 (IQR 800–3300) ml. For patients with thrombus level ≤ 2 and ≥ 3 (Mayo-level), the blood loss were 1500 (IQR 600–2875) ml and 3000 (IQR 1400–5350) ml, respectively [4]. Massive transfusion of allogeneic blood may cause bacterial infection, allergic reactions, hemolytic reactions, transfusion-related risks of acute lung injury and viral infections. An association between perioperative transfusion of allogeneic blood products and risk for recurrence has been shown in colorectal cancer in randomized trials due to transfusion related immune modulation [5, 6]. It is concerned that allogeneic transfusion may result in immunosuppression and possible adverse effects on urological cancer recurrence [7–9].

Intra-operative cell salvage (IOCS) is of great significance in saving blood and offers an efficacious, alternative technique for blood replacement. Leukocyte-depleted filter (LDF) is normally used after IOCS washing and before infusion to remove nucleated cells such as bacteria and tumor cells. There were AAGBI safety guidelines in 2009, NICE guidelines in 2005, 2008 and 2015, UK Cell Salvage Action Group consensus in 2017, National Blood Authority in Australia in 2014, uniformly stated that despite theoretical risks and benefits, there is no conclusive evidence that cell salvage can induce metastases or affect cancer prognosis. The theoretical risk of inducing metastatic spread (unproven) is offset by reduced allogeneic transfusion and immunomodulation, which is proven [10]. However, concerns regarding the increased risk of cancer recurrence or development of metastases resulting from re-infusion of malignant cells renders the reluctance of adopting IOCS–LDF. At present, there were few studies on the safety assessment of recovered blood in patients with RCC–IVC thrombus. This study intends to analyze the tumor cell eliminating effect of IOCS–LDF in patients with RCC–IVC thrombus with a novel strategy integrating negative enrichment by immunomagnetic beads and immunostaining fluorescence in situ hybridization (NE-iFISH) with probes identifying aneuploidy.

Method

Patients selection

We recruited patients with RCC–IVC thrombus underwent open/laparoscopy radical nephrectomy and IVC tumor thrombectomy from January to December, 2018 in Peking University Third Hospital. Thrombus level was defined according to Mayo classification [11]. Only RCC–IVC thrombus (Mayo-levels II–IV) were included in the study. Excluding criteria: patients with blood diseases, infectious diseases, and those who refused to participate in the study. The study was approved by the hospital ethics committee (No. M2017296). Patients and their families all signed informed consent. Patients' demographic information were recorded (Table 1).

Anesthesia and surgical methods

General anesthesia was performed. Patients' vital signs and the depth of anesthesia were closely monitored. The surgery of open/laparoscopy radical nephrectomy and IVC tumor thrombectomy were dictated by the extent and level of the tumor thrombus. The surgical technique has been described in detail by Berczi [12]. Surgical time, intraoperative blood loss, the amount of autologous

Table 1 Patients' demographic information, follow-up and tumor pathological classification

Case	Mayo-level grading	Surgical duration (min)	Tumor size (cm)	WHO/ISUP grading	Pathological diagnosis	20-mon follow-up	Tumor recurrenceor metastasis
1	II	553	7.1*5.2*4.6	G2	ccRCC	Alive	None
2[a]	III	350	–	–	ccRCC	Dead	Preoperative lung metastasis
3	II	161	12*10*6	G3	ccRCC	Alive	None
4	IV	320	5*3*2.5	G2	ccRCC	Alive	None
5	II	540	9*5*4	G3	ccRCC	Alive	None

ISUP, International Society of Urological Pathology. G2, Tumour cell nucleoli conspicuous and eosinophilic at × 400 magnification and visible but not prominent at × 100 magnification; G3, Tumor cell nucleoli conspicuous and eosinophilic at × 100 magnification

ccRCC clear cell Renal Cell Carcinoma

[a] The patient underwent radical right nephrectomy for renal cancer 3 years ago. Now he was diagnosed as inferior vena cava thrombus with lung metastasis. The patient died of emphysema 16 months after surgery

blood recovery, and the amount of allogeneic blood transfusion were recorded. Recovered blood was not re-infused as this was not allowed by the ethical committee for fear of tumor dissemination and subsequent risk of metastatic disease.

IOCS–LDF

The suction tube and blood reservoir of the IOCS machine (Cell Saver Elite, Haemonetics Corporation, MA, U.S.) was rinsed and pre-filled with 50–100 ml anti-coagulant saline (heparin saline, 500 IU/ml). The negative pressure of the suction device is set at 120–150 mmHg. The anticoagulant drip rate was adjusted to about 1 drop/second, and the flow rate was adjusted according to the amount and speed of the bleeding. All intraoperative shed blood was recovered from the skin incision to tumor removal. Recovered blood was anti-coagulated and washed with sterilized saline (1500–2000 ml for 250 ml RBC). After washing, the recruited blood was filtered through PALL® leukocyte reduction filter (SB, Haemonetics Corporation, MA, U.S.). Blood products treated with IOCS–LDF are for research use only and are not returned to patients.

Sample preparation

Blood samples were collected intraoperatively at 4 different stages and sites (S1, peripheral venous blood from internal jugular vein before skin incision; S2, blood sampled in the vena cava around the tumor thrombus during surgery; S3, IOCS blood after washing and before LDF filtering; S4, blood sampled from post-LDF filtration). Each sample contains 4.0 ml blood (Fig. 1).

Negative enrichment of CTC

The strategy of enrichment for circulating tumor cell (CTC) is performed according to manufacturer's instructions. Briefly, 4.0 ml blood samples were lysed by RBC hypotonic hemolysis. Solution was centrifuged at $300 \times g$ for 5 min. Then, the residue cell pellet was resuspended in PBS and subsequently incubated with anti-CD45 monoclonal antibody-coated magnetic beads for 30 min, followed by the separation of magnetic beads using a magnetic stand (Promega, Madison, WI, USA). Supernatants were subsequently subjected to identification.

Immunocytochemistry staining of CTCs

The identification of enriched CTCs was performed by combing the chromosome enumeration using iFISH with chromosome 7 (CEP7, green) and 8 (CEP8, orange) centromere probes (Abbott Molecular Diagnostics, Des Plaines, IL, USA) and anti-CD45 monoclonal antibody (red) (CD45-FISH). Specimens were hybridized at 37 °C for 20 min in hybridizer (DAKO). Then they were washed in 50% formamide at 43 °C for 15 min, and subsequently immersed into 2*SSC and gradient alcohol again. Specimens were washed twice with 0.2% BSA and incubated with the CD45 mixture/2% BSA conjugated to Alexa Fluor 594 (Invitrogen) for 1 h. Afterward, samples were washed again with 0.2% BSA, and covered with DAPI which contained Vectashield mounting medium [13]. CTCs were examined and identified as hyperdiploid CEP8+/DAPI+/CD45−, hyperdiploid CEP7+/DAPI+/CD45− and hyperdiploid CEP7+, 8+/DAPI+/CD45− by two independent pathologists, while cells with CD45+ were differentiated as WBC.

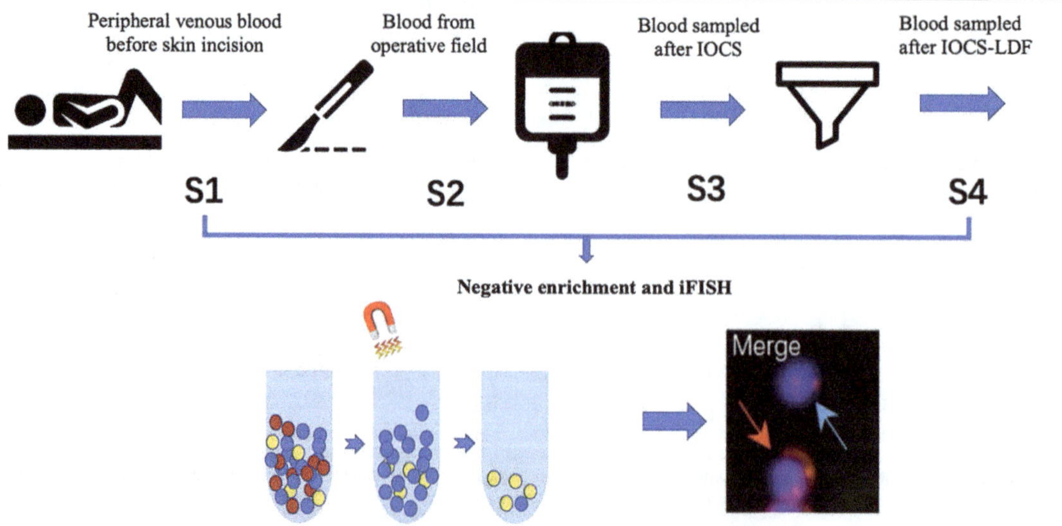

Fig. 1 Schematic plot of sample collection and processing

Statistical analysis

All data were recorded and compared among 5 RCC–IVC thrombus patients. Medians and quartiles were used to describe the amount of intraoperative blood loss, transfusion and recovered blood.

Results

Demographic information

In the current study, a total of 5 patients with RCC–IVC thrombus were included for surgical treatment. Of all these 5 patients, one (case No. 2) underwent radical nephrectomy of the right kidney due to renal cancer in local hospital 3 years ago. The patient complaint shortness of breath recently and was admitted to our hospital. His lung CT revealed multiple nodules in both lungs, indicative of metastasis (4.1 cm*3.8 cm). Abdominal CT revealed IVC thrombosis which was operated later and diagnosed from clear cell renal cell carcinoma (ccRCC) origin by pathological examination. The size of the renal tumors of the other four patients were 7.1 cm*5.2 cm*4.6 cm, 12 cm*10 cm*6 cm, 5 cm*3 cm*2.5 cm, 9 cm*5 cm*4 cm, respectively, and the WHO/ISUP grading system of the tumors were G2, G3, G2, G3, respectively [14] (Table 1). The pathological diagnosis of all 5 patients were ccRCC (Fig. 2). Post-operative follow-up showed the patient (case No. 2) with radical nephrectomy history died of emphysema 16 months after thrombectomy. Other 4 patients were closely followed up for at least 20 months and no cancer recurrence or metastasis were found till now.

Intraoperative blood loss and recovery

A total of 5 patients (ASA II–III) were enrolled, including 1 female and 4 male patients, with an average age of 58.6 years. 3 patients (2 with Mayo-levels II, and 1 with Mayo-level IV) underwent open radical nephrectomy and IVC tumor thrombectomy, 1 (Mayo-level III) with open thrombectomy, and 1 patient (Mayo-level II) received laparoscopic radical nephrectomy and IVC tumor thrombectomy. Surgical duration was 335 (IQR, 320–540) min. The total intraoperative blood loss was 10,500 ml, and median amount of 2100 (IQR, 1500–2700) ml, with one patient (Mayo-level IV) lost 4000 ml blood. The total amount of transfused allogeneic red blood cells was 8800 ml, with median amount of 2000 (IQR, 1200–2000) ml. The total amount of transfused plasma was 2800 ml. One patient (Mayo-level II) who underwent laparoscopic radical nephrectomy and IVC tumor thrombectomy did not receive allogeneic blood transfusion due to small amount of blood loss. A total amount of 5150 ml of autologous blood, with median amount of 1000 ml (750, 1300) was recovered during surgery (Table 2). One patient (Mayo-level IV) experienced major bleeding and was managed with vasoactive

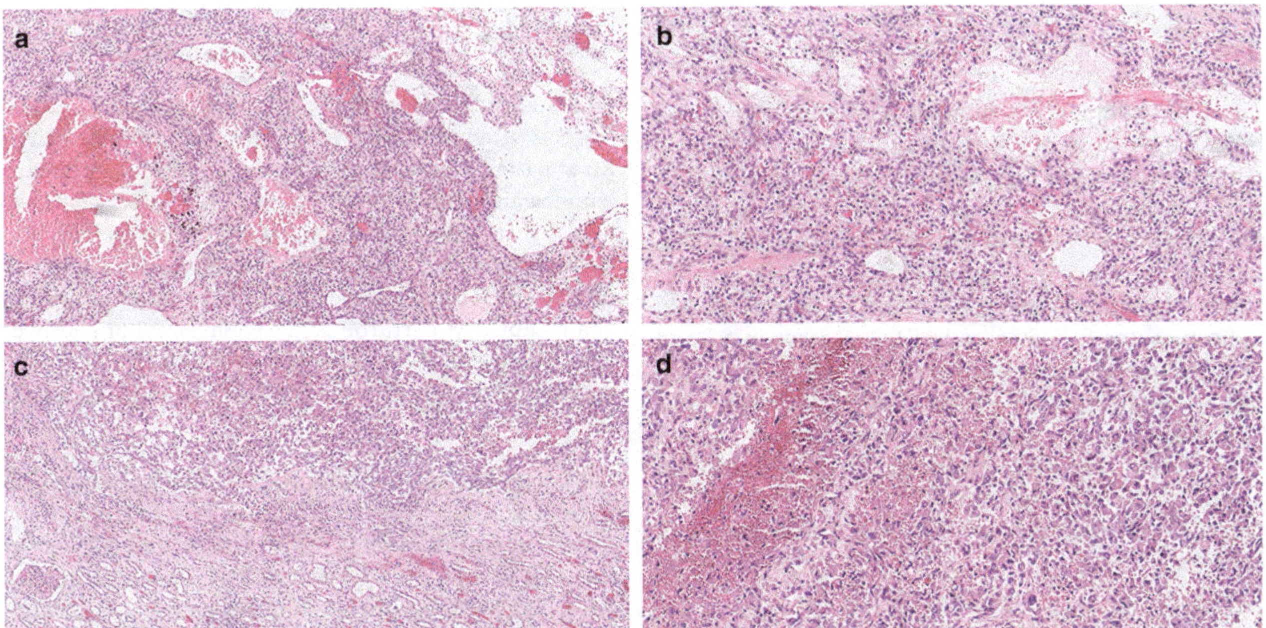

Fig. 2 Pathological examination of the dissected renal tumor and thrombus. All five patients were diagnosed as ccRCC. **a**, **b** Histological examination showing the ccRCC as WHO/ISUP grade 2 (hematoxylin and eosin, original magnification: **a** × 100; **b** × 200). **c**, **d** Histological examination showing the ccRCC as WHO/ISUP grade 3 (hematoxylin and eosin, original magnification: **c** × 100; **d** × 200)

Table 2 Intraoperative blood loss and the transfusion

Case	Total blood loss (ml)	Infused RBC (ml)	Infused plasma (ml)	Recovered blood (ml)
1	2700	2000	0	1300
2	1500	1200	400	750
3	200	0	0	100
4	2100	2000	800	1000
5	4000	3600	1600	2000
Median	2100	2000	400	1000
IQR (ml)	1500–2700	1200–2000	0–800	750–1300

IQR inter quartile range

drugs and massive blood product transfusion and fluid resuscitation. All patients' vital signs were stable during hospitalization.

Detection of tumor cells

20 blood samples from 5 RCC–IVC thrombus patients were studied. After excluding CD45+ leukocytes by immunomagnetic beads, the aneuploidy (abnormal chromosome numbers) of chromosome 8 and/or 7 were detected with iFISH examination. The aneuploidy of chromosome 8 or 7 include: trisomy 8, tetraploidy 8, polyploidy 8 (>4), trisomy 7, tetraploidy 7, polyploidy 7 (>4), aberrant number of both chromosome 8 and 7, and circulating tumor micro emboli (CTM). The negative expression of CD45 and the aneuploidy of chromosomes 8 and/or 7 (chromosome number > 2) were discriminated as CTCs (Table 3).

In all S1 samples, the number of tumor cells in the peripheral blood were 3, 4, 10, 7 and 3, respectively; and the number of tumor cells in the S2 sample were 0, 0, 2, 5 and 1, respectively; in S3 samples, the number of tumor cells decreased to 1, 0, 0, 0 and 0; and no tumor cell was found in any sample in S4 group (0, 0, 0, 0, 0) (Fig. 3).

In this preliminary study, most CTCs were of triploid of chromosome 8 (5/5 cases in S1, 2/5 cases in S2 and 1/5 cases in S3) or chromosome 7 (4/5 cases in S1, 3/5 cases in S2, and 1/5cases in S3), while only 1 case with tetraploidy of chromosome 8. The hyperdiploidy of both chromosome 7 and 8 were detected in 3 cases (2 cases of S1 and 1 case of S2). No tetraploidy of chromosome 7, or other aberrant chromosome number ≥ 4 were detected. (Table 4).

Discussion

Aneuploidy of detected viable tumor cells

Intraoperative tumor metastasis occurred when large amounts of cancer cells were shed from primary tumor focus during surgical manipulation into the blood stream, becoming circulating tumor cells (CTC) and may target distant organs and develop metastatic tumors [15]. Reinfusion of viable tumor cells from intraoperative recovered blood poses potential risks of tumor dissemination and metastasis. However, due to scarce number of residual tumor cells from vast majority of leukocytes, capturing viable tumor cells from shed blood after IOCS–LDF treatment is difficult [16–19].

Currently, the majority of the methodology of detecting CTCs are restricted to the tumor cell density, size, and charge as well as biomarkers using antigen expression profiles and specific tumor antigen–antibody interactions to distinguish and isolate CTCs from other cells. However, a large quantity of primary CTCs are of smaller cell size (≤ WBCs) which makes it difficult to separate from WBC, and the rare CTCs are inevitability lost during filtration based cell size selection strategy [20]. Moreover, it is reported that positive EpCAM expression rate ranges 37–42.3% of the various cancers with FDA-approved Cell Search system. The invasive tumor cells tend to lose their epithelial antigens by the epithelial to mesenchymal transition process, which results in loss of EpCAM on CTCs and made the capturing of CTCs more difficult [21]. On the other hand, capturing non-tumor derived epithelial cells originated from inflammation, trauma, surgery and benign epithelial hyperplasia may cause false positive results [22]. For RCC, the expression of EpCAM was absent and there is no widely acknowledged specific cell surface marker for RCC detection[23, 24]. Therefore, a promising alternative approach of EpCAM-independent enrichment strategy has been introduced [25].

In this preliminary study, detecting aberrant chromosome is attempted as a way of capturing tumor cells in RCC patients. Aneuploidy is the abnormal alternation (either gain or loss) of chromosomes in a cell. It is estimated that 90% of solid tumors exhibit aneuploidy [20]. By integrating cellular and molecular approach of NE-iFISH, which is independent of cell size variation and free of anti-EpCAM perturbing. We could simultaneously co-detecting biomarker expression qualitatively and quantitatively, as well as discovering chromosome aneuploidy [13, 26].

It is reported that chromosome 7 and 8 abnormalities were detected in RCC cases. The positive rate of chromosome 7 abnormality ranges in 9.5–36%, and CTC detection rate using CEP 8 was 86.20% with a cut-off value of 1 CTC [27–30]. In this preliminary study, aneuploidy of chromosome 8 and/or 7 were analyzed and tumor cells were differentiated (Fig. 4). In this way, we could separate CTCs from recovered blood in RCC with IVC thrombus patients. To our knowledge, this is the first time that NE-iFISH was used to capture CTCs in the recovered blood of RCC–IVE thrombus patients with encouraging result.

Table 3 CTC counts of aneuploidy of chromosome 8 and/or 7 from blood samples

Case	Sample	CTC counts									
		Triploid of chromosome 8	Tetraploid of chromosome 8	Polydiploid (>4) of chromosome 8	Triploid of chromosome 7	Tetraploid of chromosome 7	Polydiploid (>4) of chromosome 7	Polydiploidy chromosome of both 7 and 8	CTM	Sum	Total number
1	S1	3								3	
	S2										
	S3	1								1	
	S4										4
2	S1	1			2			1[a]		4	
	S2										
	S3				1					1	
	S4										5
3	S1	6	1		3					10	
	S2	1			1				1	3	
	S3										
	S4										13
4	S1	4			3					7	
	S2	3			1			1[a]		5	
	S3										
	S4										12
5	S1	1			1			1[a]		3	
	S2				1					1	
	S3										
	S4										5

Tumor cells were recognized and counted using immunostaining and fluorescence in situ hybridization technology. Only cells with CD45−/DAPI+/CEP8+ (>2), CD45−/DAPI+/CEP8+ (>2), and CD45−/DAPI+/CEP8+ and CEP7+ (hyperdiploidy) were identified as CTCs

Number 0 were not shown in the table

S1, peripheral venous blood sample from internal jugular vein before skin incision, indicative of the circulating tumor cells; S2, blood sampled in the vena cava around thrombus during surgery, indicating direct cells shedding in surgical manipulation; S3, blood after IOCS washing and before LDF filtering, which represents the tumor cell cleaning efficacy with only IOCS; S4, blood sampled after LDF filtration, meaning the actual final filtering result after IOCS–LDF

CTM circulating tumor microemboli

[a] Triploid of both chromosome 8 and 7

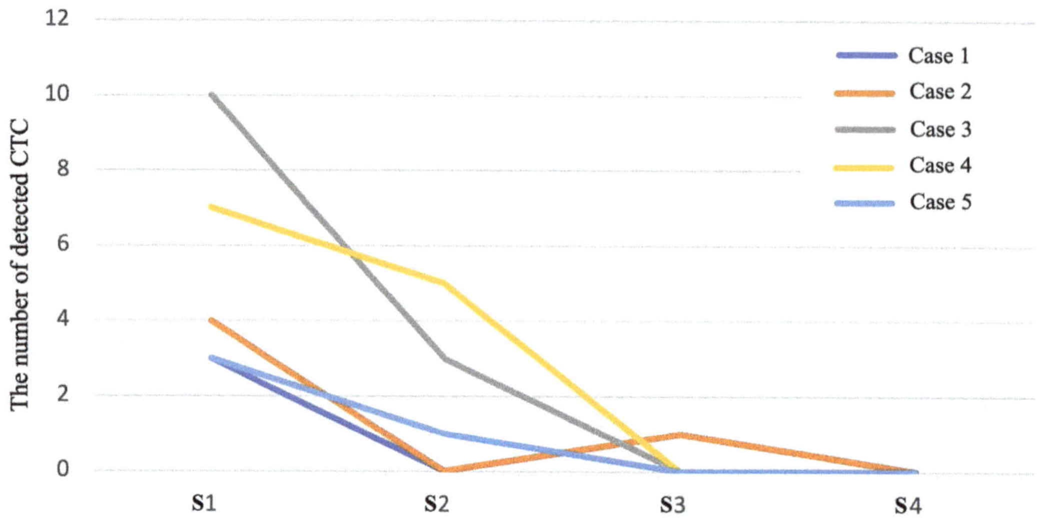

Fig. 3 Detection and numeration of CTCs in 5 RCC patients at 4 different stages and sites. Significant decrease of CTC numbers were noted in all 5 patient. S1, peripheral venous blood sample from internal jugular vein before skin incision, indicative of the circulating tumor cells; S2, blood sampled in the vena cava around thrombus during surgery, indicating direct cells shedding in surgical manipulation; S3, blood after IOCS washing and before LDF filtering, which represents the tumor cell cleaning efficacy with only IOCS; S4, blood sampled after LDF filtration, meaning the actual final filtering result after IOCS–LDF

Table 4 Case number of aneuploidy of chromosome 7 and/or 8

Sample	Case numbers			
	Chromosome 8 triploidy	Chromosome 8 tetraploidy	Chromosome 7 triploidy	Chromosome 7 and 8 hyperdiploidy
S1	5	1	4	2
S2	2		3	1
S3	1		1	
S4				
Total	8	1	8	3

Triploidy of chromosome 8 were detected in 8 cases: 5/5 cases in S1, 2/5 cases in S2 and 1/5 cases in S3; Triploidy of chromosome 7 were detected in 8 cases: 4/5 cases in S1, 3/5 cases in S2, and 1/5cases in S3; The hyperdiploidy of both chormosome 7 and 8 were detected in 3 cases: 2 cases of S1 and 1 case of S2; Only 1 case with tetraploidy of chromosome 8; No tetraploidy of chromosome 7, or other aberrant chromosome number ≥ 4 were detected

It is interesting to note that CTCs recovered from intraoperative blood in ccRCC-IVC thrombus patients have the propensity of developing trisomy of chromosome 7 or 8. This chromosome karyotype was not reported before and deserve further exploration. It may be useful for future chromosome karyotype analysis and also for further study of the clinical significance in treatment efficacy of tumor recurrence, metastasis detection and prognosis.

IOCS–LDF and RCC metastasis

Leukocyte depletion filter (LDF) is a filtering device based on a membrane-like filter material to remove leukocytes from blood. Its mechanism for removing tumor cells is physical interception and charge adsorption based on cell size. Kumar and colleagues revisited the safety of salvaged blood from the point of view of metastatic potential, and presented basic and applied science evidence regarding the innocuous nature of tumor cells that have been subjected to the cell salvage process. They believe that the current prevalent apprehensions on the usage of salvaged blood are ill-founded [31].

Radical nephrectomy and IVC tumor thrombectomy is widely acknowledged as the curative method for patients with RCC–IVC thrombus [32]. When the tumor thrombus extends to the right atrium, intraoperative establishment of extracorporeal circulation is required. Patients with Mayo-level III–IV often experienced life-threatening intraoperative major bleeding. As blood resource is limited, scheduled surgeries are always delayed. A recent meta-analysis has shown that the infusion of allogeneic blood during radical prostatectomy, radical nephrectomy and cystectomy lead to worsened prognosis for patients [33], and this may be related to transfusion-related immunomodulation [34]. The application of IOCS–LDF is an effective alternative for massive blood transfusion. A study concerning the IVC tumor thrombus extending to right atrium has shown that the use of cardiopulmonary

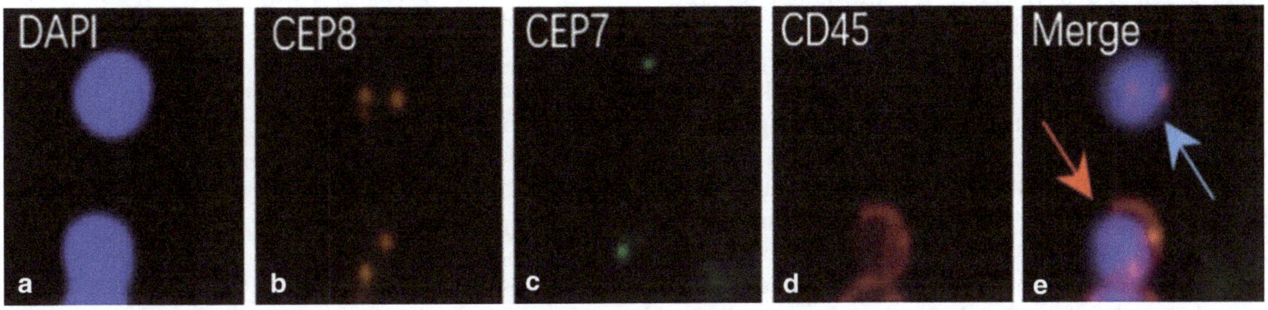

Fig. 4 Detection and identification of RCC tumor cells by NE-iFISH. CTCs (blue arrow) were examined and identified as hyperdiploid CEP8+/DAPI+/CD45−, hyperdiploid CEP7+/DAPI+/CD45− and hyperdiploid CEP7+, CEP8+/DAPI+/CD45− by two independent pathologists. Cells with CD45+ were differentiated as WBC (red arrow). CEP, centromere polyploidy

bypass and cell-saver technique in borderline situations like combined oncologic and cardiovascular surgery without increasing the risk of hematogenous tumor dissemination. Postoperative cytological investigation showed that the tumor cells were only found on the internal surface of the heart–lung machine arterial filters. No distant metastasis was found in all surviving patients [35]. There were limited clinical study concerning the safety of returning shed blood to RCC–IVC thrombus patients, and the results were inconclusive [15, 36]. Other single center studies or meta-analysis of urological tumors showed that the use of IOCS with or without LDF did not increase the post-operative complication occurrences [37–39], or medical cost [39].

In the current study, we demonstrated with NE-iFISH method, all the tumor cells in 5 patients were com pletely removed after LDF treatment, and intraoperative IOCS–LDF usage could clear all tumor cells in RCC–IVC thrombus patients with high efficiency.

IOCS–LDF for RCC–IVC thrombus tumor cell removal

In this study, 5 RCC–IVC thrombus patients were enrolled and 20 blood samples taken at different sites and stages during surgery were studied. Samples of S1 is indicative of the circulating tumor cells; S2 indicated peri-thrombus tumor cells shedding into inferior vena cava during operation; S3 represents the tumor cell cleaning efficacy with IOCS; and S4 is the actual final filtering result after LDF. Tumor cell numbers of all S4 samples were zero after IOCS–LDF treatment. This dem onstrated that IOCS–LDF is effective in removing tumor cells. To our surprise, the number of tumor cells in inter nal jugular vein in S1 is most abundant (3, 4, 10, 7 and 3, respectively), while the cell number in S2 decreased (0, 0, 2, 5 and 1).

This might be explained by the solid texture of the IVC thrombus and its smooth surface which could extend itself way up to the atrium without being flushed away by blood flow in the inferior vena cava. The chances of tumor cell embolus detachment were not common. This also indicate that intraoperative exploration of the tumor thrombus does not necessarily result in significant shedding of tumor cells which might lead to tumor dissemination. Another important reason is related with patient blood management strategy. For RCC–IVC patients, considering the possible massive bleeding in the process of renal tumor and tumor thrombus separation and resection, anaesthesiologists would prefer to pre-infuse crystalloids and colloids to expand the blood volume and achieve tolerable hemodilution to reduce the red blood cells loss. This often results in hemodilution, which may lead to a relative decrease in the number of CTCs. In some conditions, apart from hemodilution, allogeneic blood products might also be pre-infused to prevent subsequent massive bleeding in a short time interval and causing violent hemodynamic fluctuation. Therefore, the number of CTCs might be reduced as a result of dilutional effect. In the current study, the S1 was sampled from peripheral venous blood in internal jugular vein before skin incision (when hemodilution was not achieved); while S2 was sampled in the vena cava around thrombus during surgery (when large amounts of crystalloid, colloids or blood products have been pre-infused).

Our study also demonstrated that IOCS alone is not enough for tumor cell depletion as CTCs were still detected in 2/5 cases in S3. The IOCS–LDF is efficient in depleting tumor cells from recovered blood as the number of CTCs reduced to 0 in all S4 samples. Due to limited sample size, further research with enlarge sample size is needed to verify the clearance ability of IOCS–LDF in RCC–IVC thrombus cases. Considering cell size differences, the application of IOCS–LDF to other tumor types may not achieve the equivalent effect.

Moreover, we also found that there is no close correlation between the amount of blood loss and the number of CTCs from the current study, which was also stated by

Ernil Hansen in their research [40]. The number of CTCs were more prominent in patients with more advanced tumor stage and higher WHO-ISUP grading as well as Mayo-level grading. In case 3 and 4, the Mayo-level grading were II and IV, and the WHO-ISUP grading were G3 and G2, respectively. In case 3, the number of CTCs were 10 (S1) and 3 (S2), and the size of the dissected tumor is 12 cm*10 cm*6 cm; while for case 4, the number of CTCs were 7 (S1) and 5 (S2), with the size of the dissected tumor 5 cm*3 cm*2.5 cm. However, it is arbitrary to reach any definitive conclusion based on the limited sample size. Further research is warranted to verify this finding.

Conclusion

There were no definitive guidelines or experts consensus to support the use of LOCS–LDF in RCC patients. There also lack laboratory and clinical evidence of safe reinfusion of autologous blood. In this preliminary study, CTCs of all samples decreased to 0 after IOCS–LDF in all five RCC–IVC thrombus patients. Which is encouraging. More convincing conclusions are to be drawn with enlarged sample size and discovery of more specific and accurate bio-markers for tumor cells originated from RCC–IVC thrombus.

Abbreviations

IOCS: Intra-operative cell salvage; LDF: Leukocyte-depleted filter; RCC: Renal cell carcinoma; IVC: Inferior vena cava; CTC: Circulating tumor cell; NE-iFISH: Negative enrichment by immunomagnetic beads and immunostaining fluorescence in situ hybridization.

Acknowledgements

None.

Authors' contributions

Guarantor of integrity of entire study: HZ, YL, XG. Study concepts Study design: HZ, XG. Literature research: XZ, XG, JW. Clinical studies: XZ, YZ, CX, BZ, CL. Experimental studies: XZ, YG, LX. Data acquisition: XZ, LM, SZ. Data analysis/interpretation: XZ, HZ. Statistical analysis: XZ, XG, JW. Manuscript preparation: XZ, XG, JW, YG, LX, HZ. Manuscript editing and revision: HZ, XG, JW. Manuscript final version approval: HZ, XG. All authors have read and approved the final manuscript.

Author details

[1]Department of Anesthesia, Peking University Third Hospital, Huayuan 49# Rd, Haidian Dist., Beijing, China. [2]Biological Sample Bank, Peking University Third Hospital, Beijing, China. [3]Department of Urology, Peking University Third Hospital, Beijing, China.

References

1. Capitanio U, Bensalah K, Bex A, et al. Epidemiology of renal cell carcinoma. Eur Urol. 2019;75:74–84. https://doi.org/10.1016/j.eururo.2018.08.036.
2. Wein AJ, Kavoussi LR, Partin AW, Peters CA. Campbell's urology (ed 11). Malignant renal tumors. Elsevier; 2016.
3. Campi R, Tellini R, Sessa F, et al. Techniques and outcomes of minimally-invasive surgery for nonmetastatic renal cell carcinoma with inferior vena cava thrombosis: a systematic review of the literature. Minerva Urol Nefrol. 2019;71:339–58. https://doi.org/10.23736/S0393-2249.19.03396-4.
4. Lue K, Russell CM, Fisher J, et al. Predictors of postoperative complications in patients who undergo radical nephrectomy and IVC thrombectomy: a large contemporary tertiary center analysis. Clin Genitourin Cancer. 2015;14:89–95. https://doi.org/10.1016/j.clgc.2015.09.007.
5. Cata JP, Wang H, Gottumukkala V, et al. Inflammatory response, immunosuppression, and cancer recurrence after perioperative blood transfusions. Br J Anaesth. 2013;110:690–701. https://doi.org/10.1093/bja/aet068.
6. Aquina CT, Blumberg N, Becerra AZ, et al. Association among blood transfusion, sepsis, and decreased long-term survival after colon cancer resection. Ann Surg. 2017;266:311–7. https://doi.org/10.1097/SLA.0000000000001990.
7. Aning J, Dunn J, Daugherty M, et al. Towards bloodless cystectomy: a 10-year experience of intra-operative cell salvage during radical cystectomy. BJU Int. 2012;110:E608–13. https://doi.org/10.1111/j.1464-410X.2012.11338.x.
8. Soubra A, Zabell JR, Adejoro O, et al. Effect of perioperative blood transfusion on mortality for major urologic malignancies. Clin Genitourin Cancer. 2015;13:e173–81. https://doi.org/10.1016/j.clgc.2014.12.006.
9. Linder BJ, Frank I, Cheville JC, et al. The impact of perioperative blood transfusion on cancer recurrence and survival following radical cystectomy. Eur Urol. 2013;63:839–45. https://doi.org/10.1016/j.eururo.2013.01.004.
10. Klein AA, Bailey CR, Charlton AJ, et al. Association of Anaesthetists guidelines: cell salvage for peri-operative blood conservation 2018. Anaesthesia. 2018;73:1141–50. https://doi.org/10.1111/anae.14331.
11. Neves RJ, Zincke H. Surgical treatment of renal cancer with vena cava extension. Br J Urol. 1987;59:390–5. https://doi.org/10.1111/j.1464-410x.1987.tb04832.x.
12. Berczi A, Flasko T, Szerafin T, et al. Surgical management and outcome of renal cell carcinoma with inferior vena cava tumor thrombus. Urol Int. 2017;99:267–71. https://doi.org/10.1159/000464108.
13. Chen YY, Xu GB. Effect of circulating tumor cells combined with negative enrichment and CD45-FISH identification in diagnosis, therapy monitoring and prognosis of primary lung cancer. Med Oncol. 2014;31:240. https://doi.org/10.1007/s12032-014-0240-0.
14. Delahunt B, Cheville JC, Martignoni G, et al. The International Society of Urological Pathology (ISUP) grading system for renal cell carcinoma and other prognostic parameters. Am J Surg Pathol. 2013;37:1490–504. https://doi.org/10.1097/PAS.0b013e318299f0fb.
15. Chaffer CL, Weinberg RA. A perspective on cancer cell metastasis. Science. 2011;331:1559–64. https://doi.org/10.1126/science.1203543.
16. Gwak MS, Lee KW, Kim SY, et al. Can a leukocyte depletion filter (LDF) reduce the risk of reintroduction of hepatocellular carcinoma cells? Liver Transpl. 2005;11:331–5. https://doi.org/10.1002/lt.20346.
17. Li J, Shi SB, Shi WL, et al. LUNX mRNA-positive cells at different time points predict prognosis in patients with surgically resected nonsmall cell lung cancer. Transl Res. 2014;163:27–35. https://doi.org/10.1016/j.trsl.2013.09.010.
18. Kumar N, Lam R, Zaw AS, et al. Flow cytometric evaluation of the safety of intraoperative salvaged blood filtered with leucocyte depletion filter in spine tumour surgery. Ann Surg Oncol. 2014;21:4330–5. https://doi.org/10.1245/s10434-014-3950-9.
19. Kumar N, Ahmed Q, Lee VK, et al. Are we ready for the use of intraoperative salvaged blood in metastatic spine tumour surgery? Eur Spine J. 2016;25:3997–4007. https://doi.org/10.1007/s00586-015-4112-x.
20. Lin PP. Aneuploid CTC and CEC. Diagnostics (Basel). 2018;8:26. https://doi.org/10.3390/diagnostics8020026.
21. Wang H, Stoecklein NH, Lin PP, Gires O. Circulating and disseminated tumor cells: diagnostic tools and therapeutic targets in motion. Oncotarget. 2017;8:1884–912. https://doi.org/10.18632/oncotarget.12242.
22. Tanaka F, Yoneda K, Kondo N, et al. Circulating tumor cell as a diagnostic marker in primary lung cancer. Clin Cancer Res. 2009;5:6980–6. https://doi.org/10.1158/1078-0432.CCR-09-1095.
23. Spizzo G, Fong D, Wurm M, et al. EpCAM expression in primary tumour tissues and metastases: an immunohistochemical analysis. J Clin Pathol. 2011;64:415–20. https://doi.org/10.1136/jcp.2011.090274

24. Baeuerle PA, Gires O. EpCAM (CD326) finding its role in cancer. Br J Cancer. 2007;96:417–23. https://doi.org/10.1038/sj.bjc.6603494.
25. Ning N, Zhan T, Zhang Y, et al. Improvement of specific detection of circulating tumor cells using combined CD45 staining and fluorescence in situ hybridization. Clin Chim Acta. 2014;433:69–75. https://doi.org/10.1016/j.cca.2014.02.019.
26. Ge F, Zhang H, Wang DD, et al. Enhanced detection and comprehensive in situ phenotypic characterization of circulating and disseminated heteroploid epithelial and glioma tumor cells. Oncotarget. 2015;6:27049–64. https://doi.org/10.18632/oncotarget.4819.
27. Klatte T, Rao PN, de Martino M, et al. Cytogenetic profile predicts prognosis of patients with clear cell renal cell carcinoma. J Clin Oncol. 2009;27:746–53. https://doi.org/10.1200/JCO.2007.15.8345.
28. Kuroda N, Tamura M, Shiotsu T, et al. Chromosomal abnormalities of clear cell renal cell carcinoma: frequent gain of chromosome 7. Pathol Int. 2010;60:9–13. https://doi.org/10.1111/j.1440-1827.2009.02467.x.
29. Pailoor J, Rajandram R, Yap NY, et al. Chromosome 7 aneuploidy in clear cell and papillary renal cell carcinoma: detection using silver in situ hybridization technique. Indian J Pathol Microbiol. 2013;56(2):98–102. https://doi.org/10.4103/0377-4929.118688.
30. Tian D, Zhang M, Zheng G, et al. Clinical significance of phenotyping and karyotyping of detecting circulating tumor cells in renal cell carcinoma using subtraction enrichment and immunostaining-fluorescence in situ hybridization (SE-iFISH). Int Urol Nephrol. 2020;52:2281–7. https://doi.org/10.1007/s11255-020-02587-8.
31. Kumar N, Zaw AS, Kantharajanna SB, et al. Metastatic efficiency of tumour cells can be impaired by intraoperative cell salvage process: truth or conjecture? Transfus Med. 2017;5:327–34. https://doi.org/10.1111/tme.12453.
32. Shao P, Li J, Qin C, et al. Laparoscopic radical nephrectomy and inferior vena cava thrombectomy in the treatment of renal cell carcinoma. Eur Urol. 2015;68:115–22. https://doi.org/10.1016/j.eururo.2014.12.011.
33. Wang YL, Jiang B, Yn FF, et al. Perioperative blood transfusion promotes worse outcomes of bladder cancer after radical cystectomy: a systematic review and meta-analysis. PLoS ONE. 2015;10:e0130122. https://doi.org/10.1371/journal.pone.0130122.
34. Li SL, Ye Y, Yuan XH. Association between allogeneic or autologous blood transfusion and survival in patients after radical prostatectomy: a systematic review and meta-analysis. PLoS ONE. 2017;12:e0171081. https://doi.org/10.1371/journal.pone.0171081.
35. Akchurin RS, Davidov MI, Partigulov SA, et al. Cardiopulmonary bypass and cell-saver technique in combined oncologic and cardiovascular surgery. Artif Organs. 1997;21:763–5. https://doi.org/10.1111/j.1525-1594.1997.tb03738.x.
36. Moskowitz DM, Perelman SI, Cousineau KM, et al. Multidisciplinary management of a Jehovah's Witness patient for the removal of a renal cell carcinoma extending into the right atrium. Can J Anaesth. 2002;49:402–8. https://doi.org/10.1007/BF03017330.
37. Casey RG, Raheem OA, Elmusharaf E, et al. Renal cell carcinoma with IVC and atrial thrombus: a single centre's 10 year surgical experience. Surgeon. 2013;11:295–9. https://doi.org/10.1016/j.surge.2013.02.007.
38. Lyon TD, Ferroni MC, Turner RM II, Jones C, Jacobs BL, Davies BJ. Short-term outcomes of intraoperative cell saver transfusion during open partial nephrectomy. Urology. 2015;86:1153–8. https://doi.org/10.1016/j.urology.2015.09.008.
39. Kinnear N, Hua L, Heijkoop B, et al. The impact of intra-operative cell salvage during open nephrectomy. Asian J Urol. 2019;6:346–52. https://doi.org/10.1016/j.ajur.2018.06.008.
40. Hansen E, Wolff N, Knuechel R, et al. Tumor cells in blood shed from the surgical field. Arch Surg. 1995;130:387–93. https://doi.org/10.1001/archsurg.1995.01430040049007.

29

Sulfamethoxazole-induced sulfamethoxazole urolithiasis

Megan M. Roedel[1], Stephen Y. Nakada[2,3] and Kristina L. Penniston[2*]

Abstract

Background: Drug-induced urolithiasis falls into two categories: drug-induced and metabolically-induced. Certain antimicrobials are associated with each; sulfonamides are associated with drug- or metabolite-containing calculi when taken in large doses over a long period of time. Trimethoprim-sulfamethoxazole, a member of the sulfonamide family, is a rare cause of drug-induced calculi. Cases of sulfonamide urolithiasis occurring in patients with known stone disease have rarely been reported.

Case presentation: We report a case of a patient with a brief history of recurrent calcium oxalate nephrolithiasis requiring 2 ureteroscopic procedures whose existing 6 mm lower pole renal stone more than quadrupled in size to form a 4 cm renal staghorn after 4 months of high-dose treatment for *Nocardia* pneumonia with trimethoprim-sulfamethoxazole. After ureteroscopy with laser lithotripsy and basketing of fragments, the stone was found to be predominantly composed of N^4-acetyl-sulfamethoxazole, a metabolite of sulfamethoxazole.

Conclusion: Stones composed of sulfamethoxazole or its metabolites are rare but have known associated risk factors that should be considered when prescribing this antibiotic. This case report illustrates additional risk factors for consideration, including pre-existing urinary calculi that may serve as a nidus for sulfamethoxazole deposition, and reviews treatment and prevention methods.

Keywords: Drug-induced urolithiasis, Trimethoprim-sulfamethoxazole, Nocardia, Case report

Background

Drug-induced kidney stones account for up to 2% of all urinary tract calculi [1]. Typically, these drugs fall into one of two categories: (1) drugs that have high renal excretion and are poorly soluble in urine; and (2) drugs that induce metabolic changes that favor urinary stone formation. Drugs in the first category, or metabolites thereof, are identified as components of calculi whereas drugs in the second category lead to formation of calcium- and/or uric acid-containing stones. Select drugs within the drug-containing calculi category, including the antihypertensive diuretic triamterene and the nonsteroidal analgesic glafenine, are now used less frequently due to their lithogenic potential; others continue to be used due to their treatment efficacy—these include indinavir and other protease inhibitors used in the treatment of HIV [1]. Metabolically-induced calculi containing calcium can be caused by hypercalciuria from excessive calcium and vitamin D supplementation. Other metabolism-altering drugs, such as carbonic anhydrase inhibitors (e.g., acetazolamide, topiramate) contribute to calcium oxalate and calcium phosphate stone formation by dramatically lowering urinary citrate excretion. Because they significantly raise urine pH, the risk for calcium phosphate stones in particular is increased. Uric acid-containing metabolic calculi can be induced by laxative abuse or by uricosuric agents such as benzbromarone used to treat gout [1].

*Correspondence: penn@urology.wisc.edu
[2] Department of Urology, University of Wisconsin School of Medicine and Public Health, 1685 Highland Avenue, 3258 Medical Foundation Centennial Building, Madison, WI 53705-2281, USA
Full list of author information is available at the end of the article

Several antimicrobial agents are associated with urinary tract calculi [1, 2]. Some act by altering the gut microbiome and its ability to degrade oxalate [3], leading to the formation of hyperoxaluria and calcium oxalate stones. Others, especially when taken in large doses over a long period of time, are known to form urinary crystals and calculi that contain the drug itself or its metabolite(s); these include ciprofloxacin, ceftriaxone, and sulfonamides [1]. Trimethoprim-sulfamethoxazole (TMP-SMX) is a combination antibiotic of the sulfonamide family used to treat a wide variety of commonly encountered infections, including those affecting the urinary tract, respiratory system, and gastrointestinal tract. It is also indicated in the treatment and prophylaxis of opportunistic infections by *Pneumocystis carinii* and *Nocardia spp* [4]. While first-generation sulfonamides were well-known to provoke drug-induced urolithiasis, it is significantly less common with newer sulfonamides and even less common with TMP-SMX [1]. Cases of sulfonamide urolithiasis occurring in patients with known stone disease have rarely been reported.

Here we present a case of a patient with a known kidney stone who was subsequently treated with a long course of high-dose TMP-SMX for *Nocardia* pneumonia. After 4 months of TMP-SMX therapy, the patient's known renal stone more than quadrupled in size to form a 4 cm staghorn stone with an accompanying obstructive conglomerate of ureteral stones. From fragments obtained during surgical stone removal, composition was predominantly N^4-acetyl-sulfamethoxazole.

Case presentation

The patient was a 64-year-old woman with gastroesophageal reflux disease, asthma (treated with inhaled but not systemic steroids), obesity, and type II diabetes mellitus (treated with metformin extended release 500 mg and glipizide 5 mg twice daily). Her stone onset was characterized by presentation to emergency care for nausea, vomiting, diarrhea, and lower left quadrant abdominal pain. While awaiting computed tomography (CT), she acutely became febrile and tachycardic. Labs were significant for white blood cell count of 20,000 K/uL, lactate of 2.2 mmol/L, creatinine of 1.98 mg/dL (baseline 1.06), and concurrent infection on urinalysis. CT scan revealed a 1 cm obstructive proximal ureteral stone. She was diagnosed with sepsis and acute kidney injury and was admitted for decompression and antibiotic therapy; she was discharged after 3 days. Immediate left ureteroscopy (URS) was scheduled but then postponed due to the COVID-19 pandemic. Ultimately, 2 months post presentation, she underwent left URS with laser lithotripsy (LL). Stone composition was unknown. A 24-h urine collection demonstrated high oxalate and low citrate; other risk parameters were within normal limits. She initiated medical management in our multidisciplinary stone prevention clinic for these risk factors. Further assessment revealed positive family history for nephrolithiasis (sister), history of prior ascorbic acid supplementation, very low calcium intake, and high suspicion for antibiotic-induced dysbiosis. The regimen for reducing urine oxalate was to: (1) not re-start ascorbic acid supplement to protect against higher oxalate biosynthesis; (2) pair calcium-containing foods or beverages with every meal to reduce bioavailability of dietary oxalate and, hence, its urinary excretion; and (3) increase intake of prebiotics from fruits and vegetables in effort to enhance colonization and proliferation of oxalate-degrading probiotics (bacteria) in the digestive tract. The regimen for raising urine citrate was to increase intake of fruits and vegetables because they provide bicarbonate precursors that reduce renal citrate reabsorption and thus increase its excretion. Three months later she was found in follow-up to have an 8 mm left renal calculus which was removed within 2 weeks by URS with LL.

Shortly thereafter she was evaluated by infectious disease for a worsening productive cough over several months and was found to have *Nocardia* pneumonia with pulmonary nodules seen on CT scan. She was subsequently started on a six-month course of twice daily TMP-SMX 2DS and cefpodoxime 200 mg. Prior to starting the antibiotic regimen, a non-contrast CT scan showed a new 6 mm non-obstructing stone in the left lower renal pole. A repeat CT scan three months later (2 months after starting TMP-SMX) revealed interval growth of the renal stone to 9 mm; intervention with URS was scheduled. But in the interim, the patient became symptomatic and presented for emergency treatment. Physical exam was significant for mild pelvic tenderness. Labs were significant for creatinine of 1.58 mg/dL and hematuria but no infection. Her pain was managed, and she was discharged. Repeat CT, now 4 months after starting TMP-SMX, revealed a developing staghorn calculus in the left renal pelvis measuring up to 4 cm (Fig. 1) and an obstructing conglomerate of calculi in the left lower ureter measuring up to 7 mm with mild upstream hydroureteronephrosis. Within 2 days, the patient underwent left URS and LL of the renal pelvis and ureteral stones. During the procedure, stone fragments were retrieved via basket and sent for analysis; results demonstrated 80% N^4-acetyl-sulfamethoxazole with remaining constituents calcium oxalate (12% monohydrate and 5% dihydrate) and 3% calcium phosphate carbonate apatite (composition was assessed by Fourier transform infrared spectroscopy at Dianon Systems in Oklahoma City, OK). The origin of the fragments that were analyzed, whether from the larger renal pelvis stone or from the ureteral

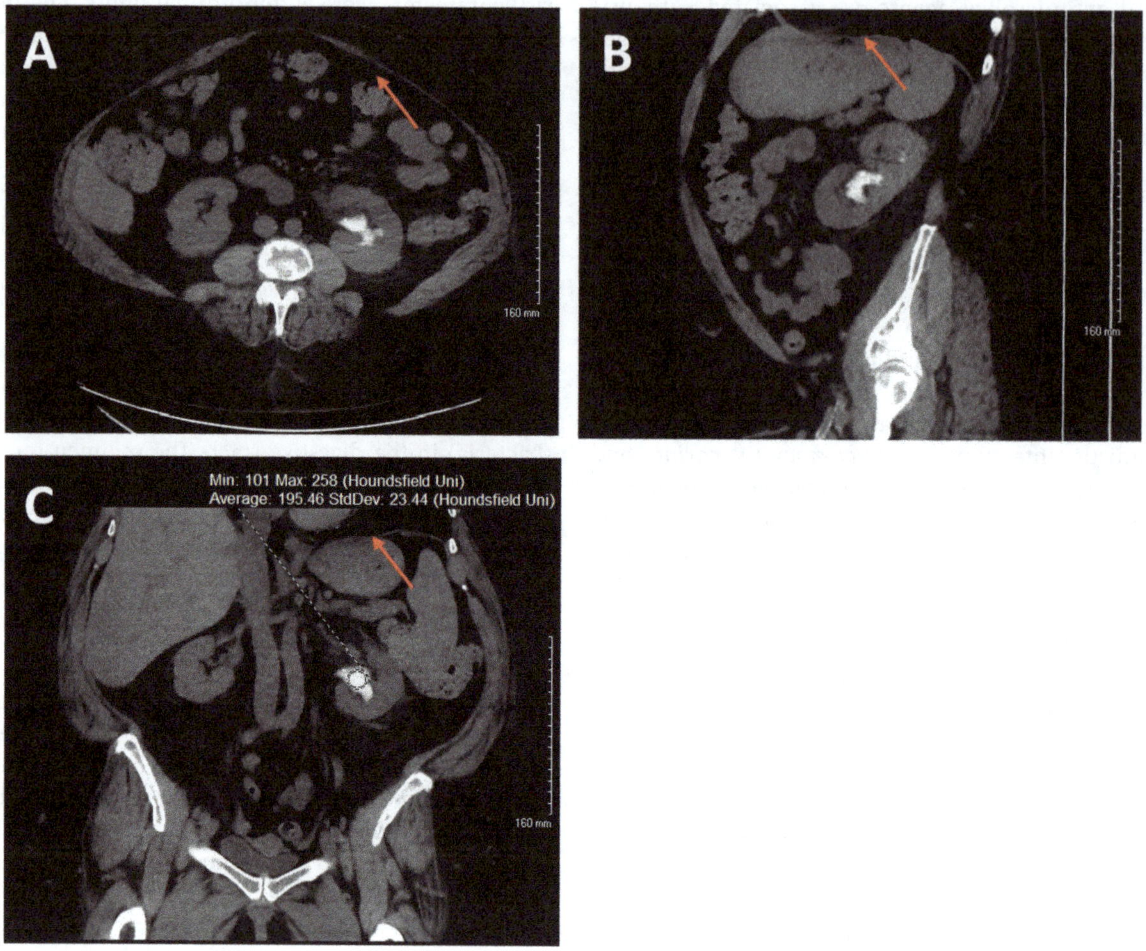

Fig. 1 Radiographic images of left renal pelvis stone (red arrow) in the axial (**a**), sagittal (**b**), and coronal (**c**) on non-contrast CT abdomen and pelvis. The stone was demonstrated on imaging to have a density of 194.46 Hounsfield Units

conglomerate of stones, was not documented and is thus unknown. Afterward, the patient passed multiple amber-colored stone fragments (Fig. 2).

The patient completed 6 months of antibiotics with resolution of lung nodules seen on CT and improvement of respiratory status to baseline. TMP-SMX and cefpodoxime were thus discontinued. A repeat CT a few months later showed clearance of post-URS fragments and no new urolithiasis bilaterally. She continues to follow in our stone prevention clinic.

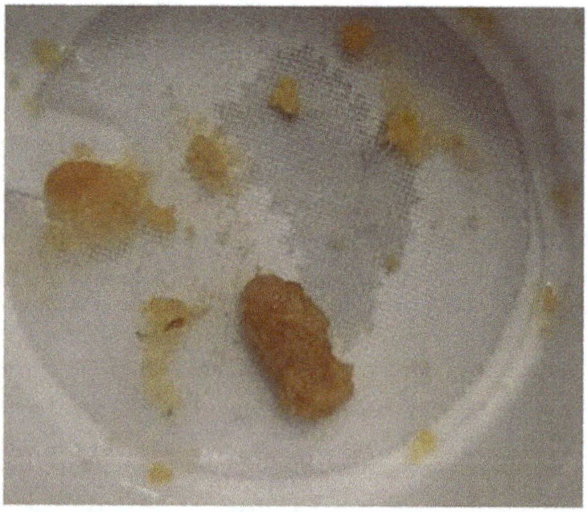

Fig. 2 Jagged, amber-colored stone fragments passed and collected by patient after ureteroscopy

Discussion and conclusions

Sulfamethoxazole is a member of the sulfonamide family, a group of short-acting antibiotics given via orally or parenterally. They are readily absorbed systemically, partially acetylated in the liver, and eliminated by the kidney [4, 5]. The first generation sulfonamides developed in the late 1930s had low urine solubility and were known to cause drug-induced crystalluria resulting in acute renal injury or obstructive urolithiasis [5]. Sulfonamides with higher urine solubility have since been developed, and sulfonamide crystalluria has become a rare occurrence. According to a study by Albala et al., sulfonamide stones make up less than 1% of all stones analyzed [2].

Sulfamethoxazole and its metabolite, N^4-acetyl-sulfamethoxazole, have particularly low lithogenic potential due to the losangic shape of the crystals, which are not readily retained in the kidney [1]. There have been few reports of N^4-acetyl-sulfamethoxazole-induced urolithiasis over time except in recent years, during which TMP-SMX has been used for long-term prophylactic treatment of HIV-associated infections [6]. According to Barnes and Kawaichi, the most important factors in urinary precipitation of sulfonamides include concentration of the drug in the urine, degree of acetylation, urinary stasis, urine pH, and urine temperature [7]. The patient in this case was undergoing prolonged treatment with TMP-SMX at high doses for *Nocardia* pneumonia, which likely led to a high urine drug concentration. Her history of type II diabetes mellitus and the associated insulin resistance may have contributed to a more acidic urine pH at baseline [8]. She also had a change in urine pH from 6.5 prior to beginning the antibiotics to 5.5 at the time of symptomatic presentation. In addition, the pre-antibiotic 6 mm lower left renal stone (which was presumably calcium oxalate) may have acted as a nidus for sulfamethoxazole crystal deposition. It is not clear if this is the case as the stone was submitted for analysis in fragment form with no discernable core.

The patient had a known renal calculus at the time of starting TMP-SMX, which is a relatively rare finding. Albala et al. identified 40 people who developed sulfonamide stones, four of whom had a history of prior urolithiasis; however, none had a known stone at the time of treatment [2]. Siegel described a patient who presented with oliguria while on a 2-week course of TMP-SMX for prostatitis who was found with bilateral ureteral stone obstruction; analysis revealed a pure N^4-acetyl-sulfamethoxazole stone on one side and a calcium oxalate stone contralaterally [9]. However, unlike our patient, he had no prior history of nephrolithiasis; presence of his stone was unknown until presentation.

The treatment and prevention of sulfonamide crystalluria and urolithiasis has not changed significantly since the 1940s and, given the rarity of cases, no standard regimen is established. The mainstays of treatment include discontinuation of the sulfonamide if possible, diuresis, and urinary alkalization, as sulfonamides have greater solubility at alkaline pH. Prevention techniques include avoiding sulfonamides if alternative treatments are available, encouraging patients to increase fluid intake when taking sulfonamides, and urinary alkalization with sodium bicarbonate or other alkali [1, 2, 5]. The presence of known renal stones or other foreign bodies such as indwelling catheters should be considered when selecting a sulfonamide for long-term use, as these may be reasons to avoid this family of antibiotics in such patients.

Stones composed of sulfamethoxazole or its metabolites are rare as they do not readily precipitate in urine. Factors such as high drug concentration in urine, urinary stasis, and low urine pH increase this risk. Findings from our report suggest that additional risk factors are prior stone history, pre-existing metabolic (urinary) risk factors, and pre-existing urinary calculi that may serve as a nidus for sulfamethoxazole deposition. Treatment and prevention include diuresis, urinary alkalization, treatment of underlying metabolic and urinary stone risk factors, and use of an alternative antibiotic if possible.

Abbreviations

CT: Computed tomography; HIV: Human immunodeficiency virus; LL: Laser lithotripsy; TMP-SMX: Trimethoprim-sulfamethoxazole; URS: Ureteroscopy.

Acknowledgements

None.

Authors' contributions

MMR analyzed the patient data and wrote the preliminary draft, SYN and KLP provided expertise and edited the manuscript. All authors read and approved the final manuscript.

Author details

[1]Wisconsin Academy for Rural Medicine, University of Wisconsin School of Medicine and Public Health, Madison, WI, USA. [2]Department of Urology, University of Wisconsin School of Medicine and Public Health, 1685 Highland Avenue, 3258 Medical Foundation Centennial Building, Madison, WI 53705-2281, USA. [3]Department of Radiology, University of Wisconsin School of Medicine and Public Health, Madison, WI, USA.

References

1. Daudon M, Frochot V, Bazin D, Jungers P. Drug-induced kidney stones and crystalline nephropathy: pathophysiology, prevention and treatment [Internet]. Drugs. Springer International Publishing; 2018 [cited 2021 Jun 1]. p. 163–201. Available from: https://doi.org/10.1007/s40265-017-0853-7
2. Albala DM, Galal HA, Prien EL. Urolithiasis as a hazard of sulfonamide therapy. J Endourol [Internet]. 1994 [cited 2021 May 8];8:401–3. Available from: https://www.liebertpub.com/doi/abs/https://doi.org/10.1089/end.1994.8.401
3. Miller AW, Orr T, Dearing D, Monga M. Loss of function dysbiosis associated with antibiotics and high fat, high sugar diet. ISME J [Internet]. Nature Publishing Group; 2019 [cited 2021 Jun 2];13:1379–90. Available from: http://www.nature.com/articles/s41396-019-0357-4
4. Cockerill FR, Edson RS. Trimethoprim-sulfamethoxazole. Mayo Clin Proc [Internet]. Mayo Clin Proc; 1991 [cited 2021 May 25];66:1260–9. Available from: https://pubmed.ncbi.nlm.nih.gov/1749295/

5. Dorfman LE, Smith JP. Sulfonamide crystalluria: a forgotten disease. J Urol. 1970;104:482–3.
6. DeMasi MS, Bernstein AP, Schulster M, Silva M V. 100% N4-acetyl-sulfamethoxazole stone induced by trimethoprim-sulfamethoxazole in an HIV patient being treated for toxoplasmosis. Urol Case Reports [Internet]. Elsevier Inc.; 2021;34:101453. Available from: https://doi.org/10.1016/j.eucr.2020.101453
7. Barnes RW, Kawaichi GK. Factors influencing the formation of sulfonamide urinary concretions. J Urol Ovid Technologies (Wolters Kluwer Health). 1943;49:324–30.
8. Maalouf NM, Cameron MA, Moe OW, Sakhaee K. Metabolic basis for low urine pH in type 2 diabetes. Clin J Am Soc Nephrol [Internet]. Am Soc Nephrol.; 2010;5:1277. Available from: /pmc/articles/PMC2893060/
9. Siegel WH. Unusual complication of therapy with sulfamethoxazole trimethoprim. J. Urol. No longer published by Elsevier; 1977. p. 397.

Permissions

All chapters in this book were first published by BioMed Central; hereby published with permission under the Creative Commons Attribution License or equivalent. Every chapter published in this book has been scrutinized by our experts. Their significance has been extensively debated. The topics covered herein carry significant findings which will fuel the growth of the discipline. They may even be implemented as practical applications or may be referred to as a beginning point for another development.

The contributors of this book come from diverse backgrounds, making this book a truly international effort. This book will bring forth new frontiers with its revolutionizing research information and detailed analysis of the nascent developments around the world.

We would like to thank all the contributing authors for lending their expertise to make the book truly unique. They have played a crucial role in the development of this book. Without their invaluable contributions this book wouldn't have been possible. They have made vital efforts to compile up to date information on the varied aspects of this subject to make this book a valuable addition to the collection of many professionals and students.

This book was conceptualized with the vision of imparting up-to-date information and advanced data in this field. To ensure the same, a matchless editorial board was set up. Every individual on the board went through rigorous rounds of assessment to prove their worth. After which they invested a large part of their time researching and compiling the most relevant data for our readers.

The editorial board has been involved in producing this book since its inception. They have spent rigorous hours researching and exploring the diverse topics which have resulted in the successful publishing of this book. They have passed on their knowledge of decades through this book. To expedite this challenging task, the publisher supported the team at every step. A small team of assistant editors was also appointed to further simplify the editing procedure and attain best results for the readers.

Apart from the editorial board, the designing team has also invested a significant amount of their time in understanding the subject and creating the most relevant covers. They scrutinized every image to scout for the most suitable representation of the subject and create an appropriate cover for the book.

The publishing team has been an ardent support to the editorial, designing and production team. Their endless efforts to recruit the best for this project, has resulted in the accomplishment of this book. They are a veteran in the field of academics and their pool of knowledge is as vast as their experience in printing. Their expertise and guidance has proved useful at every step. Their uncompromising quality standards have made this book an exceptional effort. Their encouragement from time to time has been an inspiration for everyone.

The publisher and the editorial board hope that this book will prove to be a valuable piece of knowledge for researchers, students, practitioners and scholars across the globe.

List of Contributors

Laragh L. W. Harvey-Kelly
University of Cambridge School of Clinical Medicine, Addenbrooke's Hospital, Hills Road, Cambridge CB2 0SP, UK

Hannah Harrison, Simon J. Griffin and Juliet A. Usher-Smith
The Primary Care Unit, Department of Public Health and Primary Care, University of Cambridge, Cambridge CB2 0SR, UK

Sabrina H. Rossi
Department of Oncology, University of Cambridge, Addenbrooke's Hospital, Cambridge Biomedical Campus, Hills Road, Cambridge CB2 0QQ, UK

Grant D. Stewart
Department of Surgery, University of Cambridge, Addenbrooke's Hospital, Cambridge Biomedical Campus, Hills Road, Cambridge CB2 0QQ, UK

Adi Adelman, Yaniv Shilo, Jonathan Modai and Dan Leibovici
Department of Urology, Kaplan Medical Center, 7661041 Rehovot, Israel

Ishai Dror and Brian Berkowitz
Department of Earth and Planetary Sciences, Weizmann Institute of Science, 7610001 Rehovot, Israel

Parvin Khalili
Department of Epidemiology, School of Public Health, Social Determinants of Health Research Centre, Rafsanjan University of Medical Sciences, Rafsanjan, Iran

Zahra Jamali, Ali Esmaeili-nadimi, Fatemeh Ayoobi and Alireza Nazari
Non-Communicable Diseases Research Center, Rafsanjan University of Medical Sciences, Rafsanjan, Iran

Tabandeh Sadeghi
Department of Pediatric Nursing, School of Nursing and Midwifery, Non-Communicable Diseases Research Center, Rafsanjan University of Medical Sciences, Rafsanjan, Iran

Maryam Mohamadi
Occupational Safety and Health Research Center, NICICO, World Safety Organization and Rafsanjan University of Medical Sciences, Rafsanjan, Iran

Amir Moghadam-Ahmadi
Department of Neurology, School of Medicine, Non-Communicable Diseases Research Center, Rafsanjan University of Medical Sciences, Rafsanjan, Iran

Cai Lv, Qingqing Lei and Zhenxiang Liu
Department of Urology, Haikou Municipal Hospital, Haikou 570208, Hainan, China

Yuan Huang
Department of Neurology, Haikou Municipal Hospital, Haikou 570208, Hainan, China

Shixing Shen
Department of Urology, Danzhou People's Hospital, Danzhou 571799, Hainan, China

Wenxia Si
Hubei Key Laboratory for Kidney Disease Pathogenesis and Intervention, Huangshi Central Hospital of Edong Healthcare Group, Hubei Polytechnic University School of Medicine, Huangshi, China

Jeanette E. Eckel-Passow, Huihuang Yan, Matthew L. Kosel and Paul A. Decker
Division of Biomedical Statistics and Informatics, Mayo Clinic, 200 First Street SW, Rochester, MN 55905, USA

Daniel Serie and Alexander Parker
Department of Health Sciences Research, Mayo Clinic, Jacksonville, FL, USA

Robert B. Jenkins
Department of Laboratory Medicine and Pathology, Mayo Clinic, Rochester, MN, USA

Brian Costello and Bradley Leibovich
Department of Urology, Mayo Clinic, Rochester, MN, USA

Thai H. Ho
Division of Hematology and Medical Oncology, Mayo Clinic, Scottsdale, AZ, USA

Tsung-Hsin Chang and Jen-Shu Tseng
Department of Urology, MacKay Memorial Hospital, No. 92, Sec. 2, Zhongshan N. Rd., Taipei City 10449, Taiwan

Wun-Rong Lin, Wei-Kung Tsai and Pai-Kai Chiang
Department of Urology, MacKay Memorial Hospital, No. 92, Sec. 2, Zhongshan N. Rd., Taipei City 10449, Taiwan
Mackay Medical College, No.46, Sec. 3, Zhongzheng Rd., Sanzhi Dist., New Taipei City 252, Taiwan

Marcelo Chen
Department of Urology, MacKay Memorial Hospital, No. 92, Sec. 2, Zhongshan N. Rd., Taipei City 10449, Taiwan
Mackay Medical College, No.46, Sec. 3, Zhongzheng Rd., Sanzhi Dist., New Taipei City 252, Taiwan
Mackay Junior College of Medicine, Beitou District, Nursing and Management, No.92, Shengjing Road, Taipei City 11272, Taiwan

Allen W. Chiu
Department of Urology, MacKay Memorial Hospital, No. 92, Sec. 2, Zhongshan N. Rd., Taipei City 10449, Taiwan
School of Medicine, National Yang-Ming University, No.145, Zhengzhou Rd., Datong Dist., Taipei City 10341, Taiwan

Qun Lu, Xiaozhi Zhao, Changwei Ji, Xuefeng Qiu, Guangxiang Liu, Shiwei Zhang, Xiaogong Li, Gutian Zhang and Hongqian Guo
Department of Urology, Drum Tower Hospital, Medical School of Nanjing University, Institute of Urology, Nanjing University, 321 Zhongshan Rd., Nanjing 210008, Jiangsu, People's Republic of China

Suhan Guo
School of Public Health, Nanjing Medical University, Nanjing 210029, Jiangsu, People's Republic of China

Xuebin Zhang
Department of Radiology, Drum Tower Hospital, Medical School of Nanjing University, Nanjing 210008, Jiangsu, People's Republic of China

Ruotao Xiao, Chuxiao Xu and Wei He
Peking University Health Science Centre, 100191 Beijing, People's Republic of China
Department of Urology, Peking University Third Hospital, No.49 North Garden Road, Haidian District, 100191 Beijing, People's Republic of China

Lei Liu and Hongxian Zhang
Peking University Health Science Centre, 100191 Beijing, People's Republic of China

Cheng Liu and Lulin Ma
Department of Urology, Peking University Third Hospital, No.49 North Garden Road, Haidian District, 100191 Beijing, People's Republic of China

Mingxin Zhang and Haitao Niu
Department of Urology, The Affiliated Hospital of Qingdao University, Qingdao, China

Zhilei Zhang, Yongbo Yu and Jilu Zheng
Department of Urology, The Affiliated Hospital of Qingdao University, Qingdao, China
Department of Clinical Medicine, Qingdao University, Qingdao, China

Chao Liu and Zhiyang Shang
Department of Oncology, Zhuozhou Hospital, No.129, Fanyang Road, Zhuozhou City, Hebei Province, China

Jingjing Piao
College of Nursing, Hebei University of Chinese Medicine, Shijiazhuang, Hebei Province, China

Kai Johnson, Majd Issa, Anish Parikh, Paul Monk, Ming Yin, Amir Mortazavi and Yuanquan Yang
Medical Oncology, Ohio State University James Cancer Hospital, Suite 1335 Lincoln Tower, 1800 Cannon Drive, Columbus, OH 43210, USA

Suresh de Silva
Faculty of Medicine, University of NSW, Kensington, NSW, Australia
Department of Radiology, I-MED Radiology Network, Sydney, Australia

Kathleen Rebecca Lockhart, Peter Aslan, Peter Nash, Dominic Lee and David Malouf
Department of Urology, St George Hospital, Kogarah, NSW, Australia

Anthony Hutton and James Thompson
Faculty of Medicine, University of NSW, Kensington, NSW, Australia
Department of Urology, St George Hospital, Kogarah, NSW, Australia

Paul Cozzi
Hurstville Private Hospital, Hurstville, NSW, Australia

Fiona MacLean
Department of Anatomical Pathology, Sonic Healthcare, Ryde, NSW, Australia

Kun Sirisopana, Pocharapong Jenjitranant, Premsant Sangkum, Kittinut Kijvikai, Charoen Leenanupunth, Wachira Kochakarn and Wisoot Kongchareonsombat
Division of Urology, Department of Surgery, Faculty of Medicine, Ramathibodi Hospital, Mahidol University, 270 Thanon Rama VI, Thung Phaya Thai, Ratchathewi, Bangkok 10400, Thailand

Suthep Pacharatakul
Division of Urology, Department of Surgery, Police Hospital, Bangkok, Thailand

Jiannan Wang, Xiang Li, Yixia Zhang and Xuemei Wang
Department of Ultrasound, The First Hospital of China Medical University, No. 155 NanjingBei Street, Heping District, Shenyang 110001, Liaoning Province, People's Republic of China.

Tan Li
Department of Cardiovascular Ultrasound, The First Hospital of China Medical University, Shenyang 110001, People's Republic of China

Benedikt Martin, Martin Burchardt and Uwe Zimmermann
Department of Urology, University Medicine Greifswald, Ferdinand-Sauerbruch-Str., 17475 Greifswald, Germany

Andreas Greinacher
Department of Transfusion Medicine, University Medicine Greifswald, Ferdinand- Sauerbruch-Str., 17475 Greifswald, Germany

Fabian Hammer
Department of Cardiology, KMG Clinic Guestrow, Friedrich-Trendelenburg-Allee 1, 18273 Guestrow, Germany

Andreas Hoene
Department of Vascular Surgery, University Medicine Greifswald, Ferdinand-Sauerbruch- Str., 17475 Greifswald, Germany

Robin Bülow
Department of Radiology, University Medicine Greifswald, Ferdinand-Sauerbruch-Str., 17475 Greifswald, Germany

Giovanni Liguori, Giacomo Rebez and Michele Rizzo
Azienda Sanitaria Universitaria Giuliano-Isontina, Strada di Fiume 447, 34149 Trieste, Italy

Alessandro Larcher, Carlo Trombetta and Andrea Salonia
Università Vita Salute San Raffaele, Milan, Italy

Tommaso Cai
Ospedale Santa Chiara, Trento, Italy

Alec Zhu and Peter Connolly
NewYork-Presbyterian/Weill Cornell Medical Center, 525 E 68th St, New York, NY 10065, USA

A. Ari Hakimi
Memorial Sloan Kettering Cancer Center, 1275 York Ave, New York, NY 10065, USA

Kenichi Nishimura, Noriyoshi Miura, Naoya Sugihara, Keisuke Funaki, Kanae Koyama, Yuichiro Sawada, Terutaka Noda, Tetsuya Fukumoto, Yuki Miyauchi, Tadahiko Kikugawa and Takashi Saika
Department of Urology, Ehime University, Shitsukawa, Toon, Ehime 791-0295, Japan

Masafumi Matsumura and Katsuyoshi Hashine
Department of Urology, National Hospital Organization Shikoku Cancer Center, Minamiumemoto, Matsuyama 791-0280, Japan

Mashio Taniwaki
Department of Pathology, Ehime University, Shitsukawa, Toon 791-0295, Japan

James Elander, Romaana Kapadi, Carol Stalker and Kathryn Mitchell
School of Psychology, University of Derby, Derby, UK

Emma Coyne
Nottingham University Hospitals NHS Trust, Nottingham, UK

Maarten W. Taal and Nicholas M. Selby
Centre for Kidney Research and Innovation, University of Nottingham, Derby, UK

Adili Keranmu, Yajian Li, Feiya Yang, Wasilijiang Wahafu, Dong Chen, Kaopeng Guan and Nianzeng Xing
State Key Laboratory of Molecular Oncology, National Cancer Center/ National Clinical Research Center for Cancer/Cancer Hospital, Chinese Academy of Medical Sciences and Peking Union Medical College, Beijing 100021, People's Republic of China
Department of Urology, National Cancer Center/ National Clinical Research Center for Cancer/ Cancer Hospital, Chinese Academy of Medical Sciences and Peking Union Medical College, No. 17, Panjiayuan South Li, Chaoyang District, Beijing 100021, People's Republic of China

Mingshuai Wang
State Key Laboratory of Molecular Oncology, National Cancer Center/ National Clinical Research Center for Cancer/Cancer Hospital, Chinese Academy of Medical Sciences and Peking Union Medical College, Beijing 100021, People's Republic of China
Department of Urology, National Cancer Center/ National Clinical Research Center for Cancer/ Cancer Hospital, Chinese Academy of Medical Sciences and Peking Union Medical College, No. 17, Panjiayuan South Li, Chaoyang District, Beijing 100021, People's Republic of China
Department of Urology, Institute of Urology, Beijing Chaoyang Hospital, Capital Medical University, Beijing 100020, People's Republic of China

Jing Liang
Department of Pathology, National Cancer Center/ National Clinical Research Center for Cancer/Cancer Hospital, Chinese Academy of Medical Sciences and Peking Union Medical College, Beijing 100021, People's Republic of China

Jiaxing Ma, Wei Sun, Weiwei Qian, Jie Min, Tao Zhang and Dexin Yu
Department of Urology, The Second Affiliated Hospital of Anhui Medical University, 678 Furong Rd, Hefei 230032, Anhui, People's Republic of China

Brent Cleveland and Michael Borofsky
University of Minnesota, 420 Delaware St. S. E., MMC 394, Minneapolis, MN 55455, USA

Desie Kasew, Setegn Eshetie and Feleke Moges
Department of Medical Microbiology, School of Biomedical and Laboratory Sciences, College of Medicine and Health Sciences, University of Gondar, Gondar, Ethiopia

Abeje Diress and Zerubabiel Tegegne
Department of Radiology, School of Medicine, College of Medicine and Health Sciences, University of Gondar, Gondar, Ethiopia

Yujie Liu and Xuemei Liang
Department of Geriatric Medicine, The Affiliated Hospital of Southwest Medical University, Luzhou 646000, China

Xing Hu
Department of General Practice, The Affiliated Hospital of Southwest Medical University, Luzhou 646000, China

Liang Hu
Department of Cardiovascular Surgery, The General Hospital of Western Theater Command, Chengdu 610083, China

Changjing Xu
Department of Pharmacy, The Affiliated Hospital of Southwest Medical University, Luzhou 646000, China

Masaki Kobayashi, Yuichi Fukuda, Yusuke Kohno, Keizo Kawano and Shinji Morimoto
Department of Urology, Tsuchiura Kyodo General Hospital, Tsuchiura, Japan

Junichiro Ishioka, Yoh Matsuoka, Soichiro Yoshida, Minato Yokoyama and Yasuhisa Fujii
Department of Urology, Tokyo Medical and Dental University, Tokyo, Japan

Rie Muta, Motohiro Fujiwara, Naoko Kawamura and Tetsuo Okuno
Department of Urology, JA Toride Medical Center, Toride, Japan

Rumi Suda and Ryota Saiki
Department of Information and Communications Engineering, Tokyo Institute of Technology, Tokyo, Japan

Kenji Suzuki and Itsuo Kumazawa
Laboratory for Future, Interdisciplinary Research of Science and Technology, Institute of Innovative Research, Tokyo Institute of Technology, Tokyo, Japan

Chenglu Wang and Min Zheng
Reproductive Medicine Center, Department of Reproductive Endocrinology, Affiliated People's Hospital, Zhejiang Provincial People's Hospital, Hangzhou Medical College, No.158 Shangtang Road, Hangzhou 310014, Zhejiang, People's Republic of China

Lu Jin, Xinyang Zhao and Boxin Xue
Department of Urology, Second Affiliated Hospital of Soochow University, Suzhou, Jiangsu, People's Republic of China

Kazumi Taguchi, Shuzo Hamamoto, Atsushi Okada, Yutaro Tanaka, Teruaki Sugino, Rei Unno, Taiki Kato, Ryosuke Ando, Keiichi Tozawa and Takahiro Yasui
Department of Nephro-urology, Nagoya City University Graduate School of Medical Sciences, Kawasumi 1, Mizuho-cho, Mizuho-ku, Nagoya 4678601, Japan

Xiaoqing Zhang, Xiangyang Guo, Yanan Zong, Chuanya Xu, Jilian Wang, Bin Zhang, Chang Liu, Yi Li and Hong Zeng
Department of Anesthesia, Peking University Third Hospital, Huayuan 49# Rd, Haidian Dist., Beijing, China

Yueqing Gong and Lixiang Xue
Biological Sample Bank, Peking University Third Hospital, Beijing, China

Lulin Ma and Shudong Zhang
Department of Urology, Peking University Third Hospital, Beijing, China

Megan M. Roedel
Wisconsin Academy for Rural Medicine, University of Wisconsin School of Medicine and Public Health, Madison, WI, USA

Kristina L. Penniston
Department of Urology, University of Wisconsin School of Medicine and Public Health, 1685 Highland Avenue, 3258 Medical Foundation Centennial Building, Madison, WI 53705-2281, USA

Stephen Y. Nakada
Department of Urology, University of Wisconsin School of Medicine and Public Health, 1685 Highland Avenue, 3258 Medical Foundation Centennial Building, Madison, WI 53705-2281, USA
Department of Radiology, University of Wisconsin School of Medicine and Public Health, Madison, WI, USA

Index

www.ingramcontent.com/pod-product-compliance
Lightning Source LLC
LaVergne TN
LVHW082159200926
848484LV00008B/2189
* 9 7 9 8 8 8 7 4 0 2 2 5 3 *